Multiple Sclerosis: Clinical Challenges and Controversies

MULTIPLE SCLEROSIS: CLINICAL CHALLENGES AND CONTROVERSIES

Edited by

Alan J Thompson MD FRCP FRCPI
Consultant Neurologist and Reader
Institute of Neurology
University of London
London UK

Chris Polman MD PhD
Professor of Neurology
Department of Neurology
Academisch Ziekenhuis
Vrije Universiteit
Amsterdam, The Netherlands

Reinhard Hohlfeld MD
Professor
Klinikum Grosshadern
Neurologishce Klinik
München, Germany

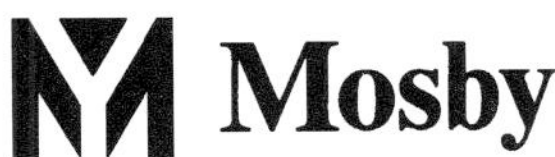

St. Louis Baltimore Boston Carlsbad Chicago Naples New York Philadelphia Portland
London Madrid Mexico City Singapore Sydney Tokyo Toronto Wiesbaden

MARTIN DUNITZ

First published in the United Kingdom in 1997 by
Martin Dunitz Ltd
The Livery House
7-9 Pratt Street
London NW1 0AE

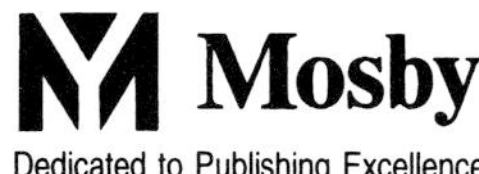 **Mosby**
Dedicated to Publishing Excellence

A Times Mirror Company

Distributed in the U.S.A. and Canada by
Mosby–Year book
11830 Westline Industrial Drive
St. Louis, Missouri 63146

Times Mirror Professional Publishing Ltd.
130 Flaska Drive
Markham, Ontario L6G 1B8

A CIP catalogue record for this book is available from the British Library

ISBN 1-85317-4289

Composition by Wearset, Boldon, Tyne and Wear
Printed and bound in Great Britain by Cambridge University Press.

CONTENTS

Contributors

Cécile Azais-Vuillemin MD
Service de Neurologie, CHU Hopital
Purpan, Place du Docteur Baylac, 31059
Toulouse, France

Frederik Barkhof MD MR
Radiologist, Centre for Multiple Sclerosis
Research, Department of Diagnostic
Radiology, Vrije Universiteit Hospital,
1007 MB Amsterdam, The Netherlands

Michel Clanet MD
Professor of Neurology, Service de
Neurologie, CHU Hopital Purpan, Place du
Docteur Baylac, 31059 Toulouse, France

Leo Cohen PhD
Department of Psychology, Vrije
Universiteit, van der Boechorstraat 7,
1081 BT Amsterdam, The Netherlands

Alastair Compston PhD FRCP
Professor of Neurology, Department of
Neurology, Addenbrooke's Hospital, Hills
Road, Cambridge CB2 2QQ, UK

Cesare Fieschi MD
Department of Neurological Sciences,
Universita degli Studi di Roma 'La
Sapienza', V. le dell' Universita 30, 00185
Roma, Italy

Clare Fowler MBBS FRCP
Senior Lecturer and Consultant in
Uroneurology, Department of
Uroneurology, The National Hospital for
Neurology and Neurosurgery, Queen
Square, London WC1N 3BG, UK

Jennifer A Freeman B Appl Sci
Physiotherapist, Neurorehabilitation
Unit, The National Hospital for
Neurology and Neurosurgery, Great
North Road, East Finchley, London
N2 0NW, UK

Claudio Gasperini MD PhD
Department of Neurological Sciences,
Universita degli Studi di Roma 'La
Sapienza', V. le dell' Universita 30, and
Department of Neurology, San Camillo
Hospital, 00185 Roma, Italy

Robert J Goodwin MA FRCS
Registrar and Honorary Lecturer,
Department of Uroneurology, The
National Hospital for Neurology and
Neurosurgery, Queen Square, London
WC1N 3BG, UK

Jan Hatch
Welfare Director, The Multiple Sclerosis
Society of Great Britain and Northern
Ireland, 25 Effie Road, London SW6 1EE,
UK

Jeremy C Hobart BSc MRCP
Lecturer, The National Hospital for
Neurology and Neurosurgery, Queen
Square, London, and Department of
Clinical Neurology, Institute of
Neurology, Health Services Research
Unit, Department of Public Health
and Policy, London School of Hygiene
and Medicine, London WC1E 7HT,
UK

Reinhard Hohlfeld MD
Professor of Neurology, Department of
Neurology, Klinikum Grosshadern,
University of Munich,
D-81366 München, Germany

Michael Hutchinson MB FRCP
Consultant Neurologist, St. Vincent's
Consultants Private Clinic, Herbert
avenue, Merrion Road, Dublin 4,
Eire

Jane Johnson MSc RGN
Clinical Nurse Specialist,
Neurorehabilitation Unit, Great North
Road, East Finchley, London N2 0NW,
UK

Lauren Krupp MD
Associate Professor of Neurology,
Department of Neurology, State
University of New York, Stony Brook
Health Sciences Building, T12-020, Stony
Brook, NY 11794-8121, USA

Dawn Langdon PhD
Clinical Psychologist, Neurorehabilitation
Unit, The National Hospital for
Neurology and Neurosurgery, Great
North Road, East Finchley, London
N2 0NW, UK

Fred D Lublin MD
Professor of Neurology, Allegheny
University of the Health Sciences, 3300
Henry Avenue, Philadelphia PA-19129,
USA

Roland Martin MD
Chief of Cellular Immunology,
Neuroimmunology Branch, National
Institutes of Neurological Diseases
and Stroke, National Institutes of
Health, Building 10, 10 Center DR
MSC 1400, Bethesda MD 20892-1400,
USA

W Ian McDonald PhD FRCP
Profesor of Neurology, Department of
Clinical Neurology, Institute of
Neurology, The National Hospital for
Neurology and Neurosurgery, Queen
Square, London WC1N 3BG, UK

David H Miller MD FRCP
Professor of Clinical Neurology,
Department of Clinical Neurology,
Institute of Neurology, The National
Hospital for Neurology and
Neurosurgery, Queen Square, London
WC1N 3BG, UK

Xavier Montalban MD
Unit of Neuroimmunology, Hospital
General Universitari 'Vall d'Hebron',
Servei de Neurologia, Pg Vall d' Hebron,
119/129, 08035 Barcelona, Spain

John H Noseworthy MD FRCPC
Professor and Chair, Department of
Neurology, Division of
Neuroimmunology, Mayo Clinic, 200
First Street Southwest, Rochester MN
55905, USA

Hillel Panitch MD
Maryland Center for Multiple Sclerosis,
Department of Neurology, University of
Maryland Hospital, Baltimore MD 21201,
USA

Lilian EMA Pfennings MSc
Professor of Medical Psychology,
Department of Medical Psychology, Vrije
Universiteit, van der Boechorstraat 7,
1081 BT Amsterdam, The Netherlands

Chris H Polman PhD MD
Professor, Department of Neurology, Vrije
Universiteit Hospital, De Boelelaan 1117,
Po Box 7057, 1007 MB Amsterdam, The
Netherlands

Ronald A Remick MD FCPP
Department of Psychiatry, St. Pauls
Hospital, Vancouver BC, Canada V6T 1Z3

Neil Robertson MD
Clinical Lecturer in Neurology,
Department of Neurology, Addenbrooke's
Hospital, Hills Road, Cambridge CB2
2QQ, UK

Trond Riise PhD
Associate Professor, Department of Public
Health, University of Bergen, Bergen,
Norway

Giovanni Ristori MD PhD
Department of Neurological Sciences,
Universita degli Studi di Roma 'La
Sapienza', V. le Dell' Universita 30,
00185, Roma, Italy

A Dessa Sadovnick PhD
Associate Professor, Department of
Medical Genetics, University of British
Columbia, 222 Wesbrook Building, 6174
University Boulevard, Vancouver BC,
Canada V6T 1Z3

Stephen Sawcer MD
Specialist Registrar in Neurology,
Department of Neurology, Addenbrooke's
Hospital, Hills Road, Cambridge CB2
2QQ, UK

Randall T Schapiro MD
The Fairview Multiple Sclerosis Center,
701-25th Avenue South, Minneapolis MN
55454, USA

William A Sibley MD
Professor of Neurology, Department of
Neurology, Arizona Health Sciences
Centre, Tucson AZ 85724, USA

Norbert Sommer MD
Eberhard-Karls Universität Neurologische
Klinik, Kliniken Schnarrenberg, Abteilung
Allgemeine Neurologie, Tübingen–72076,
Germany

Alan J Thompson MD FRCP
Consultant Neurologist and Reader,
Institute of Neurology, University of
London, The National Hospital for
Neurology and Neurosurgery, Queen
Square, London WC1N 3BG, UK

Henk van der Ploeg PhD
Professor of Medical Psychology,
Department of Medical Psychology, Vrije
Universiteit, van der Boechorststraat 7,
1081 BT Amsterdam, The Netherlands

Preface

Multiple sclerosis is a variable, unpredictable condition of unknown aetiology and poorly understood pathogenesis. It places a huge burden, physical, psychological, social and financial on those affected by it (people with multiple sclerosis, their carers, families and friends) and those who attempt to treat it. There remains a huge number of unanswered questions but recent developments have resulted in exciting, new information becoming available in the areas of basic research, treatment and management. Advances in one area frequently stimulate or guide research activity in another. It is particularly important that those involved in basic or laboratory based research are aware of the advances in clinical and applied research. It is for this reason that we have addressed issues which are either challenging or controversial across the whole spectrum of multiple sclerosis in this book. It is essential that developments continue in parallel in all of these areas so that improved understanding of the underlying mechanisms of disease activity will rapidly lead to improved treatment.

Acknowledgements

On behalf of my co-editors and myself, I would like to thank all the contributors who responded so promptly and with such enthusiasm to yet another demand on their limited time and for tolerating the gentle pressure exerted by Alan Burgess.

We would also like to acknowledge Dr Nicholas Losseff for the design on the front cover which is based on the study of the disease classification in multiple sclerosis carried out by Fred Lublin and Steve Reingold in 1966.

We owe a great debt of gratitude to our editor Yasmin Khan-Chowdhury, at Martin Dunitz Ltd, who has overseen the production of this book. Finally I would like to thank my secretary, Mrs Priscilla Pode, for coordinating efforts at my end.

AJT

1

Is the incidence of multiple sclerosis increasing?

Trond Riise

Introduction

Multiple sclerosis (MS) is a serious neurological disorder which has a major impact on those affected and the people around them. Yet – to the researcher – this disease is highly intriguing with its many unpredictable and mysterious features. The impression emerges that a complicated and forceful set of unknown mechanisms is determining the outbreak, appearance and course of this disease. One of the most intriguing aspects of the disease is the seemingly odd pattern of its occurrence, viewed both in time and geographically.

Many reports of the incidence of 'clusters' of MS cases have prompted the question: is the disease completely randomly distributed in the population throughout time and space, or is the occurrence of disease actually showing real biological variations?[1] There is now little doubt that there are differences in the frequency of the disease between various areas around the world, and such geographical variations might have a number of explanations, including a difference in genetic susceptibility and less exciting explanations related to differences in methods for case ascertainment.[2,3] But, do we also see variation over time within geographical areas in a stable population? Furthermore, are we – in line with the observations of many clinicians – facing a general increase in the incidence of this disease?

The answer to this key question might hold important clues to the search for the causes of this devastating disease. The observation of an increased number of cases in a stable population with a well-established health care system is more likely to be explained by changes in methods for case ascertainment than geographical differences. Since the aetiology is still rather unclear, the hope is that the study of such variations in the distribution might reveal the unknown causes of the disease. This is fundamental for epidemiological research nicely expressed by Fox in 1970:[4]

'The basic premise of epidemiology is that the disease does not occur randomly, but in patterns which reflect the operation of the underlying causes.'

Numerous studies have been performed to describe the distribution of MS in time and space.[5] And although we still lack evidence of specific agents some consistent information has been obtained.

However, in order to be able to properly interpret the observations reported in the literature, let us first look at some basic principles which need to be applied in such descriptive research.

How to study the frequency of the disease

Case ascertainment

Several major problems arise when trying to determine the frequency of MS in a population. The most serious problem in achieving an accurate case ascertainment is probably related to the definition and diagnosis of the disease. There is no simple diagnostic test for the disease, and various sets of clinical criteria have been used to establish the diagnosis. These criteria have gone through several modifications and have recently been supported by laboratory tests, such as cerebrospinal fluid and neurophysiological examinations, with the introduction of magnetic resonance imaging (MRI) criteria as the most recent addition.[6] Obviously, the number of cases included in the reported frequency number in a study will depend on the criteria used, and the comparisons of studies are therefore complicated by the change of criteria employed and by the lack of a standard set of criteria which uniquely define the disease. As more refined and sensitive criteria have been developed, it is likely that a generally higher percentage of those who have the disease have been included which also complicates the comparisons between time periods in the same population.

Since the disease usually shows an initially slow progression and one is still basically in need of clinical information to establish the diagnosis, it means that there is usually a substantial time lag between the clinical onset of the disease and the date when a firm diagnosis can be made. This lag period creates particular problems when trying to estimate the disease frequency, as many cases can only be included in the computation of occurrence data several years after they experienced their first symptoms of the disease. The median lag period in many studies has been around 3–5 years,[7] but in recent studies applying diagnostic criteria, which include laboratory tests, a marked reduction has been obtained.

The main point for achieving reliable data on the occurrence is, of course, to ensure that all potential cases in the area and period in question really are being traced. This point becomes more crucial the larger the area or population being surveyed. The optimal design would be to screen the whole population repeatedly by a door-to-door survey using trained field workers to identify possible cases who at a later stage can be thoroughly scrutinized by neurologists. This is not a practicable design, for obvious reasons, but it has been used in some areas where there have been little or no previous studies of this disease, or where it is likely that a significant number of cases have not been in contact with the public health service.[8,9] The basis for the majority of studies, at least in countries with a well-developed health system, has been to rely on the assumption that most cases with MS will sooner or later get in touch with the health service. Therefore, by scrutinizing all available medical records from neurological departments and other relevant specialist departments, such as ophthalmological departments, private neurologists, and general practitioners, one might assume that the majority of the cases in the population in question will be found. Several studies have in addition also examined files at community nursing services and patient societies. The system for including cases developed by the Mayo Clinic in Rochester might serve as a good model.[7] The reliability of data based on such designs is consequently dependent on the quality of the medical files and the health care system in general. An improvement of this system including the use of more refined diagnostic criteria will lead to better case ascertainment and might bias the longitudinal results of a single study if it includes periods where such a change has taken place.

Measures of frequency

The most intuitive and also most informative measure of disease frequency is the *incidence rate* which is simply the number of new cases within a period, i.e. one year, divided by the number of individuals at risk of developing the disease during the same period:

$$\frac{\text{number of new cases during a year}}{\text{number of individuals at risk during the same year}}$$

Usually it is expressed as the number of cases per 100,000 population. This rate is the best estimate of the risk of developing the disease in the population under study. A basic requirement for obtaining such meaningful estimates is the ability to determine a well-defined area or population from which one can assume that all new cases will be ascertained. Furthermore, the case ascertainment in an incidence study should ideally be done prospectively; i.e. when a proper system for case ascertainment is established one may register, for each year, the number of new cases. However, when doing this, there is an immediate problem in relation to the previously mentioned time lag between the date of clinical onset and date of diagnosis. Although the goal is to find the number of cases who developed the disease during each year, the only figure which might be observed during a year is the number of cases who have received a diagnosis. Only a few cases will receive their diagnosis during the same year as they first experienced symptoms of the disease. The rest will be observed during the following years. Reliable data on the number of new cases in a particular year can therefore only be produced several years later, and the most recent years will be grossly underestimated. This is reflected in the 'dip' of every curve drawn on incidence rates which are calculated close to the end of the follow-up period (study date). Some investigators have tried to estimate this bias based on an expected distribution of this time lag,[10] but such calculations may easily produce false results if the crucial assumptions on the distribution of the time lag

are violated. And, in fact, due to improved diagnostic criteria there seems in most studies to be a continuous shortening of this time lag. The important implication of this lag time is that one can always expect that the incidence rate of the most recent years will prove to be higher than the figures suggest.

Another major problem when doing incidence studies is that, since MS is a relatively rare disease, only a few new cases will appear every year even in large populations. Therefore, in order to achieve stable estimates of the incidence quite a large number of years need to be included.

Because of the problem with small numbers and the problem with time lag between the date of onset of disease and the date of diagnosis, a real prospective incidence study would only produce incidence rates which are good estimates of the risk of the disease in the population after some 5–10 years. Therefore, most incidence studies have been done retrospectively, often based on repeated surveys of all possible files. This design produces new problems since the longer the period in the past being investigated, or the longer the period between the surveys, the greater the risk of missing cases. Older files may be of less quality, increasing the risk of misclassification, and deceased cases and cases who have moved out of the region under study are more likely to be missed. To avoid the influence of shift in diagnostic criteria the best design would be to apply the same criteria for the whole period. But if the diagnostic criteria applied have changed during the period investigated, in a retrospective design there might not be enough information in the files to apply the same criteria for the whole period, again with biased rates as the result.

In conclusion, the generation of reliable incidence data on MS is related to a number of difficulties and therefore most studies investigating the frequency of the disease have aimed only at ascertaining all patients who have the disease at the particular date of study. This gives the *prevalence rate*, which is defined as the number of cases in a population who, at some fixed point in time, have the disease relative to the total population at the time of study. The prevalence rate is easier to obtain, since it can be calculated directly based on present information and needs no follow-up period. However, the major drawback of the prevalence rate is that it is not a very good measure of the risk of developing the disease in the population under study, since it is strongly influenced by other factors not related to the risk, such as survival and migration in the population. It is also directly influenced by the time lag between onset and diagnosis. This means that the comparison of prevalence rates for determining differences in the risk between areas and time periods is subject to a number of factors which potentially can bias the results. In other words, the fact that a prevalence rate in one study is higher than the rate found in a study of the same population a number of years earlier does not directly imply that the risk of developing the disease has increased.

The frequency of disease might also be surveyed by indirect measures such as *mortality rates* and *disability pensioning rates* recorded at the country's Central Office of Health Statistics or at the National Insurance Registry. Such measures involve a number of specific problems, which renders them of limited value when looking at variation over time. Both measures will underestimate the true frequency of the disease to a degree that is dependent on mechanisms in the recording system of the medical files in question, which probably differ between areas and probably also change over time. As mentioned earlier the prevalence rate is influenced by disease duration in general, and this is even more so for mortality rates. The mortality rate reflects the incidence rate from 20 to 40 years earlier in a highly mixed fashion, and improved survival will automatically give a decreased rate. Such indirect measures might in the best case be used to investigate non-temporal geographical differences between sub-areas in a region with a homogeneous administrative and medical practice.

Standardization of rates

Since all rates of disease frequency are calculated using the total population number in the denominator, these rates will be influenced by the age distribution of the population in question. What we essentially want to estimate is the frequency of the disease among those individuals who are at risk of developing the disease, and since the onset of the disease is limited to individuals mainly between 20 and 45 years of age, the rates will be influenced by the proportion of population within this age group. Therefore, all rates should be age-standardized, especially when comparing rates across areas. Also, when estimating incidence rates over a substantial period of time, a change in the age distribution might significantly influence the rates. The age-standardization involves the use of a standard population, and what is usually used in this latter situation is the age distribution at the beginning or the end of the study period, or some average distribution of the population in question. A better choice would be to use international standard populations which are developed and frequently used for comparison, i.e. cancer rates.[11] These standard populations might also easily be used for MS as has already been done in some studies.[12–15] A more widespread use of age-standardization according to international standard populations would significantly increase the value of comparing rates between areas and between time periods.

Review of recent studies

What is the situation now at the end of the twentieth century? What are the most recent data on the incidence of MS? No other neurological disease has been more extensively studied regarding the occurrence, and the majority of variations reported during the last two decades have been in the direction of an increased frequency.[16,17] Unfortunately, due to the aforementioned reasons, most of the descriptive studies on MS have aimed only at estimating the prevalence of the disease, and the trends of increased frequency are mostly based on observations of differences in prevalence rates. Since the incidence rate more directly reflects changes in frequency of the disease, this document will focus in some detail on some recent studies which have been aimed at investigating possible changes in incidence directly.

North America

Olmstead county is the geographical area in the USA which has been most carefully studied regarding the frequency of MS. The Mayo Clinic has a highly developed case-finding system as the source of all the data from this area. In a report of the most recent investigation of the incidence in this area the authors conclude, after a careful evaluation of possible methodological issues, that a real increase in incidence can be observed in this area.[7]

Two recent studies from the neighbouring counties of Westlock[18] and Barrhead[19] in Alberta, Canada, show marked increases in incidence rate. However, only cases alive on prevalence day January 1st 1991 and 1990 were included, resulting in a total of 17 and 11 cases respectively, making it difficult to

intercept the changes in rates because of selection bias and statistical uncertainty.

A marked increase in incidence is also reported in a recent study from Mexico,[20] which is traditionally characterized as a low prevalence area.[21] The number of patients admitted to the National Institute of Neurology and Neurosurgery increased from only 9 patients in the 13-year period from 1964 to 1976, to 263 patients in the following 16-year period 1977 to 1992. There are numerous potential sources for bias in the case ascertainment of this study, and it is likely that much of this increase in the number of diagnosed patients is due to improvement of case finding. The authors of this report conclude that the increase at least partly reflects a real increase in incidence. They argue that if the incidence of MS had been stable in this period one would have expected a higher proportion of chronic patients with a long duration of disease among patients diagnosed early in the study period compared to the more recent periods, but this was not found. The areas previously considered as low prevalence areas are often going through major environmental changes and are therefore of great potential epidemiological interest.

Sardinia

The Mediterranean area has been carefully studied during recent decades. Studies in Spain and Italy suggest that the disease is much more common than previously assumed, according to the traditionally accepted general north–south gradient.[16,22] One area where significant changes in incidence have been shown is Sardinia. The occurrence of MS among the inhabitants on this island, during the last 20 years, has been investigated through several studies of selected areas, including the most recent thorough study of about 270,000 inhabitants in a well-defined region of north-west Sardinia.[23] An almost 2½-fold increase in the incidence rate, from an average of about 2 per 100,000 in the period 1962 to 1971 to 5 for the period 1977 to 1991, was shown. This finding is in contrast to other carefully studied areas on the mainland of Italy using similar methodology, where the increase in the prevalence rate is mainly ascribed to longer survival and the incidence rates are considered to be relatively stable over time.[24,25]

United Kingdom

In the UK the focus has for a long time been on an apparently striking north–south gradient with a high occurrence in some carefully studied areas in the north-east mainland and off-shore islands of Scotland to a much lower occurrence in England, indicated by several mortality studies and some morbidity studies reporting prevalence figures only. A recent review indicates a temporal trend of generally increased rates except for the previously high prevalence areas in the northern part, again inferred from differences in repeated prevalence studies and trends in mortality.[26] The authors of this review point to the limited epidemiological value of all the studies which have been done regarding aetiological hypothesis. They ascribe this to a shaky epidemiological foundation of these studies, and conclude that much of the increased trend may be ascribed to improvement in the methods of case ascertainment.

Evidently, in order to determine whether there is a real increase in the risk of developing MS in England one needs a good study which carefully aims at investigating the incidence in a smaller area directly. Some data from such a study in Cambridgeshire, initiated in 1990, have recently been published – again showing an increase in the prevalence rate in 1993 compared to the rate in 1990.[27] But since there are still no interpretable incidence data avail-

able, due to time lag between onset and diagnosis, one is once again left with rather indirect data in the discussion on whether the increased prevalence rate is due to variation in case ascertainment rather than being an expression of a biological increase. A repeated follow-up study of this area in a few years (maybe also including incidence calculations for some five to ten years before 1990), would constitute a potential for more definite conclusions.

Scandinavia

A high prevalence area stretching across Scandinavia and Finland, defined as the so-called Fenno-Scandinavian focus by Kurtzke in 1968,[28] has undergone several investigations. Denmark has the only country-wide MS registry including more than 7700 patients with onset since 1948. This registry probably represents the most reliable source for data on changes in incidence. The most recent report from Denmark, presenting data up to 1982, shows that there has been a steady decrease in the rate from 1950 to the mid 1960s, followed by an increase, although less marked.[10] An updated study covering the most recent years is in process and will be needed to tell us whether there is a continuing increase in this country.

While the rates in Denmark seem to be rather evenly distributed throughout the country, some striking geographical differences in incidence trends are found in Norway. The frequency of the disease in this country was first studied by Swank *et al.*, who found that the eastern part of the country, consisting of inland areas and valleys, had a markedly higher incidence than the coastal area in the western and northern parts of the country.[29] This difference in frequency was further confirmed in prevalence studies in one county in the eastern part, Vestfold,[30] and two counties in the western part, Hordaland[31] and Møre of

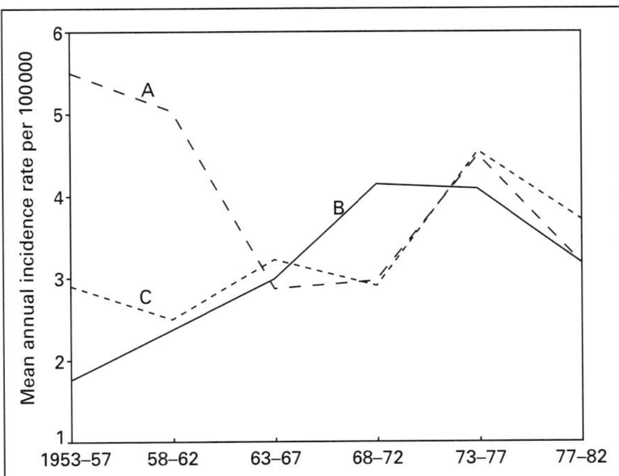

Fig. 1.1

Age-adjusted incidence rates in the Norwegian counties of (A) Vestfold, (B) Hordaland and (C) Møre og Romsdal including patients diagnosed before January 1st 1983 in Vestfold and Hordaland and January 1st 1994 in Møre og Romsdal.

Romsdal.[32] A mortality study covering the whole country confirmed this difference.[33] These three counties have recently been re-investigated for calculation of prevalence and incidence rates.[12–15] The results from these investigations are shown in *Fig. 1.1*.

The incidence rates for the beginning of this period in these three counties are in accordance with what has previously been shown. The following trends are very similar for the two counties in Western Norway with a marked increase in rate during the decades of 1970 and 1980. Vestfold shows an opposite trend with decreasing rates during the 1960s and early 1970s. The pattern in Vestfold, with a decline during the late 1950s and the 1960s, is remarkably similar to what is observed in

the region of Gothenburg in Western Sweden located at the opposite side of the Oslo Fjord[34] and in Denmark located south of Norway.[10] The development of the health care system has been very similar in the three Norwegian counties with the establishment of the only neurological department in two of these counties, Tønsberg in Vestfold and Bergen in Hordaland, at the same time in 1953. It is therefore very unlikely that the difference in these incidence patterns can be solely a result of methodological differences in case ascertainment. A study examining the migration of the patients' ancestors showed that the different trends could not be explained by a shift in genetic composition of the populations caused by migration between these areas (personal communication). This same study also includes an update of the material of Hordaland including all cases diagnosed before January 1st 1996 and showing an even steeper increase with a mean rate for the period 1983–93 now reaching 6.5 per 100,000. Since it is unlikely that these changes simply reflect changes in case ascertainment, these observations represent compelling evidence for the existence of real changes in incidence which cannot be explained by a corresponding change in genetic composition of the population. The most reasonable explanation for such variations is a similar change in the distribution of causal exogenous agents in this population.

Discussion

The most recent studies investigating the incidence of MS show either a stable or increasing incidence. An increasing trend is also suggested by most studies examining time trends by comparison of prevalence rates. This can be interpreted as an argument that these changes are due to variation in case ascertainment. It is likely that the case ascertainment generally has been enhanced along the trends of improved diagnostic tools, more interest and better knowledge of the disease among neurologists and practitioners and a generally better health care system. Therefore, one could argue that the only change in incidence which would be convincingly interpreted as a real biological change would be a decrease in a stable population with an unchanged system for case finding. And, in fact, such decreased trends have been shown in several areas, with the Faeroe Islands,[35] Orkneys,[36] Denmark,[10] and the counties of Gothenburg in Sweden[34] and Vestfold in Norway[15] as some good examples. The epidemic-like increase in the occurrence on the Faeroe Islands after World War II, also represents one of the most distinct increases observed.[35]

The distribution of the delay period between clinical onset of disease and diagnosis is the main obstacle for receiving valid data on the most recent period. This time lag directly influences the prevalence rate and leads to an underestimate of the incidence rates of the most recent years. On the other hand, an examination of the distribution of this time lag might give some information regarding other problems related to case ascertainment. Most studies investigating time lag report a decreased trend.[13,23] If this is a result of a more active and aggressive case ascertainment, it could imply better case finding, with an artificially increased incidence rate as the result. However, a reduction of this time lag could also simply be due to a change in diagnostic practice, where new diagnostic tools facilitate an earlier diagnosis. Such an effect will only lead to a lesser underestimate of the most recent years.

In any event, many of the benign cases potentially missed by one survey will later develop symptoms eventually bringing them to the attention of the health service, where a diagnosis can be established and their real onset of disease estimated. Since the incidence rates are calculated according to year of onset and not according to year of diagnosis, this means that a change in the delay caused by methodological issues will have little effect on the rates in the long run. One might, of course, question the ability to correctly estimate the clinical onset retrospectively. It is likely that the longer the period from onset to diagnosis the less accurate this estimate will be; that is, it is more likely that early episodes might be missed. This is consistent with an observed higher mean age at onset in earlier series reported in one study.[13]

Another indirect measure of methodological changes in case ascertainment is the distribution of the clinical picture or the severity of the cases. If there is a tendency to an increasing proportion of benign cases this could also be an indication of a change in diagnostic practice. Such an interpretation is of course based on the assumption that there is no real biological change in the appearance of the disease. In any case, if there is no marked change in the distribution of severity of the cases, then it is less likely that changes in the incidence rate are due to shift in case ascertainment. No such marked change was found in the series from Mexico. A prognostic study of the material in Olmstead county showed no increased survival among the patients diagnosed during the most recent decades,[7] while a similar study of the patients in Møre and Romsdal, Norway, actually showed a slightly poorer prognosis among the most recent cases (onset after 1970).[37] This argues against the view that the increased incidence rates observed in these countries are the result of a more complete inclusion of benign cases caused by improved case ascertainment at the end of the study period.

Conclusion

There is now sufficient evidence to conclude that the risk of developing MS in a population may vary over time. Fluctuations in the incidence rate have been shown in stable populations where the health care system has been good enough to ensure a reasonable quality of the case-finding methods employed, and furthermore the migration in the population has been at a level such that a change in genetic mixture of the population could not have explained the trend in the incidence. These observations represent, together with the observations in migration studies,[38] imposing evidence for the existence of important exogenous aetiological agents.

The majority of the studies investigating the most recent period have reported an increased rate. However, the true answer to what the trend is today can only be given in the future. Because of the delay period between onset and diagnosis valid data on the incidence rate for a particular period may only be constructed after several years of additional follow-up. Some areas, such as Sardinia, Western Norway, and some parts of the world which earlier were considered as low prevalence areas, like Mexico, are probably going through a phase of increased risk. The recent reports covering Olmstead county in New York State suggest that the disease is increasing also in this part of the world. The evidence of a changing rate is less convincing in many other parts of the world. Despite a number of studies in many areas, reliable data on the incidence rate are often lacking. This means that since we now have new and improved diagnostic tools and many centres have well developed systems for case finding, there is a great potential for getting new and better data on the real frequency of MS. A good example of this is England where the incidence rate is suspected to be on the increase, but where too much of the evidence relies on indirect measures of disease frequency.

Improved treatment and the development of any prophylactic strategy for MS will require increased insight into the aetiology of the disease. When studying the variation in disease frequency for aetiological purposes, the goal is to relate changes in the risk in a population to corresponding changes in the exposure to putative risk factors in the same population. Since we do not know the time of disease initiation, the closest we can get is the time of clinical onset, although the latency period between disease initiation and clinical onset probably varies and makes the inference difficult.[39] The relationship between variation in exposure to risk factors and measures which even more indirectly estimate the risk, such as prevalence rate and mortality rate, would be further blurred and this might explain the somewhat disappointing results in the search for aetiological clues despite considerable effort in determining changes in the disease occurrence.

Therefore, since there already exist a number of aetiological hypotheses which are still neither accepted nor rejected, an important step might be to move from occurrence research, which in the best case can only generate hypotheses, to more analytical epidemiological studies where specific hypotheses might be tested. Such designs are case-control studies, historical cohort studies and ecological studies. The methodological requirements for doing meaningful analytical studies, however, are at least as high as for descriptive epidemiological studies, i.e. choice of study population and controls, uniform diagnostic criteria, delay, statistical methods and design, including the number of cases to be included.[40] The lack of necessary methodological rigour including size of studies might explain much of the seemingly conflicting results from the various analytical studies which have been conducted.[41] The need for well designed studies becomes even more important when considering the possibility of a strong multifactorial aetiology with additional interactions between genetic factors and exogenous factors. This requires stratified analysis of subgroups and demands an even higher number of cases to be included in order to avoid inconclusive results. Such a mixture of aetiological factors is also compatible with the seemingly confusing picture of the distribution of the disease.

Finally, whether there is a general biological increase in the risk of acquiring MS or not, it is a fact that most neurological departments are experiencing an increased number of patients for consultations and treatment. This puts an increasing burden on the health care system and society in general, considering both the expense of current therapy and also the general burden of care of chronically ill patients. There is at present no indication that the disease will diminish in frequency, and this disease therefore represents a major future challenge for our health system.

References

1. Riise T. Cluster studies in multiple sclerosis. In: Riise T, Wolfson C, eds. The Epidemiologic Study of Exogenous Factors in the Etiology of Multiple Sclerosis: Guidelines for Future Analytical Research. *Neurology* 1997; **49** (suppl 2): S29–S34.

2. Kurtzke JF. MS epidemiology world wide. One view of current status. *Acta Neurol Scand* 1995; **161** (suppl): 23–33.

3. Ebers GC, Sadovnick AD. The geographic distribution of multiple sclerosis: a review [editorial]. *Neuroepidemiology* 1993; **12**: 1–5.

4. Fox JP. *Epidemiology, Man and Disease*, Toronto: The Macmillan Company 1970.

5. Martyn C. The epidemiology of multiple sclerosis. In: Matthews WB, Compston A, Allen IV, Martyn CN, eds. *McAlpine's Multiple Sclerosis*, Edinburgh: Churchill Livingstone 1990.

6. Kurtzke JF. Multiple sclerosis: what's in a name? *Neurology* 1988; **38**: 309–314.

7. Wynn DR, Rodriguez M, O'Fallon WM *et al.* A reappraisal of the epidemiology of multiple sclerosis in Olmsted County, Minnesota. *Neurology* 1990; **40**: 780–786.

8. Bian HJ, Xin ZZ. Prevalence of multiple sclerosis: a door-to-door survey in Lan Cang La Hu Zu Autonomous County, Yunnan Province of China. *Neuroepidemiology* 1992; **11**: 52.

9. al Rajeh S, Bademosi O, Ismail H *et al.* A community survey of neurological disorders in Saudi Arabia: the Thugbah study. *Neuroepidemiology* 1993; **12**: 164–178.

10. Koch-Henriksen N, Brønnum-Hansen H, Hyllested K. Incidence of multiple sclerosis in Denmark 1948–1982: a descriptive nationwide study. *Neuroepidemiology* 1992; **11**: 1–10.

11. Waterhouse J, Muir C, Correa P *et al. Cancer Incidence in Five Continents*, Vol. 3, IARC Scientific Publications No 15. Lyon: International Agency for Cancer Research 1976.

12. Larsen JP, Aarli JA, Nyland H *et al.* Western Norway, a high risk area for multiple sclerosis. A prevalence/incidence study in the county of Hordaland. *Neurology* 1984; **34**: 1202–1207.

13. Grønning M, Riise T, Kvåle G *et al.* Incidence of multiple sclerosis in Hordaland, Western Norway: a fluctuating pattern. *Neuroepidemiology* 1991; **10**: 53–61.

14. Midgard R, Riise T, Svanes C *et al.* Incidence of multiple sclerosis in Møre and Romsdal, Norway from 1950 to 1991. *Brain* 1996; **119**: 203–211.

15. Edland A, Nyland H, Riise T, *et al.* The epidemiology of multiple sclerosis in the county of Vestfold, Eastern Norway. *Acta Neurol Scand* 1996; **93**: 104–109.

16. Rosati G. Descriptive epidemiology of multiple sclerosis in Europe in the 1980s: a critical overview. *Ann Neurol* 1994; **36** (suppl 2): S164–S174.

17. Weinshenker BG. Epidemiology of multiple sclerosis. *Neurol Clin* 1996; **14**: 291.

18. Warren S, Warren KG. Prevalence incidence and characteristics of multiple sclerosis in Westlock, Alberta, Canada. *Neurology* 1993; **43**: 1760–1763.

19. Warren S, Warren KG. Prevalence of multiple sclerosis in Barrhead County, Alberta, Canada. *Can J Neurol Sci* 1992; **19**: 72–75.

20. Gonzalez O, Sotelo J. Is the frequency of multiple sclerosis increasing in Mexico? *J Neurol Neurosurg Psychiatry* 1995; **59**: 528–530.

21. Alter M, Olivares L. Multiple sclerosis in Mexico. An epidemiologic study. *Arch Neurol* 1970; **23**: 451–459.

22. Granieri E, Casetta I, Tola MR. Epidemiology of multiple sclerosis in Italy and in southern Europe. *Acta Neurol Scand* 1995; **91** (suppl 161): 60–70.

23. Rosati G, Aiello I, Pirastru MI *et al.* Epidemiology of multiple sclerosis in Northwestern Sardinia: Further evidence for higher frequency in Sardinians compared to other Italians. *Neuroepidemiology* 1996; **15**: 10–19.

24. Granieri E, Malagu S, Casetta I *et al.* Multiple sclerosis in Italy. A reappraisal of incidence

and prevalence in Ferrara. *Arch Neurol* 1996; **53**: 793–798.

25. Guidetti D, Cavalletti S, Merelli E *et al*. Epidemiological survey of multiple sclerosis in the provinces of Reggio Emilia and Modena, Italy. *Neuroepidemiology* 1995; **14**: 7–13.

26. Robertson N, Compston A. Surveying multiple sclerosis in the United Kingdom [editorial]. *J Neurol Neurosurg Psychiatry* 1995; **58**: 2–6.

27. Robertson N, Deans J, Fraser M *et al*. Multiple sclerosis in south Cambridgeshire: incidence and prevalence based on a district register. *J Epidemiol Community Health* 1996; **50**: 274–279.

28. Kurtzke JF. A Fennoscandinavian focus of multiple sclerosis. *Neurology* 1968; **18**: 16–20.

29. Swank RL, Lerstad O, Strøm A *et al*. Multiple sclerosis in rural Norway. *N Engl J Med* 1962; **246**: 721–728.

30. Oftedal SI. Multiple sclerosis in Vestfold, Norway. *Acta Neurol Scand* 1965; **41** (suppl 16): 3–62.

31. Presthus J. Report on multiple sclerosis investigations in West-Norway. *Acta Psychiat Neurol Scand* 1960; **35** (suppl 147): 88–92.

32. Presthus J. Multiple sclerosis in Møre and Romsdal county, Norway. *Acta Neurol Scand* 1996; **42** (suppl 19): 12–18.

33. Westlund K. Recent statistical data on multiple sclerosis and some other diseases in Norway. *Nordic Counsil Arct Med Res Rep* 1982; **32**: 19–29.

34. Svenningsson A, Runmarker B, Lycke J *et al*. Incidence of MS during two fifteen-year periods in Gothenburg region of Sweden. *Acta Neurol Scand* 1990; **82**: 161–168.

35. Kurtzke JF, Hyllested K, Heltberg A. Multiple sclerosis in the Faroe Islands: transmission across four epidemics. *Acta Neurol Scand* 1995; **91**: 321–325.

36. Cook SD, Cromarty JI, Tapp W *et al*. Declining incidence of multiple sclerosis in the Orkney Islands. *Neurology* 1985; **35** (suppl 4): 545–551.

37. Midgard R, Albrektsen G, Riise T *et al*. Prognostic factors for survival in multiple sclerosis. A longitudinal, population-based study in Møre and Romsdal, Norway. *J Neurol Neurosurg Psychiatry* 1995; **58**: 417–421.

38. Gale CR, Martyn CN. Migrant studies in multiple sclerosis. *Prog Neurobiol* 1995; **47**: 425–448.

39. Wolfson C, Wolfson DB. The latent period of multiple sclerosis: a critical review. *Epidemiology* 1993; **4**: 464–470.

40. Riise T, Wolfson C. The Epidemiologic Study of Exogenous Factors in the Etiology of Multiple Sclerosis: Guidelines for Future Analytical Research. Part I. Methodology. *Neurology* 1997; **49** (suppl 2): S6–S34.

41. Riise T, Wolfson C. The Epidemiological Study of Exogenous Factors in the Etiology of Multiple Sclerosis: Guidelines for Future Analytical Research. Part II. Selected Reviews. *Neurology* 1997; **49** (suppl 2): S44–S77.

2

Genetic epidemiology of multiple sclerosis

Stephen Sawcer, Neil Robertson and Alastair Compston

Introduction

A role for genes in the aetiology of multiple sclerosis (MS) was proposed in the late nineteenth century and was prompted by the observation of familial clustering which has since been acknowledged as one of the cardinal epidemiological features of the disease. Eichorst first labelled MS as an 'inherited, transmissible disease'.[1] Although the pendulum of professional opinion has since swung regularly between nurture and nature as the dominant aetiological force,[2] few would now doubt a significant contribution from a gene or genes involved in conferring susceptibility. The supporting epidemiological evidence was at first based on studies showing the variable distribution of MS depending on ethnicity. Later, patterns of disease recurrence within different family structures provided greater insight into the character of the genetic effect, and these have recently been the catalyst for application of novel molecular genetic techniques in the search to identify and characterize relevant genes. Evidence for a genetic contribution to disease aetiology can therefore be divided into that derived from epidemiological and from molecular genetic studies.

Epidemiological evidence

Racial susceptibility and disease frequency in genetically isolated populations

In a cursory examination of the geographical distribution of disease, it is striking that those areas with the highest prevalence of MS are all places of origin or common destinations for the emigration of northern Europeans. The origin of this phenomenon may stretch back over 2,000 years and relates to the observation that populations in the North Atlantic islands having a high prevalence of MS were founded by immigrants from the west coast of Norway (Vikings) which led to a high concentration of Nordic genes in many northern European communities. A further dissemination of northern Europeans and their genes occurred in the 19th century and led to popular emigration especially from the British Isles to North America, South Africa, Australasia and the Indian subcontinent (*Fig. 2.1*). The hypothesis that the pool of susceptibility genes for MS originated from Scandinavia prompted early researchers to match patterns of disease prevalence with population movements from northern European countries which were originally influenced by Scandinavian drift.

Disease susceptibility between racial groups can be examined by comparing disease frequency in indigenous populations with those who have migrated from a country of origin

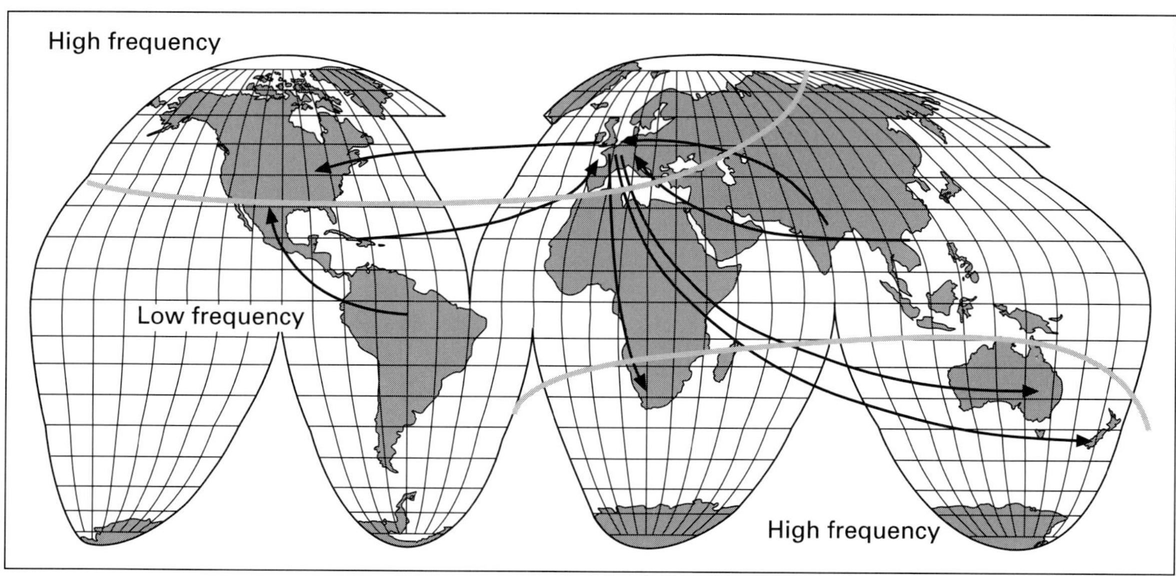

Fig. 2.1
*Patterns of migration from and to northern
Europe in the 19th century. Arrows denote major
migration patterns from and to northern Europe
during the nineteenth century and are compared
with observed disease distribution.*

with a noticeably different prevalence of MS. However, lessons to be learnt from these transcultural studies may only become apparent in successive generations. One of the first systematic examinations of ethnicity was by Davenport who suggested, on the basis of mortality and morbidity statistics, that the distribution of MS in North America reflected patterns of immigration from Scandinavia.[3] These observations were given further credence by Ebers and Bulman[4] who re-examined the veterans data derived by Kurtzke[5] and showed that the pattern of disease distribution closely parallels the proportion of the population in North American states with northern

European, particularly Scandinavian, ancestry. They concluded that associations with certain genetic markers simply reflect ethnic origin rather than linkage to specific MS susceptibility genes. Swingler and Compston correlated the prevalence of MS within the United Kingdom to regional variations in the frequency of previously identified markers of disease susceptibility in northern Europeans.[6] In Europe, Sutherland had previously suggested that Orcadians with Nordic descendants have a higher risk of developing the disease than Celts,[7] and in New Zealand Skegg, taking an unusual approach, related the regional frequency of disease to the proportion of

Racial group	Reference
Japanese-Americans	Detels et al 1977[16]
Latin-Americans	Enstrom and Operskalski 1978[15]
Hutterites	Hader 1989[96]
Lapps	Gronning and Mellgren 1985[97]
Central European Gypsies	Palffy et al 1993[98]
Black South Africans	Dean 1949[11]
American Blacks	Kurtzke 1985[99]
Chinese	Yu et al 1989[39]
Asians	Bharucha et al 1988[100]
Maoris	Skegg et al 1987[8]
Yakutes	Popov 1983[101]
Inuit	Hader et al 1988[102]
Saudis	Yaqub and Daif 1988[103]

Table 2.1
Racial groups with low prevalence.

Macs/M^cs in the phone book concluding that this reflected Scottish ancestry.[8]

In relating the frequency of disease to these populations, certain exceptions are apparent in areas where genetic isolates exist for historical or social reasons. In some situations, these peoples exhibit a low disease prevalence despite living in areas of recognized high prevalence suggesting the exclusion of disease susceptibility genes whereas in others they appear to be concentrated (*Table 2.1*). It is worth pointing out that these communities frequently have cultural traditions that may expose them to different environmental influences and modify disease frequency for other than genetic reasons.

Migration studies

Migration studies are conceptually easy but difficult to perform. They are based on comparing incidence or prevalence in population(s) migrating between areas of differing disease risk. An environmental aetiological factor is implicated if groups moving from areas of low to high prevalence, and *vice versa*, show a disease frequency which approximates to the indigenous population. However, in order for these studies to be valid, a number of important factors should be considered; the most important is that the migrant group should be entirely representative of their original population and after migration they should distribute themselves in a random fashion. It is unlikely that, in practice, either of these points hold up to close examination in any of the migrant studies, and this will confound interpretations of the relationship of latitude to prevalence. In addition, many population migrations have been prompted by religious or sectarian conflicts and the migrant cohort may be further selected by age, health, economics or physical phenotype.

Alter[9] suggested a number of additional

criteria that should be met if migration studies are to provide meaningful information: the migrant population must be of sufficient size (>100,000) and have access to good medical facilities; demographic data should be available for the migrant population and a well matched control population is needed. A good example of a migrant study in which little notice appears to have been taken of these pitfalls was that performed on Vietnamese immigrants to France.[10] The risk amongst immigrants appeared to increase, but all had at least one French parent, the principal characteristic that made immigration possible, unlike those remaining in Vietnam who were used as the control group.

One of the most influential migration studies in MS was performed in South Africa by Dean,[11] who noticed the relative paucity of the disease amongst the South African-born white population and initially published his observations in 1947. Later he identified 281 white South Africans with MS from a population of 3 million and showed that amongst South African born affected individuals, the rate was 3.5 times higher in the English-speaking than Afrikaaner population but both were lower than the rate for individuals born in northern Europe.[12] It is worth pointing out that the actual numbers in any single informative group were small (not exceeding 46) and, in the absence of census data, control information was derived from manipulations of available immigrants requiring assumptions to be made concerning subsequent mortality rates within that population. The observation of a steep gradient in the prevalence of MS amongst cohorts from the same genetic stock suggests that the predominant aetiological factor is environmental and acquired in infancy. Dean postulated that this may well be a virus.[11,12] He proposed that the excess of female patients amongst English speaking

South Africans is also relevant and because of cultural differences in the behaviour of male and female children suggested that very early infection is protective. Another explanation for the apparent relationship to age at migration might be that adults in whom the first symptoms of the disease had already manifested, as well as those who were already disabled, might choose not to emigrate.

Later, Dean began a series of studies in the UK that examined disease frequency of migrants from low to high risk areas, and subsequently in successive generations of these ethnic groups. The first considered MS among immigrants in greater London[13] by examining the records of 7,000 patients who had been admitted to hospital and attempted to determine their place of birth. They were then segregated into those from different regions and age-adjusted incidence rates were compared between groups. The incidence of admission to hospital for the Old Commonwealth countries (Australia, South Africa etc.) approximated to the rate observed for native Londoners, but was reduced in those born in the new Commonwealth countries (West Indies), and even lower if both parents had been born in these countries compared with those having native European parents. This study, like many before, suffers from lack of numbers; the group demonstrating the most marked reduction (new Commonwealth immigrants) has only 16 patients; in addition there is no comment on racial characteristics so that it may be that some immigrants with both parents born in the new Commonwealth are of Caucasian stock. Despite this, it does seem apparent that migrating to England from low risk parts of the world increases the risk of developing MS. As the 1971 census included a question on place of birth of parents it subsequently became possible to compare the incidence and prevalence of United Kingdom born children of immigrants from the Indian sub-continent, Africa and the West Indies. The rates are comparable to those expected amongst similar age groups calculated from figures for prevalence in the London Borough of Sutton. The methodological difficulties of case finding, misdiagnosis, ethnic as opposed to geographical origin, and the small numerator were all acknowledged by the investigators but the evidence suggests that the increase in disease frequency amongst this group implicates an acquired environmental susceptibility.

The Israeli policy of offering citizenship to Jewish people irrespective of place of birth provides an opportunity to study prevalence in a number of different ethnic groups domiciled within this country. The observations of Alter *et al.* following a nationwide survey between 1960 and 1966 were first published in 1971[9] and demonstrated that MS is three times more prevalent among Jewish immigrants from Europe or America than in immigrants from Africa or Asia. The rate in native born Israelis of Euro–American parentage was also slightly higher than in native born Israelis of Afro–Asian parentage. This work was later repeated analysing all patients who were hospitalized or who died with a diagnosis of MS or related disease from 1955–82, in both a nationwide and Jerusalem population and morbidity statistics were prudently adjusted for age.[14] The authors found that prevalence and incidence of MS in native born Israelis of European/American ancestry was as high or higher than that found previously in immigrants from Europe and America; amongst native born Israelis of Asian/African ancestry the prevalence was significantly higher than in Asian/African immigrants. Although the early Israeli studies appeared to indicate quite strongly the effect of environment, the later work showing differential rates in native born, second generation groups now provides sub-

stantial support for the role of genetic susceptibility. In contemplating these results, it seems valid to point out that like many other migration studies the impact on our understanding of disease susceptibility is substantially reduced by the lack of molecular genetic evidence for population homogeneity. In addition, the wanderings of the Jewish race are complicated, and it would be naïve to think that even if the original migrants to Africa, Europe and America were entirely representative of the indigenous population, which in itself is doubtful, no genetic admixing occurred with the native populations over the considerable period of their exile.

Apart from the US army related epidemiological studies of Kurtzke, two migration studies are worthy of mention. The first was the study in 1978[15] of disease amongst Spanish-surnamed Californians who have a similar genetic heritage to those from Latin America although they experience a different diet, culture and socio-economic environment. Using information from the 1970 USA census and mortality statistics, Enstrom and Operskalski[15] reported an age adjusted MS death rate of $0.27/10^5$ based on 48 MS deaths between 1966 to 1975, compared to $0.83/10^5$ for white Californians. These figures again suggest either an effect of genes or local environment as disease modifying factors, although the two cannot be separated. A similar study was performed[16] investigating the prevalence of disease amongst Japanese Americans in King and Pierce Counties, Washington, and Los Angeles County, California and an age and sex adjusted rate of $5.9/10^5$ was found despite the difference in latitude. This was felt to be the result of lower racial susceptibility to disease amongst Orientals.

The migration studies to Australia and New Zealand are of interest; although these countries are noted to have a somewhat lower prevalence than northern Europe, their genetic stock is largely similar since until recently no cases amongst Aboriginals were reported and this ethnic group constitutes only a minority of the population. The early study by Sutherland et al.[17] identified 128 cases in Queensland born either in Australia, the UK and Ireland or other parts of Europe. He reported prevalences of 9, 15 and 6/10^5, respectively, figures that failed to demonstrate a significant difference depending on country of origin. Hammond et al.[18] in a more extensive epidemiological study of Australia examined disease frequency in migrant populations from the UK and Ireland, 70 per cent of whom were 15 years of age at migration. They compared latitudinal trends in disease frequency within this population and native Australians and found similarities suggesting that factors modifying risk are operative after migration. Furthermore, they observed a trend of decreasing risk with increasing duration of Australian residence and the results of a case control study appeared to indicate that contrary to other interpretations, the age of risk for acquisition of MS is likely to extend well into adulthood. The only constraint on this well performed study is that age at onset and migration were derived from a point prevalence study and therefore one is unable to take account of incident cases who died or moved out of the area prior to prevalence day.

Migration studies were initially viewed as powerful evidence in support of an environmental aetiology, but, ironically, as the history of the world's migrant populations and their uneven distribution through host countries is incorporated into knowledge derived from wider epidemiological studies, their impact is dwindling. Furthermore, studies of second generation immigrants are providing some support for racial susceptibility, although the extent to which these peoples are incorporated into, and adopt the living patterns of their new country is difficult to assess. Migration studies are therefore inescapably linked to those of geographical distribution and racial susceptibility since it is only with comparison of disease frequency within groups in similar geographic areas that differences become apparent.

Clusters and putative epidemics

One of the most important observations in support of an environmental contribution to disease aetiology comes from reports of putative epidemics in the North Atlantic islands showing abrupt increases in incidence. Attempts have been made to associate these clusters with specific events in the social history of those populations. The first report of this nature was by Kurtzke and Hyellsted.[19] from the Faroe Islands. Before 1972 only informal assessments by visiting neurologists had been made of disease frequency in 1960 and 1966, and on both occasions the observation was made that MS is rare. Kurtzke and his colleagues began a more intensive retrospective survey in 1972 and documented 32 native Faroese with clinical onset of disease between 1943 and 1973. Since no patients were found with onset prior to 1940 they conclude that the disease was introduced by a common source which may have been British troops, resulting in a cyclical pattern of incidence representing four separate epidemics involving 20, 9, 6 and 7 patients, respectively.

It is difficult to accept these observations unreservedly as representative of an epidemic without making some comments on the nature of the data. First it is clear that the standard of medical care on the Faroes, especially with respect to neurological disease, has changed dramatically over the century, and Kurtzke's observation that no cases of MS were reported prior to 1940 may simply reflect the lack of neurological expertise. Indeed a retrospective review of death certificates by Fog in 1966[20] identified two islanders in whom MS was the stated cause of death. Although no hospital records survive for these individuals, he suggests that the diagnoses should be accepted since hospital access to Copenhagen, the closest neurological centre, was considerably restricted during the German occupation of Denmark. Also, it may not be appropriate to compare medical notes from more than 90 years ago with more contemporary records. It is probably inappropriate to consider the Faroe Islands as a virgin receptacle for propagation of a novel disease since the Faroese were, and continue to be, a mobile population, with up to 25 per cent at any one time to be found in Denmark or Iceland, both already recognized as areas of high prevalence for MS at that time. Lastly, the number of patients involved must be put into some perspective since a direct comparison between confidence intervals of the highest and lowest recorded incidence is barely significant and is given added inaccuracy by the retrospective manner in which year-of-onset was assigned.

After initial suboptimal disease surveys in the 1950s and 1960s[21,22] Iceland was also subjected to an intensive survey by Kurtzke *et al.*,[23] who found a similar pattern of a post war increase in incidence which was felt both to mirror and support the findings within the neighbouring Faroe Islands. A recent review of this work along with more detailed prospective data has now provided further insight into the temporal distribution of the disease in Iceland and sheds some doubt on the relevance of the original conclusions.[24] Initial increases in incidence coincided with the arrival of the first neurologists on the island; subsequent increases were related to cross sectional surveys and a further increase in the complement of neurologists. Incidence rates after 1975

appear to have stabilized, although (despite the variability in new cases and because of the small number involved) no statistically significant difference in incidence was observed from the beginning of the century. Analysis of the latency between year of onset and year of diagnosis by Benedikz suggests that this fell after 1940; he argues that 'It is difficult to escape the conclusion that this long latent period before diagnosis resulted in many missed patients, particularly those mildly affected.' Application of an onset-adjusted prevalence (OAP) substantially reduces the effect of a sudden rise in incidence which spawned the epidemic theory, and Benedikz postulates that the change in prevalence and incidence over time was similar to that which one might expect with serial and prospective survey. In addition, disease incidence was rising rapidly before the arrival of British troops, and the geographical distribution of disease frequency, although showing some local clustering, was unrelated to the location of army billets during the occupation.

In contrast to the single putative epidemic in the Faroes[20] and the series of epidemics in Iceland,[23] the Orkney Islands have consistently experienced one of the highest disease frequencies in the world.[25] It was proposed that within these islands MS may, in some instances, have been caused by canine distemper virus (CDV), either directly or through an autoimmune process. Exposure of susceptible individuals, possibly those with inadequate immunity to the measles virus or to CDV would then result in expression of disease at a variable time thereafter. Although controversial, the mapping of outbreaks of CDV appeared to coincide with clusters of disease in Iceland and Alaska. Personal observations by veterinarians practising in the Orkneys suggested that CDV was endemic until around 1960 when a preventative vaccine was introduced. The fall in frequency of CDV as well as the increased uptake of measles vaccination which has seen a reduction in the reported cases has coincided with an apparent decrease in the incidence of MS with only 12 patients having disease onset between 1965 and 1982 compared to the expected number of 33. It is, of course attractive to develop a theory involving a single environmental agent to explain the pattern of incidence in the Orkneys, and certainly the morbilliform viruses or herpes viruses which have neurotropic effects are good candidates. However, these patterns are not supported by any serological data, and are not reflected by a similar fall in incidence throughout the rest of northern Europe following the introduction of CDV vaccine; indeed the prevalence of disease continues to rise.

Finally, as well as serial surveys and the genetic consequences of geographical or social isolation, it is important to consider the effect of concentrated attention in small well defined populations which lend themselves to more complete case ascertainment in the analysis of MS clusters. It is noteworthy that two such clusters reported in Finland and France may well not be due to environmental factors; in the former study historical pedigree analysis demonstrated that of the 33 patients identified (prevalence 253 per 100,000) 22 were related, albeit distantly, and in the latter HLA typing 'demonstrated a high kinship coefficient' compared with controls suggesting a high degree of inbreeding.

Family studies

Twins

The determination of disease concordance in twins is a classical method for estimating the genetic contribution to aetiology. Concordance rates of 100 per cent in monozygotic twin pairs suggest pure genetic aetiology, whereas rates of less than 100 per cent suggest incomplete penetrance, or an interplay with the environment, and indicate that genetic factors alone are not sufficient for clinical expression of the disease. Comparison of concordance in monozygotic and dizygotic twins provides indication of the relative contribution made by genetic and environmental factors. Twin surveys, however, should not be viewed as an infallible method for assessing these factors since increased monozygous concordance has also been observed in diseases with a pure infective aetiology. Twin studies also depend heavily on methodology which must be examined critically in each study.

Collecting adequate numbers of twins with MS to produce meaningful results is difficult because of their relative rarity and, investigators have therefore attempted either to extend their population base or canvas many sources for notifications – thereby introducing a recruitment bias. In addition, inaccurate assignment of zygosity, falsely low concordance related to variable age at onset and failure to recognize mild or subclinical forms of the disease can also influence results. Longitudinal data which allow for this are of particular value but these have rarely been incorporated in twin studies. Only one study offers longitudinal data[26] and this saw the concordance rise from 26 to 31 per cent in monozygous twins and from 2 to 5 per cent in the dizygous pairs over a period of 7.5 years.[27]

Popular methods of recruitment have been from twin registers,[28–30] advertisement,[31–34] or from clinic populations.[26,27] Most demonstrate an increased concordance rate in monozygous twins of between 21 and 50 per cent compared with 0–17 per cent in dizygous twins (*Table 2.2*). The largest studies are remarkably consistent with monozygous concordance of around 25 per cent; magnetic resonance

				Concordance rates				
Reference	Year	DZ*/MZ†	Recruitment	MZ†			DZ*	
Bobowick[28]	1978	0.8	Twin register	2/5	40.0%		0/4	0%
Williams[31]	1980	1.0	Advertisement	6/12	50.0%		2/12	17%
Heltberg[29]	1982	1.5	Twin register	4/19	21.1%		1/28	4%
Kinnunen[30]	1987	0.9	Twin register	2/7	28.6%		0/6	0%
Uitdehaag[32]	1989	0.8	Advertisement	0/4	0.0%		0/3	0%
Ebers[36]	1983	1.6	Clinic	7/27	25.9%		1/43	2%
Sadovnick[35]	1988	1.2	Clinic	5/19	26.3%		0/23	0%
Mumford[34]	1994	1.4	Advertisement	11/44	25.0%		2/61	3%
French Research Group[33]	1992	2.2	Advertisement	1/17	5.9%		1/37	3%
Total		1.4		40/153	26.1%		8/217	4%

*DZ = dizygous twins; †MZ = monozygous twins.

Table 2.2
Twin studies.

demonstrates abnormalities consistent with MS in a further 14 per cent of unaffected monozygotic co-twins.[26,34]

Two studies are at odds with the general trend. The first reported on only 7 twins of which 4 were monozygotic and included no concordant pairs; however complementary cranial magnetic resonance scanning revealed changes compatible with MS in 75 per cent of clinically unaffected monozygotic co-twins.[32] A large study by the French Research Group on Multiple Sclerosis[33] which employed a national recruitment campaign from appeal on public television identified 116 pairs and reported concordance that was independent of zygosity in 54 twinships. This is the largest study failing to produce evidence for an effect of zygosity but over half the cohort could not be fully evaluated and the 95 per cent confidence limits (0–17.1 per cent) are not significantly different from those of the larger Canadian study (13.0–42.5 per cent).[26]

Taken together, despite the method of recruitment, three of the largest twin studies achieved monozygotic:dizygotic ratios of >1:1.3 and sex ratios of 2:1 F:M, which are close to those expected in an unselected group of patients with MS, thereby providing some validity to the varying methods of recruitment. The excess of monozygotic concordance in all large contemporary studies (with the exception of the French Research Group) provides very powerful support for a genetic contribution to disease aetiology, although genetic factors appear neither sufficient nor necessary for disease expression.

General recurrence risks

Three measurements of recurrence risk are commonly quoted and it is essential to understand the basis for each in interpretation of published literature. The familial recurrence risk is the proportion of families of probands with a second affected family member; the crude recurrence risk is the proportion of affected relatives within a designated group; and the age adjusted recurrence risk provides a statistical correction for crude risks to estimate the number of relatives likely to be affected if all were followed throughout life. Direct comparison of studies has previously been made difficult by methodological differences relating to the definition of probands and the extent to which first and second degree relatives have been investigated.

Comparison of recurrence rates for MS reveals substantial differences between geographically and ethnically distinct populations that cannot be explained by study methodology alone and may well represent differences in the genetic contribution to disease aetiology within different populations. Sadovnick *et al.* reported a familial recurrence risk of 21.9 per cent[35] in first, second or third degree relatives for a clinic based population in Vancouver; in London, Ontario only 12.9 per cent of patients in a similar clinic had an affected relative;[36] the frequency in an epidemiological study from Iceland was 14.9 per cent[22] and 19 per cent in Cambridgeshire. For contemporary cross sectional epidemiological studies in northern Europe, a figure of around 15 per cent seems agreed, although small studies of genetically stable populations whose genealogical associations have been extensively investigated show figures as high as 29 per cent[37] and even 66 per cent.[38] The low disease frequency in populations not dominated by northern European genetic stock may also be mirrored by decreased familial incidence.[39]

Three studies with substantial populations have been sufficiently robust to provide meaningful recurrence risks which can reliably be used for counselling in a clinical setting. Two of these are based on consecutive patients attending MS clinics providing 815 probands in Vancouver[35] and 674 in Flanders. One study of 674 probands in the United Kingdom is derived from population based prevalence data.[40] All are consistent in demonstrating age adjusted risks of around 2 per cent for children and parents and 2–4 per cent for siblings with lower rates in second and third degree relatives. Increased recurrence is seen even in distant relatives who have not shared a common environment. Overall, there is no preferential recurrence for maternal or paternal inheritance. These studies are summarized in *Table 2.3* as well as combined results based on the proportional numerical representation of probands although it should be understood that risks such as these cannot necessarily be grouped across geographically distinct populations albeit each of northern European extraction.

Disease in non-biological relatives

One of the most convincing pieces of evidence for the role of genetic factors in familial disease is provided by the Canadian Collaborative Study group who identified 260 patients with MS who had been adopted at or soon after birth. Having established recurrence risks in biological relatives the effect of environment was quantified in the nonbiological family. If familial disease is the result of shared environment then recurrence rates in the close nonbiological relatives would approximate to those found in biological relatives. However, if familial disease results from a genetic effect then recurrence risks in the non-biological relatives will be no greater than the background population risk. In 238 adoptees, 2/1201

Relative	Cambridge 1996				Flanders 1997				British Columbia 1988		
	n	Pop	CR (%)	AAR (%)	*n*	Pop	CR (%)	AAR (%)	*n*	Pop	CR (%)
Probands	674				674				815		
Parent	25	1,237	2.02	2.05	21	1,323	1.59	1.61	28	998	2.81
Sibling	43	1,347	3.19	3.82	33	1,836	1.80	2.10	54	1,886	2.86
Child	6	1,056	0.57	1.83	6	994	0.60	1.73	7	1,268	0.55
Nephew/Niece	10	1,770	0.56	1.64	5	3,261	0.15	0.45	10	2,789	0.36
Aunt/Uncle	21	2,580	0.81	0.87	26	4,071	0.64	0.66	38	2,051	1.85
First Cousin	23	3,401	0.68	0.88	35	9,553	0.37	0.44	41	3,142	1.30
Total	128	11,391	1.12		126	21,038	0.60		178	12,134	1.47

n = number of affected relatives; Pop = total population; CR = crude risk; AAR = age adjusted recurrence risk.

Table 2.3
*Meta-analysis of major published studies on crude and age
adjusted recurrence risks for relatives of probands with MS.*

affected relatives were identified (expected 51) demonstrating that their risk is no greater than for the general population.[41] A subsequent study of half siblings found predictably intermediate results in that 18/1839 (0.98%) half-siblings of probands also had MS.[42]

Conjugal disease

The study of conjugal pairs with complex traits provides valuable information regarding disease transmissibility, and the genetic contribution to disease frequency and clinical course. Despite an apparent increase in the prevalence of MS over the past 20 years,[43] reports of conjugal MS remain rare and only 38 examples (most are single case reports) have previously been reported. The low reported frequency of conjugal MS has generally been used as evidence against an infective agent.

The only systematic study of conjugal disease is based on 45 pairs included in a national register of familial disease in the United Kingdom.[44] This study found no evidence for clinical concordance, clustering at year of onset, or distortion of the expected pattern of age at onset in the second affected spouse from 33 pairs in whom both partners could be assessed, to suggest disease transmissibility and no increase in expected prevalence of conjugal pairs. However, an examination of recurrence risks in 86 offspring of the 45 pairs revealed that 5 (5.8 per cent) were concordant for MS; a further 4 (4.7 per cent) reported isolated episodes of neurological dysfunction and two out of 39 (5 per cent) clinically unaffected offspring studied by cranial magnetic resonance imaging had abnormalities which fulfilled radiological criteria for the diagnosis of MS.

The observed crude (1:17) recurrence risk in this group appears significantly higher than equivalent population based recurrence risks

for offspring of single affected parents (1:200). This would seem to indicate that the risk for developing MS is evidently inherited from both parents and argues against the concept of genetic heterogeneity.

Molecular genetic evidence

The epidemiological evidence described above has fuelled a considerable worldwide molecular genetic effect which until recently has been confined to searching for association or linkage to candidate genes. However, the advent of new technologies has enabled the completion of the first whole genome screens which have significantly changed understanding of the genetics of MS.

Candidate genes

The major histocompatibility complex

Allelic association with products of the major histocompatibility complex (MHC) on chromosome *6p21* was first reported over 20 years ago and remains the only consistently observed feature in the genetics of the disease.[45] Since then, MS in northern Europeans has also been shown to be associated with HLA-B7, -DR15 (DRB1*1501, DRB5*0101) and -DQ6 (DQA1*0102, DQB2*0602).[46–49] In common with most other autoimmune diseases, the strongest associations are seen with the class II antigens. The extensive linkage disequilibrium which occurs in the MHC means that the association extends for a substantial genetic distance and this makes it very difficult to establish which of the many genes encoded in the MHC is the primary determinant of susceptibility. Several alternative MHC candidates have been investigated, the most promising being genes for the cytokines tumour necrosis factor (TNF-α) and lymphotoxin (LT); these are closely linked and arranged tandemly between the class I and class III loci.[50] Early investigations gave mixed results[51,52] but more recently, strong evidence for association with these genes has been found both in Northern Ireland[53] and German populations.[54] Other MHC alternative candidates have not been as promising with investigators finding no consistent evidence for association to the peptide transporter genes TAP 1 or TAP 2,[55–57] the DP genes[58,59] or the class III genes.[60,61]

Non-MHC candidates

The principal non-MHC candidates investigated include the T-cell receptor alpha[62–66] and beta[67–73] chain genes, the immunoglobulin heavy chain genes[74–76] and the gene for myelin basic protein.[77–79] None of these has provided consistent evidence for a role in determining susceptibility although some, such as the immunoglobulin heavy chain variable region, remain as potential candidates.

Mitochondrial genes

In 1992 Harding *et al*.[80] identified 8 female patients with Leber's hereditary optic neuropathy who went on to develop an MS-like illness with demyelination outside the visual system. These cases all had a mutation at position 11778 in their mitochondrial DNA and were the first examples of the clinical syndrome we now refer to as Harding's disease. In a subsequent review of Leber's hereditary optic neuropathy Riordan-Eva *et al*,[81] reported that 45 per cent of 24 female patients with the 11778 mutation had an MS-like illness.

Several groups have searched without success for pathological mitochondrial mutations in unrelated, randomly selected MS patients,[82–84] making it unlikely that a susceptibility gene for MS is encoded within the mitochondrial genome.

In considering the candidate gene studies discussed above it is important to remember that the small size of most studies means that they have almost no power to detect anything other than a very major effect, and therefore caution should be used in interpreting marginal results.

The genome screens

Three broadly comparable whole genome screens have now been completed in MS.[85–87] Some of the basic experimental features of these studies are shown in *Table 2.4*. All three of the screens were performed in a staged fashion, in which the whole genome was initially screened in a moderately-sized population (stage 1) and then further families were typed only in those regions showing potential linkage (stage 2). The failure of any one of the screens to identify a major susceptibility locus indicates that it is very unlikely that a major gene exists; the probability that it would be missed in all three studies is very low. On the other hand, all of the studies identified more low threshold lod scores than would be expected by chance alone, implying that at least some of these are probably genuine.

The United Kingdom screen[85]

A multipoint linkage analysis was performed in this screen using the computer program MAPMAKER/SIBS.[88] This program calculates a maximum lod score (MLS) value at each point in the genome on the basis of all the available genotypes, and thereby generates MLS profiles along each chromosome. Any positive MLS value indicates potential linkage but the peaks in these profiles, which may be referred to as 'hits', identify the most likely locations of disease susceptibility genes. To overcome the problem of multiple testing, computer simulations were used to establish both the pointwise and genomewide significance of the observed hits.[89]

A total of twenty hits (regions where the

	UK	American/ French*	Canadian[†]
Stage 1			
Families	129	52	61
Sib Pairs	143	81	100
Total Individuals	447	471	320
Total Affected	265	129	137
Markers	311	443	261
Stage 2			
Families	98	23	114
Sib Pairs	108	45	122
Total Individuals	322	172	327
Total Affected	201	63	232
Markers[‡]	46	3	8

*This group performed traditional linkage analysis and an affected relative pair analysis in addition to a sib pair analysis. Their families had 58 alternative relative pairs in stage 1 and 30 alternative relative pairs in stage 2, in addition to those sib pairs shown.
[†]There were 257 markers in the index set used in stage 1 of this screen. However, a further 4 markers (flanking D5S406) were subsequently added giving a total of 261 markers typed in the stage 1 families.
[‡]All groups are typing additional markers in other regions in their stage 2 families.

Table 2.4
Comparison of the principal experimental details used in the three MS genome screens.

MLS profile exceeded the nominal 5 per cent significance level) was identified in the stage 1 screen, the most significant being on chromosome *5q* (MLS = 2.7). Markers from nine of these hits were typed in the stage 2 families after which the lod score increased in only three regions (*6p21*, *17q22* and X) and decreased in all others. It should be noted that even after addition of the stage 2 families no region reached an MLS value of more than 2.8, which is well short of the MLS level associated with a 5 per cent genomewide significance (MLS $\geqslant$3.2). Evidence for linkage disequilibrium was sought in the two best supported regions (*6p21* and *17q22*) using a transmission disequilibrium test. Only the TNF-α marker showed significant evidence for transmission disequilibrium with $\chi^2_{df3} = 10.2$

($p < 0.017$); this was confined almost exclusively to excess transmission of the 121 base pair allele, for which $\chi^2_{df1} = 10.1$ ($p < 0.001$).

The American/French screen[86]

These investigators typed extended pedigrees as well as sib pair families, and maximized their information extraction by typing considerably more markers than either of the other two groups.

For each marker in stage 1, the authors performed a single point sib pair analysis (IBD), an affected relative pair analysis (IBS) and four traditional lod score analyses using different models. Although testing for linkage in several ways increases the number of tests performed, this effect is offset by two other factors. First, each of the 3 main types of test (sib pair, affected relative pair and lod score) uses a slightly different, although overlapping, sample. Second, and more importantly, the authors required a positive result in more than one type of test for the marker to be declared a hit. A total of 19 regions met the authors' criteria for consideration as a stage 1 hit, the most promising of these was on chromosome *7q21–22*.

Only one region, the MHC, was further investigated in stage 2. Using all the data from both stages for the three markers D6S273, tumour necrosis factor (TNF) and HLA-DR the authors performed a multipoint analysis which produced a peak MLS of 3.6, strongly supporting the importance of the MHC region in MS and representing the highest multipoint lod score seen in any of the three screens.

The Canadian screen[87]

In stage 1 of the Canadian screen, marker D5S406 gave a single point lod score of 4.24 (the highest single point score seen in any of the screens); unfortunately the multipoint analysis of all the data on chromosome 5

reduced this value to just 1.8. This difference is important as in general, a multipoint analysis gives a more accurate estimate of the sharing probabilities in a sample of sib pairs, suggesting that the single point analysis may have exaggerated the extent of excess sharing in the region. The greater accuracy of multipoint analysis results from its ability to estimate the sharing of alleles inherited from homozygous parents by using the results in flanking markers; a single point analysis cannot extract any information from such parents and therefore generates estimates that are biased in favour of the sharing observed in those pairs that happen to be informative for the marker considered.

Although the Canadian stage 1 data provide little direct evidence for linkage in the MHC region, the authors tested their 3 markers from this region for evidence of linkage disequilibrium using a transmission disequilibrium test (TDT)[90] and demonstrated excess transmission of the 13 allele of the marker D6S461 ($\chi^2_{df1} = 10.8$), a result which was significant even after Bonferroni correction.

In stage 2 of the Canadian screen additional families were typed in the MHC and the region on chromosome *5p* showing evidence for linkage in stage 1. Considering all their data together, the final MLS values on chromosome *5p* and in the MHC region, were 1.6 and 0.7 respectively. However, the final χ^2_{df1} for the TDT of the 13 allele of marker D6S461 was 14.4 ($p < 0.0001$) indicating considerable evidence for linkage disequilibrium in the region of that marker. This is clearly the most significant result seen in any of the screens. It is important to remember that a TDT only gives positive results for a locus that is both in linkage disequilibrium and linked, and therefore it can be viewed as a test for both linkage and association, as pointed out by Spielman.[90]

Conclusions

The epidemiological evidence

Although the impact of epidemiological studies performed towards the middle of this century concerning migration studies and analyses of clusters indicating a dominant environmental aetiology may have been overshadowed by more modest genetic analyses, they remain valid. It is therefore not helpful for more recent investigators attempting to uncover the relative importance of aetiological factors in this disease to pursue one view to the exclusion of others and without an historical perspective. The simple answer to the size of genetic contribution is around 35 per cent (based on monozygotic twin concordance) and there is no reason why genes and environment should not sit comfortably together in explaining disease expression.

Much of the recent impetus into investigating the genetic effect was prompted by novel family studies and it is worth passing a critical eye over these as well. The analysis of familial recurrence in MS depends on the accurate assignment of disease status. The recall of probands and their knowledge of disease status in relatives has to be relied on heavily. Extended studies of concordant sibling pairs also indicate that the risk to relatives may not be spread evenly amongst families and high

	Highest MLS value in the region		
Region	Cambridge	American/ French*	Canadian
1p	1.2	–	1.0
3q	–	1.4	1.0
5q	2.6	1.1	–
6p	0.8†	2.0	0.2†
6q	0.8	2.4	–
7p	1.8	–	0.9
7q	–	1.1	0.7
19q	1.6	1.6	0.7

*This group only provided *p* values for the results of their sibpair and affected pair analyses and therefore where these were the most significant the asymptotic MLS values with the equivalent significance are shown.
†Both these studies demonstrated evidence for linkage disequilibrium in this region using a TDT.

Table 2.5
Stage 1 regions of agreement.

risk pedigrees may exist that have different or more potent susceptibility genes.[91] Furthermore the relevance of radiological lesions compatible with MS seen in clinically unaffected twins,[92] siblings within multiplex families[93] and offspring of conjugal pairs is not yet clear; whether this finding genuinely represents pre-clinical disease will only become apparent with time.

Perhaps the most important proviso is that recurrence rates can only be applied generally to the population under study if it is considered that the disease is aetiologically homogeneous. The clinical and radiological differences between primary progressive and relapsing-remitting disease[94] and geographical differences in phenotype[95] hint at the possibility of disease heterogeneity. If proven, the impact of this on the interpretation of studies into variable distribution and familial recurrence could be considerable.

The molecular genetic evidence

Taking the three genome screens together, it is clear that the only region which is well supported in each is the MHC region on chromosome *6p21*. The only other region in which some evidence for linkage is found in all three studies is the region on chromosome *19q*. Given the size of these studies it is to be expected that small effects will not necessarily be detected in each, thus the regions which are matched in two studies but not the third may well indicate genuine effects and certainly warrant further investigation (see *Table 2.5*). Continued molecular genetic efforts over the next few years will no doubt increase our understanding of the susceptibility to MS.

References

1. Eichorst H. Uber infantile und hereditare multiple sclerose. *Virchows Arch* 1896; **146:** 173–193.
2. Compston DAS. The dissemination of multiple sclerosis. The Langdon–Brown lecture 1989. *J R Coll Physicians Lond* 1990; **24:** 207–218.
3. Davenport CB. Multiple sclerosis from the standpoint of geographic distribution and race. *Arch Neurol Psychiatry* 1922; **8:** 51–58.
4. Ebers GC, Bulman D. The geography of MS reflects genetic susceptibility. *Neurology* 1986; **36:** 108.
5. Kurtzke JF, Beebe JW, Norman JE. Epidemiology of multiple sclerosis in US veterans. Part I. Race, sex and geographic distribution. *Neurology* 1979; **29:** 1228–1235.
6. Swingler RJ, Compston DAS. The distribution of multiple sclerosis in the United Kingdom. *J Neurol Neurosurg Psychiatry* 1986; **49:** 1115–1124.
7. Sutherland JM. Observations on the prevalence of multiple sclerosis in northern Scotland. *Brain* 1956; **79:** 635–654.
8. Skegg DCG, Corwin PA, Craven RS *et al.* Occurrence of multiple sclerosis in the north and south of New Zealand. *J Neurol Neurosurg Psychiatry* 1987; **50:** 134–139.
9. Alter M, Kahana E, Loewenson R. Migration and risk of multiple sclerosis. *Neurology* 1971; **28:** 1089–1093.
10. Kurtzke JF, Bui QJ. Multiple sclerosis in a migrant population. Part II. Half orientals immigrating in childhood. *Neurology* 1980; **8:** 256–260.
11. Dean G. Disseminated sclerosis in South Africa. *Br Med J* 1949; **1:** 842–845.
12. Dean G. Annual incidence, prevalence and mortality of multiple sclerosis in white South-African born and in white immigrants to South Africa. *Br Med J* 1967; **2:** 724–730.
13. Dean G, McLoughlin H, Brady R *et al.* Multiple sclerosis among immigrants in Greater London. *Br Med J* 1976; **1:** 861–864.
14. Kahana E, Zilber N, Abramson JH *et al.* Multiple sclerosis: Genetic versus environmental aetiology: Epidemiology in Israel updated. *J Neurol* 1994; **241:** 341–346.
15. Enstrom JE, Operskalski EA. Multiple sclerosis among Spanish-surnamed Californians. *Neurology* 1978; **28:** 434–438.
16. Detels R, Visscher BR, Malmgren RM *et al.* Evidence for lower susceptibility to multiple sclerosis in Japanese-Americans. *Am J Epidemiol* 1977; **105:** 303–310.
17. Sutherland JM, Tyrer JH, Eadie MJ *et al.* The prevalence of multiple sclerosis in Queensland Australia. A field survey. *Acta Neurol Scand* 1966; **42:** 57–67.
18. Hammond SR, McLeod JG, Millingen KS *et al.* The epidemiology of multiple sclerosis in three Australian cities: Perth, Newcastle and Hobart. *Brain* 1987; **111:** 1–25.
19. Kurtzke JF, Hyellsted K. Multiple sclerosis in the Faroe Islands. *Ann Neurol* 1979; **5:** 6–21.
20. Fog T, Hyellsted K. The prevalence of disseminated sclerosis in the Faroes, the Orkneys and Shetland. *Acta Neurol Scand* 1966; **42** (suppl 19): 9–11.
21. Gudmundsson KR, Gudmundsson G. Multiple sclerosis in Iceland. *Acta Neurol Scand* 1962; **38** (suppl 2): 1–63.
22. Gudmundsson KR. Clinical studies of multiple sclerosis in Iceland. *Acta Neurol Scand* 1971; **47** (suppl 48): 1–78.
23. Kurtzke JF, Gudmundsson KR, Bergmann S. Multiple sclerosis in Iceland. Evidence of a post war epidemic. *Neurology* 1982; **32:** 143–150.
24. Benedikz J, Magnusson H, Gudmundsson G. Multiple sclerosis in Iceland, with observations on the alleged epidemic in the Faroe islands. *Ann Neurol* 1994; **39** (suppl 2): S175–179.
25. Poskanzer DC, Prenny LB, Sheridan JL *et al.* Multiple sclerosis in the Orkney and Shetland Islands. I Epidemiology, clinical factors and

methodology. *J Epidemiol Comm Health* 1980; **34**: 229–239.

26. Ebers GC, Bulman DE, Sadovnick AD *et al*. A population based study of multiple sclerosis in twins. *N Engl J Med* 1986; **315**: 1638–1642.

27. Sadovnick AD, Armstrong H, Rice GPA *et al*. A population based study of multiple sclerosis in twins: updated. *Ann Neurol* 1993; **33**: 281–285.

28. Bobowick A, Kurtzke JF, Brody JA *et al*. Twin study of multiple sclerosis: an epidemiologic inquiry. *Neurology* 1978; **28**: 978–987.

29. Heltberg A, Holm NV. Concordance in twins and recurrence in sibships in multiple sclerosis. *Lancet* 1982; **1**: 1068.

30. Kinnunen E, Koskenvuo M, Kaprio J *et al*. Multiple sclerosis in a nationwide series of twins. *Neurology* 1987; **37**: 1627–1629.

31. Williams A, Eldridge R, McFarland H *et al*. Multiple sclerosis in twins. *Neurology* 1980; **30**: 1139–1147.

32. Uitdehaag BMJ, Polman CH, Valk J *et al*. Magnetic resonance imaging studies in multiple sclerosis twins. *J Neurol Neurosurg Psychiatry* 1989; **52**: 1417–1419.

33. French Research Group on Multiple Sclerosis. Multiple sclerosis in 54 twinships: concordance rate is independent of zygosity. *Ann Neurol* 1992; **32**: 724–727.

34. Mumford CJ, Wood NW, Kellar-Wood HF *et al*. The British Isles survey of multiple sclerosis in twins. *Neurology* 1994; **44**: 11–15.

35. Sadovnick AD, Baird PA, Ward RH. Multiple sclerosis: updated risks for relatives. *Am J Med Genet* 1988; **29**: 533–541.

36. Ebers GC. Genetic factors in multiple sclerosis. *Neurol Clin* 1983; **1**: 645–654.

37. Wikstrom J, Tienari PJ, Sumelahti ML *et al*. In: *Multiple Sclerosis in Europe – An epidemiological update*. Darmstadt: Leuchtturm-Verlag/LTV Press 1993, 73–78.

38. Binzer M, Forsgren L, Holmgren G *et al*. Familial clustering of multiple sclerosis in a northern Swedish rural district. *J Neurol Neurosurg Psych* 1994; **57**: 497–499.

39. Yu YL, Woo E, Hawkins BR *et al*. Multiple sclerosis amongst chinese in Hong Kong. *Brain* 1989; **112**: 1445–1467.

40. Robertson NP, Fraser M, Deans J *et al*. Age adjusted recurrence risks for relatives of patients with multiple sclerosis. *Brain* 1996; **119**: 449–455.

41. Ebers GC, Sadovnick AD, Risch NJ *et al*. A genetic basis for familial aggregation in multiple sclerosis. *Nature* 1995; **377**: 150–151.

42. Sadovnick AD, Ebers GC, Dyment DA *et al*. Evidence for genetic basis of multiple sclerosis. *Lancet* 1996; **347**: 1728–1731.

43. Robertson NP, Compston DAS. Surveying multiple sclerosis in the United Kingdom. *J Neurol Neurosurg Psychiatry* 1995; **58**: 2–6.

44. Robertson N, O'Riordan J, Clayton D *et al*. Conjugal multiple sclerosis. *J Neurol* 1995; **242**: S8.

45. Jersild C, Svejgaard A, Fog T. HL-A antigens and multiple sclerosis. *Lancet* 1972; **1**: 1240–1241.

46. Jersild C, Fog T, Hansen GS *et al*. Histocompatibility determinants in multiple sclerosis, with special reference to clinical course. *Lancet* 1973; **2**: 1221–1225.

47. Olerup O, Hillert J. HLA class II-associated genetic susceptibility in multiple sclerosis: A critical evaluation. *Tissue Antigens* 1991; **38**: 1–15.

48. Spurkland A, Roniningen K, Vandvik B *et al*. HLA-DQA1 and HLA-DQB1 genes may jointly determine susceptibility to develop multiple sclerosis. *Hum Immunol* 1991; **30**: 69–75.

49. Kellar-Wood H, Wood NW, Holmans P *et al*. Multiple sclerosis and the HLA-D region: linkage and association studies. *J Neuroimmunol* 1995; **58**: 183–190.

50. Udalova IA, Nedospasov SA, Webb GC *et al*. Highly informative typing of the human TNF locus using six adjacent polymorphic markers. *Genomics* 1993; **16**: 180–186.

51. Roth MP, Nogueira L, Coppin H *et al*. Tumour necrosis factor polymorphisms in multiple sclerosis: no additional association independent of HLA. *J Neuroimmunol* 1994; **51**: 93–99.

52. Sandberg-Wollheim M, Ciusani E, Salmaggi A *et al*. An evaluation of tumour necrosis factor microsatellites in genetic susceptibility to multiple sclerosis. *Multiple Sclerosis* 1995; **1**: 181–185.

53. Kirk CW, Droogan AG, Hawkins SA *et al.* Tumour necrosis factor microsatellites show association with multiple sclerosis. *J Neuro Sci* 1997; **147**: 21–25.

54. Epplen C, Jackel S, Santos EJM *et al.* Genetic predisposition to multiple sclerosis as revealed by immunoprinting. *Ann Neurol* 1997; **41**: 341–352.

55. Kellar-Wood H, Powys S, Gray J *et al.* MHC encoded TAP1 and TAP2 dimorphisms in multiple sclerosis. *Tissue Antigens* 1994; **43**: 129–132.

56. Spurkland A, Knutsen I, Undlien DE *et al.* No association of multiple sclerosis to alleles at the TAP2 locus. *Hum Immunol* 1994; **39**: 299–301.

57. Middleton D, Megaw G, Cullen C *et al.* TAP1 and TAP2 polymorphisms in multiple sclerosis patients. *Hum Immunol* 1994; **40**: 131–134.

58. Moen T, Stein R, Bratlie A *et al.* Distribution of HLA SB antigens in multiple sclerosis. *Tissue Antigens* 1984; **24**: 126–127.

59. Olerup O, Hillert J, Fredrikson S. The HLA-D region associated MS susceptibility genes may be located telomeric to the HLA-DP subregion. *Tissue Antigens* 1990; **35**: 37–39.

60. Fielder AHL, Batchelor JR, Vakarelis BN *et al.* Optic neuritis and multiple sclerosis; do factor B alleles influence progression of disease? *Lancet* 1981; **2**: 1246–1248.

61. Bulman DE, Armstrong H, Ebers GC. Allele frequencies of the third component of complement (C3) in MS patients. *J Neurol Neurosurg Psychiatry* 1991; **54**: 554–555.

62. Martell M, Marcadet A, Strominger J *et al.* T cell receptor alpha genes might be involved in multiple sclerosis genetic susceptibility. *CR Acad Sci* 1987; **304**: 105–110.

63. Oksenberg JR, Sherritt M, Begovich AB *et al.* T cell receptor V alpha and C alpha alleles associated with multiple sclerosis and myasthenia gravis. *Proc Natl Acad Sci USA* 1989; **86**: 988–992.

64. Hashimoto LL, Mak T, Ebers GC. T-cell receptor alpha-chain polymorphisms in multiple sclerosis. *J Neuroimmunol* 1992; **40**: 41–48.

65. Hillert J, Leng C, Olerup O. T-cell receptor alpha chain germline polymorphisms in mul-

66. Eoli M, Wood NW, Kellar-Wood HF *et al.* No linkage between multiple sclerosis and the T cell receptor alpha chain locus. *J Neurol Sci* 1994; **124**: 32–37.

67. Beall SS, Concannon P, Charmley P *et al.* The germline repertoire of T-cell beta chain genes in patients with progressive multiple sclerosis. *J Neuroimmunol* 1989; **21**: 59–66.

68. Seboun E, Robinson MA, Doolittle TH. A susceptibility locus for multiple sclerosis is linked to the T cell receptor beta chain complex. *Cell* 1989; **57**: 1095–1100.

69. Charmley P, Beall SS, Concannon P *et al.* Further localisation of a multiple sclerosis susceptibility gene on chromosome 7q using a new T-cell receptor β chain polymorphism. *J Neuroimmunol* 1991; **32**: 231–240.

70. Fugger L, Sandberg-Wollheim M, Morling N *et al.* The germline repertoire of T-cell receptor beta chain genes in patients with relapsing remitting multiple sclerosis or optic neuritis. *Immunogenetics* 1990; **31**: 278–280.

71. Hillert J, Leng C, Olerup O. No association with germline T-cell receptor beta-chain gene alleles or haplotypes in Swedish patients with multiple sclerosis. *J Neuroimmunol* 1991; **31**: 141–147.

72. Lynch SG, Rose JW, Petajan JH *et al.* Discordance of T-cell receptor beta-chain genes in familial multiple sclerosis. *Ann Neurol* 1991; **30**: 402–410.

73. Wood NW, Sawcer SJ, Robertson N *et al.* The T-cell receptor beta locus and susceptibility to multiple sclerosis. *Neurology* 1995; **45**: 1859–1863.

74. Gaiser CN, Johnson MJ, Delange G *et al.* Susceptibility to multiple sclerosis associated with an immunoglobulin gamma 3 restriction length polymorphism. *J Clin Invest* 1987; **79**: 309–313.

75. Walter MA, Gibson WT, Ebers GC *et al.* Susceptibility to multiple sclerosis is associated with the proximal immunoglobulin heavy chain region. *J Clin Inv* 1991; **87**: 1266–1273.

76. Wood NW, Sawcer SJ, Kellar-Wood HF *et al.* Susceptibility to multiple sclerosis and the immunoglobulin heavy chain variable region. *J Neurol* 1995; **242**: 677–682.

77. Tienari P, Wikstrom J, Sajantila A *et al.* Genetic susceptibility to multiple sclerosis linked to the myelin basic protein gene. *Lancet* 1993; **340**: 987–991.

78. Rose J, Gerken S, Lynch S *et al.* Genetic susceptibility in familial multiple sclerosis not linked to myelin basic protein gene. *Lancet* 1993; **341**: 1179–1181.

79. Wood NW, Holmans P, Clayton D *et al.* No linkage or association between multiple sclerosis and the myelin basic protein gene in affected sibling pairs. *J Neurol Neurosurg Psychiatry* 1994; **57**: 1191–1194.

80. Harding AE, Sweeney MG, Miller DH *et al.* Occurrence of multiple sclerosis-like illness in women who have a Leber's hereditary optic neuropathy mitochondrial DNA mutation. *Brain* 1992; **115**: 979–989.

81. Riordan-Eva P, Sanders MD, Govan GG *et al.* The clinical features of Leber's hereditary optic neuropathy defined by the presence of pathogenic mitochondrial DNA mutation. *Brain* 1995; **118**: 319–337.

82. Kellar-Wood H, Robertson N, Gorvan GG *et al.* Leber's hereditary optic neuropathy mitochondrial DNA mutations in multiple sclerosis. *Ann Neurol* 1994; **36**: 109–112.

83. Kalman B, Lublin FD, Alder H. Mitochondrial DNA mutations in multiple sclerosis. *Multiple Sclerosis* 1995; **1**: 32–36.

84. Nishimura M, Obayashi H, Ohta M *et al.* No association of the 11778 mitochondrial DNA mutation and multiple sclerosis in Japan. *Neurology* 1995; **45**: 1333–1334.

85. Sawcer SJ, Jones HB, Feakes R *et al.* A genome screen in multiple sclerosis reveals susceptibility loci on chromosomes 6p21 and 17q22. *Nat Genet* 1996; **13**: 464–468.

86. Haines JL, Ter-Minassian M, Bazyk A *et al.* A complete genomic screen for multiple sclerosis underscores a role for the major histocompatibility complex. *Nat Genet* 1996; **13**: 469–471.

87. Ebers GC, Kukay K, Bulman DE *et al.* A full genome search in multiple sclerosis. *Nat Genet* 1996; **13**: 472–476.

88. Kruglyak L, Lander ES. Complete multipoint sib-pair analysis of qualitative and quantitative traits. *Am J Hum Genet* 1995; **57**: 439–454.

89. Sawcer SJ, Jones HB, Judge D *et al.* Genome Screen simulations to establish empirical genomewide significance levels. *Genet Epidemiol* 1997; **14**: 223–229.

90. Spielman RS, McGinnis RE, Ewens WJ. Transmission test for linkage disequilibrium: The insulin gene region and insulin-dependent diabetes mellitis (IDDM). *Am J Hum Genet* 1993; **52**: 506–516.

91. Doolittle TH, Myers RH, Lehrich JR *et al.* Multiple sclerosis sibling pairs: clustered onset and familial predisposition. *Neurology* 1990; **40**: 1546–1552.

92. Thorpe JW, Mumford CJ, Compston DAS *et al.* British Isles survey of multiple sclerosis in twins: MRI. *J Neurol Neurosurg Psychiatry* 1994; **57**: 491–496.

93. Tienari PJ, Salonen O, Wikstrom J *et al.* Familial multiple sclerosis: MRI findings in clinically affected and unaffected siblings. *J Neurol Neurosurg Psychiatry* 1992; **55**: 883–886.

94. Thompson AJ, Kermode AG, Wicks D *et al.* Major differences in the dynamics of primary and secondary progressive multiple sclerosis. *Ann Neurol* 1991; **29**: 53–62.

95. Shibasaki H, MacDonald WI, Kuroiwa Y. Racial modification of clinical picture of multiple sclerosis: Comparison between British and Japanese patients. *J Neurol Sci* 1981; **49**: 253–271.

96. Hader WJ. MS in Canadian Indians and Hutterites. *Proceedings of a workshop on genes and susceptibility to multiple sclerosis.* Cambridge. Cited in Lachman PJ, McFarlin D. *Nature* 1989; **347**: 693.

97. Gronning M, Mellgren SI. Multiple sclerosis in the two northernmost counties of Norway. *Acta Neurol Scand* 1985; **72**: 321–327.

98. Palffy G, Czopf J, Gyodi E. In: *Multiple sclerosis in Europe – An epidemiological update.* Darmstadt: Leuchtturm-Verlag/LTV Press 1993, 274–278.

99. Kurtzke JF, Beebe JW, Norman JE. Epidemiology of multiple sclerosis in US veterans. III. Migration and the risk of MS. *Neurology* 1985; **35**: 672–678.

100. Bharucha NE, Bharucha EP, Wadia NH *et al.* Prevalence of multiple sclerosis in the Parsis of Bombay. *Neurology* 1988; **38**: 727–729.

101. Popov VS. Clinical picture and epidemiology of disseminated sclerosis. *Zh Nevropatol Psikhiatr* 1983; **83**: 1330–1334.
102. Hader WJ, Elliott M, Ebers GC. Epidemiology of multiple sclerosis in London and Middlesex County, Ontario, Canada. *Neurology* 1988; **38**: 617–621.
103. Yaqub BA, Daif AK. Multiple sclerosis in Saudi Arabia. *Neurology* 1988; **38**: 621–623.

3

How many kinds of multiple sclerosis are there?

W Ian McDonald and Alan J Thompson

The question posed by the title of this chapter is often repeated. Formerly of primarily scientific interest, it has assumed a more pressing importance now that the possibility of modifying the course of multiple sclerosis (MS) is coming closer to reality. The question arises because the neurologist sees patients with widely differing patterns and course of disease – relapsing–remitting, secondary progressive, primary progressive, benign and rapidly fatal – and there appear to be differences in the relative frequency of clinical manifestations in different racial groups. It is natural to ask, therefore, whether these various forms of the disease show distinctive pathological features, whether their pathogenesis differs and, most fundamentally, whether they have a different aetiology. The last question cannot yet be answered, but the others are at least worth examining, as we do in this chapter.

The clinical variants of MS

The commonest clinical expression of MS is the relapsing–remitting disease which, in approximately two thirds, evolves into a steadily progressive illness with or without superimposed relapses. The time from clinical onset to the development of progression varies widely, but is on average between 10 and 15 years.[1–3] What happens pathologically when the phase of insidious progression develops is still obscure. There may well be a change in

emphasis in the different elements of the pathological process (for example: axon degeneration may become relatively more important), but given that relapses do continue in many patients and gadolinium-diethylene triamine pentaacetic acid (Gd-DTPA)-enhancement continues to occur in patients with secondary progressive disease, there is no reason to suppose that there is a fundamental change in the pathogenetic mechanism.

Benign MS

The first variant of this pattern for which the question of a separate disease entity arises is so-called 'benign' MS in which there is little or no disability after 15 years.[4] But most patients with such a course ultimately do develop significant and progressive disability: in one cohort followed up,[5] although 32 per cent were classified as having little disability at 16–20 years, at over 25 years only 14 per cent were in this category. Although there is no description of the post mortem findings in patients who at death had had a long history but minimal impairment due to MS, the pathological manifestations detectable by standard magnetic resonance imaging (MRI) techniques are indistinguishable from those in cases running a shorter and more severe course. The frequency of Gd-DTPA enhancement in serial studies is, as expected, lower than in patients early in the course of relapsing–remitting disease, although it is seen in both groups, probably indicating that inflammatory activity is present.[6,7] The volume of T_2-weighted abnormality (principally reflecting gliosis) is often not different between patients with mild and severe impairment[8] although there is evidence derived from special techniques for greater atrophy and axonal loss in more disabled patients.[9,10] The possibility that patients with a benign course have a greater potential for remyelination is a real one,[11,12] but relevant data are lacking. Remyelination cannot be detected by present nuclear magnetic resonance (NMR) techniques, either imaging or spectroscopy; but its presence can be inferred from a shortening of latency in serially recorded evoked potentials.[13] It would be interesting to determine whether there was a greater frequency of normalization of evoked potentials in a cohort of patients with long-standing benign disease than in an appropriately matched cohort of patients with more rapidly progressive disease.

Taken together the clinical and MRI evidence suggests that benign disease is merely a temporal variant of relapsing–remitting–secondary progressive disease and is unlikely to be distinct pathologically or pathogenetically.

Malignant MS

At the other extreme of the temporal scale are the rare patients who die within a year of onset, sometimes referred to as having the Marburg form of MS.[14,15] At post mortem, these patients have changes indistinguishable from those of relapsing–remitting–secondary progressive disease except that many lesions in the former appear by histological criteria to be of a more similar age than is usual in the latter. While some of these patients have no remissions, others do, with subsequent relapse. It seems likely that these latter patients too have the same disease as the patients with a

longer time course. Whether those patients with rapid inexorable progression to death have the same disease must remain an open question at present.

Primary progressive MS

A third clinical variant of MS in which the question of a specifically different pathogenesis arises is that in which the illness is progressive from onset without a history of a clear-cut relapse or remission. This variant has been reviewed recently and only the main points will be summarized here.[16]

Patients with this variant tend to be older, and the usual female preponderance is less marked.[2] Prognosis is poorer, the time taken to reach EDSS6 being approximately six years, which is similar, however, to the interval between the onset of the progressive phase after the preceding years of relapses and remissions in the majority of patients.

MRI reveals significantly less T_2-weighted abnormality in the brain than in relapsing–remitting–secondary progressive MS.[17] The brain may indeed appear normal. The extent of lesions in the spinal cord is similar in primary and secondary progressive disease.[18] New lesions in the brain are less frequent than in other forms of MS and of particular note is the observation that they enhance much less frequently (5 per cent versus 80–90 per cent). The latter observation led to the suggestion that primary progressive MS may be less inflammatory than secondary progressive disease, and this has been confirmed pathologically.[19]

The possibility that a genetic difference might determine the distinctive course of primary progressive MS is an attractive one. In what is probably the most comprehensive study to date, Olerup *et al.*[20] found, in a Swedish cohort, that primary progressive MS was associated with DQB1. The same investigators, however, did not find this association in a Norwegian cohort,[21] although in relapsing–remitting disease in both cohorts DRw17 and DQw2 were five times more common than in primary progressive disease. Other associations have been found in other populations (see review by Thompson *et al.*[16]); a consistent pattern has not emerged.

Turning to the question of possible immunological differences, here too the evidence is not conclusive, not least because it has been usual to lump together cases of primary and secondary progressive MS as 'chronic progressive' disease in published reports. A few have made this distinction, but the number of patients studied and the number of investigations performed are rather small. Differences in the intrathecal synthesis of immunoglobulin G (IgG), impairment of the blood–brain barrier permeability, autoantibody production, pro- and anti-cytokine production and the presence of soluble endothelial adhesion molecules, have been reported but not yet confirmed.[22–25]

In summary, the present evidence does not justify the conclusion that primary progressive MS is a separate disease. The present data favours its belonging to a spectrum with the other forms of the disease; but the question remains open.

Asian MS

At first sight the case for a distinct form of MS is strongest in relation to the disease as it afflicts Japanese (for whom there is the largest amount of data) and other oriental populations. It has long been noted that severe neurological impairment attributable to lesions of the anterior visual pathways and spinal cord is more common in orientals than in occidentals; such cases have often been designated Devic's disease or syndrome. The frequent emphasis on this 'optic-spinal' form of the disease in the

orient has tended to obscure the fact that most such patients do have symptoms attributable to lesions elsewhere,[26] and indeed although the most extensive and severe lesions at post mortem are usually in the optic nerves and spinal cord, most cases do have lesions in other structures of the central nervous system.[27]

Turning to the histopathology, the lesions in Asian MS tend to have more axon loss, less gliosis, and less cellular infiltration even in lesions known from the history to be just a few months old.[27] Necrotic changes with marked damage to vessel walls and even haemorrhage are also more frequent. The frequency of finding oligoclonal bands in the cerebro-spinal fluid (CSF) is also lower (approximately 50 per cent versus approximately 95 per cent in Caucasians).[28] Nevertheless, lesions exhibiting what are often considered to be characteristic features of the Asian form of the disease can be found in patients of northern European descent, and *vice versa*.

The most striking distinction between the oriental and Western forms of the disease lies in the recently reported HLA associations. Western MS is consistently associated with HLA-DR15 (formerly HLA-DR2) and in particular with the haplotype HLA-DRB1*1501-DQA1*0102-DGB1*0602.[29] Kira *et al.*,[30] working in Kyushu in southern Japan, have recently investigated 57 Japanese patients with MS; 34 had the 'Western' type of MS and 23 the 'Asian' type. The DR2 associated DRB1*1501 (and also DRB5*0101) was found in 41.2 per cent of the Western type MS compared with 14.2 per cent of controls and 0 per cent of the Asian type.

These observations provide some support for the view that genetic factors influence the clinical and pathological expression of the disease, but do not in themselves establish that the Asian form of the disease is fundamentally different in nature. Once again, the question remains open.

Patterns of pathological change

The possibility of distinct pathological changes and pathogenetic mechanisms in different clinical forms of MS has been mentioned already. Here we consider rather more systematically what is known of the variations in pathology of the disease. Recent pathological studies of MS lesions taken at biopsy and at post mortem have led to an appreciation that there is a greater diversity of pathological picture than had previously been appreciated. The application of modern histochemical and immunochemical methods validated in experimental studies has led to a better understanding of the timing of different morphological features of the evolving plaque. Luccinetti *et al.*[31] are currently engaged in a study based on 82 cases derived from the pooled resources of the Mayo Clinic, the Institute of Neuropathology in Gottingen and the Institute of Neurology in Vienna. They have observed five patterns of pathology of the lesions

- demyelination with little or no oligodendrocyte loss
- demyelination with concomitant destruction and loss of oligodendrocytes
- primary demyelination with a gradient of oligodendrocyte loss towards the inactive plaque centre
- destructive plaques
- demyelinating plaques with oligodendrocyte destruction in the periplaque normal appearing white matter.

They have rejected the hypothesis that these different patterns can be accounted for on the basis of differences in timing and severity of a single pathogenetic mechanism on the following grounds.

Timing

They observed no correlation between the observed pattern of pathology and the stage of demyelination within the lesion as determined from the expression of macrophage activation markers or myelin degradation products.

Severity

Severity alone cannot explain (*a*) why in some MS lesions oligodendrocytes are destroyed completely and selectively, whereas in others they are partly preserved, even in areas where the remaining cellular elements are destroyed; (*b*) why there are two alternative patterns of oligodendrocyte destruction seen in different lesions – apoptosis or necrosis; and (*c*) the differential pattern of oligodendrocyte death within areas of demyelination in some lesions or in periplaque white matter in others.

To date, correlation of the different patterns of pathology described by Lucchinetti *et al.*[31] with different clinical subtypes is limited, but three interesting points have emerged

- similar patterns of pathology tended to be seen in different lesions from the same individual patient, although this finding was not absolute
- destructive lesions were particularly prominent in cases of Marburg's acute MS
- three cases of primary progressive MS were characterized by the presence of demyelinating plaques with oligodendrocyte destruction both within the plaque and also in a narrow rim of normal appearing white matter around it; at the latter site there was no demyelination.

These appearances were not exclusive to primary progressive cases, however, having been seen in rare instances in biopsy specimens from early bouts of the disease. We eagerly await the further data needed to determine whether these associations are informative.

Other evidence for pathological and pathophysiological differences between primary and secondary progressive MS come from sources which have already been mentioned, i.e. serial MRI and a systematic comparison of primary and secondary progressive MS at post mortem. There is clear evidence that the lesions in primary progressive MS are less inflammatory than those in secondary progressive disease.[19]

The question now arises whether the significance of the inflammation is the same in the two groups? It is generally assumed that the primary event in the evolution of the new lesion in MS is the development of focal, immune-mediated inflammation which leads to myelin breakdown. This interpretation is supported by analogy with experimental allergic encephalomyelitis in which lymphocyte adherence to post-capillary venules is followed by migration across the endothelium into the parenchyma, and then demyelination.[32,33] These early events are accompanied by an increase in permeability of the blood–brain barrier detectable by (amongst other methods) Gd-DTPA enhanced MRI.[34] In MS perivascular inflammatory infiltrates are typically present in areas of recent myelin breakdown and there is an associated local up-regulation of class 2 antigens, cytokines, adhesion molecules and chemokines.[31] There is an associated increase in permeability of the blood–brain barrier identified pathologically by leakage of immunoglobulins and damage to the vessel walls. Serial MRI in patients with relapsing–remitting and secondary progressive disease shows that relapse is associated with focal impairment of the blood–brain barrier as shown by Gd-DTPA enhancement. The latter

may precede the onset of relevant symptoms.[35] Magnetic resonance spectroscopy reveals that demyelination occurs in the period of increased permeability of the blood–brain barrier and probably quite early in it, although the precise timing is unknown. Electrophysiological evidence also suggests that demyelination is an early event in the development of the new lesion: a delay in the VEP can be detected within 24 hours of the initial symptoms in acute optic neuritis (S Jones, unpublished observations).

On the other hand, it must be remembered that there are some discrepancies in this story. Inflammatory cells are not always present in areas of active demyelination.[36–38] computed tomography (CT) and MRI enhancement correlates with extensive macrophage infiltration, not lymphocytic invasion.[39] New lesions may appear without apparent impairment of the permeability of the blood–brain barrier, although the problem of sensitivity of the MRI methods used to detect it has not yet been fully resolved.[40,41] The up-regulation of MHC class II expression in active lesions is not restricted to immune-mediated conditions, but may be seen in disorders not dependent on immune-mediated mechanisms such as trauma, infarcts and Alzheimer's disease.[31]

If the observation of Lucchinetti *et al.*,[31] that oligodendrocyte death can occur in normal appearing white matter around the lesion, proves to be a general and distinctive finding in primary progressive MS, the possibility that the inflammatory reaction may be secondary to the myelin breakdown (an inevitable consequence of oligodendrocyte destruction) will have to be seriously considered. It must be stressed, however, that the number of observations on which this conjecture is based is still very small and it is inappropriate to speculate further on details of possible different pathogenetic mechanisms in primary progressive and the other forms of MS until more data are available.

Conclusion

How then are we to answer the questions with which this chapter opened? That there are distinct clinical subgroups based on the pattern of involvement of the nervous system, the course of the illness and race, in which the prognosis differs, is undoubted. Whether these different forms of clinical expression depend on specifically different pathogenetic mechanisms is another matter. Although Lucchinetti *et al.*[31] have argued for the existence of several distinct pathogenetic mechanisms, it is not quite clear what this means. They raise the possibility that some of their data may indicate that 'several pathogenetic mechanisms were operating in parallel in the same lesion. However, in the majority of lesions examined, individual patients followed distinct pathogenetic pathways of lesion formation.' They further suggest that 'the primary target of the demyelinating process may vary between individual patients and thus may reflect distinct immunopathogenetic mechanisms operating in different MS patients.' Whether such patients belong to specific categories (e.g. primary progressive MS) is not stated although, as mentioned above, they do suggest elsewhere that this is possible. Until we know more about the details of pathogenesis – the factors which determine the presence and severity of inflammation, whether the latter is primary or secondary (or always just one of these); the factors which determine the intensity of gliosis; and what the mechanisms of axonal destruction are – it is not possible to conclude that there is more than one distinctive pathogenetic mechanism producing the different clinical forms of MS. There may be; the evidence simply does not allow us to decide at the present time.

This conclusion has implications for research on treatment. First, given that there may be more than one form of pathogenesis, it remains prudent to keep the clinical subgroups separate in therapeutic trials. Contamination of a cohort with patients unresponsive to a putative treatment because it has no effect on the specific mechanism which determines the symptomatology, may lead to a useful therapeutic effect for the remainder of the cohort being missed. Secondly, it remains impossible to predict whether a treatment that modifies the course of the disease in one clinical subgroup will have a similar effect in another. Separate therapeutic trials in homogeneous groups of patients clinically defined are, for the time being, essential.

References

1. Confavreux C, Aimard G, Devic M. Course and prognosis of multiple sclerosis assessed by the computerised data processing of 349 patients. *Brain* 1980; **103**: 281–300.
2. Runmarker B, Andersen O. Prognostic factors in a multiple sclerosis incidence cohort with twenty-five years of follow-up. *Brain* 1993; **116**: 117–134.
3. Weinshenker BG, Bass B, Rice GPA *et al*. The natural history of multiple sclerosis: a geographically based study. 1. Clinical course and disability. *Brain* 1989; **112**: 133–146.
4. Lublin FD, Reingold SC. Defining the clinical cause of multiple sclerosis: results of an international survey. *Neurology* 1996; **46**: 907–910.
5. Miller DH, Hornabook RW, Purdie G. The natural history of multiple sclerosis: a regional study with some longitudinal data. *J Neurol Neurosurg Psychiatry* 1992; **55**: 341–346.
6. Kidd D, Thompson AJ, Kendall BE *et al*. The benign form of multiple sclerosis: MRI evidence for less frequent and less inflammatory disease activity. *J Neurol Neurosurg Psychiatry* 1994; **57**: 1070–1072.
7. Katz D, Taubenberger JK, Cannella B *et al*. Correlation between magnetic resonance imaging findings and lesion development in chronic, active multiple sclerosis. *Ann Neurol* 1993; **34**: 661–669.
8. Thompson AJ, Kermode AG, MacManus DG *et al*. Patterns of disease activity in multiple sclerosis: a clinical and magnetic resonance imaging study. *Br Med J* 1990; **300**: 631–634.
9. Losseff NA, Webb SW, O'Riordan JI *et al*. Spinal cord atrophy and disability in MS: a new reproducible and sensitive MRI method to monitor disease progression. *Brain* 1996; **119**: 701–708.
10. Losseff NA, Wang L, Lai HM *et al*. Progressive cerebral atrophy in multiple sclerosis: a serial MRI study. *Brain* 1996; **119**: 2009–2020.
11. Prineas JW, Barnard RO, Kwon EE *et al*. Multiple sclerosis: Remyelination of nascent lesions. *Ann Neurol* 1993; **33**: 137–151.
12. Prineas JW, Barnard RO, Revesz T *et al*. Multiple sclerosis. Pathology of recurrent lesions. *Brain* 1993; **116**: 681–693.
13. Healy MA, McManus BG, Walsh JC *et al*. Visual evoked responses and ophthalmological examination in optic neuritis: a follow-up study. *J Neurol Sci* 1986; **75**: 275–283.
14. Marburg O. Die sogenannte 'akute Multiple Sklerose'. *Jahrb Psychiatrie* 1906; **27**: 211–312.
15. Ozawa K, Suchanek G, Breitschopf H *et al*. Patterns of oligodendroglia pathology in multiple sclerosis. *Brain* 1994; **117**: 1311–1322.
16. Thompson AJ, Polman CH, Miller DH *et al*. Primary progressive multiple sclerosis. A review. *Brain* 1997; **120**: 1088–1096.
17. Thompson AJ, Kermode AG, Wicks D *et al*. Major differences in the dynamics of primary and secondary progressive multiple sclerosis. *Ann Neurol* 1991; **29**: 53–62.
18. Kidd DK, Thorpe JW, Thompson AJ *et al*. Spinal cord MRI using multi-array coils and fast spin echo II: findings in multiple sclerosis. *Neurology* 1993; **43**: 2632–2637.
19. Revesz T, Kidd D, Thompson AJ *et al*. A comparison of the pathology of primary and secondary progressive multiple sclerosis. *Brain* 1994; **117**: 756–765.
20. Olerup O, Hillert J, Fredrikson S *et al*. Primarily chronic progressive and relapsing/remitting multiple sclerosis: Two immunogenetically distinct disease entities. *Proc Natl Acad Sci USA* 1989; **86**: 7113–7117.
21. Hillert J, Grönning M, Nyland H *et al*. An immunogenetic heterogeneity in multiple sclerosis. *J Neurol Neurosurg Psychiatry* 1992; **55**: 887–890.
22. Thompson AJ, Hutchinson M, Brazil J *et al*. A clinical and laboratory study of benign multiple sclerosis. *Q J Med* 1986; **225**: 69–80.
23. Chalon MP, Sindic CJM, Laterra EC. Serum and CSF levels of soluble interleukin-2 receptors in MS and other neurological diseases: a

reappraisal. *Acta Neurol Scand* 1993; **87**: 77–82.

24. Acarin N, Rio J, Fernandez AL *et al*. Different anti ganglioside antibody pattern between relapsing/remitting multiple sclerosis. *Acta Neurol Scand* 1996; **93**: 99–103.

25. Giovannoni G, Thorpe JW, Kidd D *et al*. Soluble E-selectin in multiple sclerosis: raised concentrations in patients with primary progressive disease. *J Neurol Neurosurg Psychiatry* 1996; **60**: 20–26.

26. Shibasaki H, McDonald WI, Kuroiwa Y. Racial modification of clinical picture of multiple sclerosis: comparison between British and Japanese patients. *J Neurol Sci* 1981; **49**: 253–271.

27. Tabira T, Tateishi J. Neuropathological features of MS in Japan. In: Kuroiwa Y, Kurland LT, eds. *Multiple Sclerosis East and West*, Japan: Kyushu University Press 1982; 273–295.

28. Yu YL, Woo E, Hawkins BR *et al*. Multiple sclerosis amongst Chinese in Hong Kong. *Brain* 1989; **112**: 1445–1467.

29. Compston A, Kellar-Wood H, Wood N. Multiple sclerosis. In: *Balliere's Clinical Neurology*. London: Balliere Tindall 1994; **3**: 353–371.

30. Kira J-i, Kanai T, Nishimura Y *et al*. Western versus Asian types of multiple sclerosis: immunologenetically and clinically distinct disorders. *Ann Neurol* 1996; **40**: 569–574.

31. Lucchinetti CF, Brück W, Rodriguez M *et al*. Distinct patterns of multiple sclerosis pathology indicates heterogeneity in pathogenesis, *Brain Path* 1996; **6**: 259–274.

32. Lampert PW, Carpenter S. Electron microscope studies on the vascular permeability and the mechanisms of demyelination in experimental allergic encephalomyelitis. *J Neuropath Exp Neurol* 1965; **29**: 11–24.

33. Raine CS. The Dale E McFarlin memorial lecture. The immunology of the multiple sclerosis lesion. *Ann Neurol* 1994; **36**: S61–S72.

34. Hawkins CP, Munro PMG, MacKenzie F *et al*. Duration and selectivity of blood–brain barrier breakdown in chronic relapsing experimental allergic encephalomyelitis studied using gadolinium-DTPA and protein markers. *Brain* 1990; **113**: 365–378.

35. Barratt HJ, Miller D, Rudge P. The site of lesion causing deafness in multiple sclerosis. *Scand Audiol* 1988; **17**: 67–71.

36. Dawson JW. The histology of disseminated sclerosis. *Trans Roy Soc Edinburgh* 1916; **5**: 517–740.

37. Guseo A, Jellinger K. The significance of perivascular infiltrations in multiple sclerosis. *J Neurol* 1975; **211**: 51–60.

38. Rodriguez M, Scheithauer BW, Forbes G *et al*. Oligodendrocyte injury is an early event in lesions of multiple sclerosis. *Mayo Clin Proc* 1993; **68**: 627–636.

39. Nesbit GM, Forbes GS, Scheithauer BW *et al*. Histopathologic and MR and/or CT correlation in 37 cases at biopsy and 3 cases at autopsy. *Radiology* 1991; **180**: 467–474.

40. Filippi M, Yousry T, Campi A *et al*. Comparison of triple dose versus standard dose gadolinium-DTPA for detection of MRI enhancing lesions in patients with MS. *Neurology* 1996; **46**: 379–384.

41. Silver NC, Good CD, Barker GJ *et al*. Sensitivity of contrast enhanced MRI in multiple sclerosis: effects of gadolinium dose, magnetisation transfer contrast and delayed imaging. *Brain* 1997 **120**: 7.

4

The role of magnetic resonance imaging in diagnosis of multiple sclerosis

Frederik Barkhof

Introduction

Magnetic resonance imaging (MRI) is a cross-sectional imaging technique that became widely available in the mid-1980s. Immediately after its introduction, it became obvious that MRI showed superior image contrast in the central nervous system and was more sensitive in detecting white matter lesions than computed tomography (*Fig. 4.1*). The first MRI study in multiple sclerosis (MS) showed ten times as many lesions as were detected with computed tomography (CT).[1]

MRI soon became the major confirmatory test for MS, showing multiple lesions in the brain in the vast majority of patients. This of course shed new light on the disease process in MS. Apparently, many clinically silent lesions occur before the first symptom. On the one hand this shows that many brain areas are either difficult to assess neurologically, or are not quite as relevant; however, silent MS lesions occur in the optic nerves and spinal cord as well. On the other hand, it illustrates how poorly defined the onset of MS is, and that disease duration is not an accurate parameter; while some patients show only 5–10 lesions at first presentation, others have well over 100.

Recently, new developments in the treatment of MS have taken place. Several drugs have become available, which seem to alter the initial course of the disease to some extent.

One could argue that those who are likely to gain most from treatment are those who have not yet developed irrecoverable deficit. This means a shift will be needed in the position of MRI; whereas its most important role previously was to exclude a diagnosis of MS, it will in the near future be used more and more to actively support the diagnosis. In the former situation sensitivity (and hence negative predictive value) is important, while in the latter specificity (and hence positive predictive value) is relevant.

In this chapter the role of MRI in the diagnosis of MS will be discussed. After having reviewed the clinical diagnostic criteria and pathology of MS, we will look at MRI criteria for MS. The sensitivity of MRI will be discussed, and its differential diagnosis, as well as criteria which might be more specific. Flow charts illustrating the diagnostic work-up with MRI will be presented, based on *a priori* classification and predictive value.

The clinical diagnosis of MS

MS can only be diagnosed with certainty at autopsy, but criteria have been developed in order to make a clinical diagnosis of MS. The criteria by Schumacher *et al.*[2] require that symptoms and signs be attributable to more than one central nervous system (CNS) lesion (*dissociation in place*) and that there has been

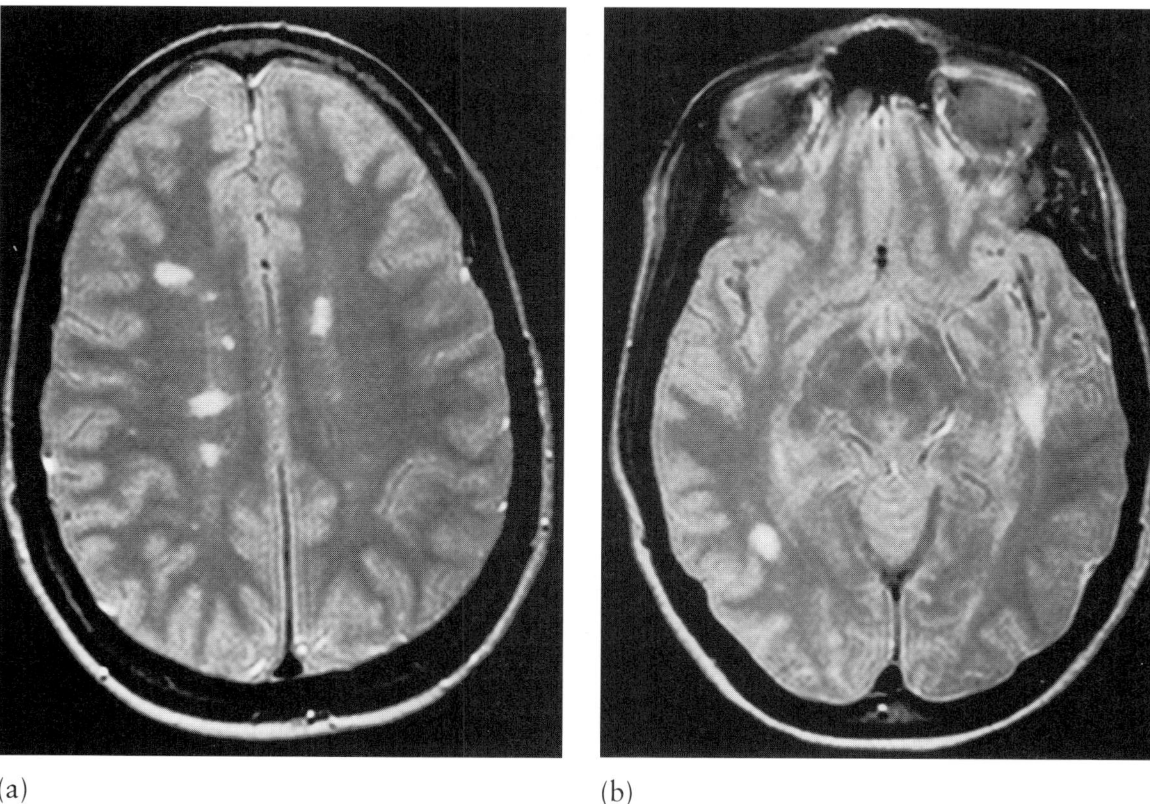

(a) (b)

Fig. 4.1
Dissociation in space. *Mildly T_2-weighted images (a,b) showing multiple high signal lesions, demonstrating dissociation of the disease in space. Note that several periventricular lesions in (a) are located in the corpus callosum, and have an ovoid or elliptical shape. Also note characteristic location of lesions in the occipital and temporal lobe (b).*

more than one period of signs or symptoms, or progression over more than half a year (*dissociation in time*).

The criteria of Poser *et al.*[3] are at present the most widely used (*Table 4.1*). The major difference with the Schumacher criteria is the introduction of the use of paraclinical tests –

CSF oligoclonal banding (OB) or increased immunoglobulin G (IgG) production, evoked responses, computed tomography and MRI – in addition to clinical signs and symptoms.

One should bear in mind that clinical misdiagnosis of MS occurs in 9–12 per cent of patients, while 4–5 per cent of MS patients

Category	Attacks	Clinical evidence		Paraclinical evidence	CSF (OB/IgG)
A. Clinically definite MS					
CDMS A1	2	2			
CDMS A2	2	1	and	1	
B. Laboratory-supported definite MS					
LSDMS B1	2	1	or	1	+
LSDMS B2	1	2			+
LSDMS B3	1	1	and	1	+
C. Clinically probable MS					
CPMS C1	2	1			
CPMS C2	1	2			
CPMS C3	1	1	and	1	
D. Laboratory-supported probable MS					
LSPMSD1	2				

Table 4.1
Diagnostic criteria for MS by Poser et al.[3]

will at first not be diagnosed as having MS.[4] The latter group may be larger, as autopsy series have found many cases of unsuspected MS. In one autopsy series of 2450 patients 5 unsuspected cases were found. This suggests an actual prevalence higher than the observed prevalence.[5] In another study, 18 per cent of the MS cases found at autopsy had not been identified clinically.[6] The experience of most authors is that about 5–20 per cent of MS cases remain clinically silent.

Table 4.1 indicates how and when paraclinical evidence can be used in the diagnosis of MS. Paraclinical evidence of a subclinical lesion can be obtained using evoked potentials or neuroimaging. MRI is the most sensitive paraclinical parameter for demonstration of dissemination in space and is more sensitive than the appropriate evoked potential.[7–10] None of the paraclinical tests is specific for MS, particularly when taken in isolation. When MRI is abnormal in the presence of oligoclonal bands, however, very few other diagnoses need to be considered (for example, acute disseminated encephalomyelitis, neuroborreliosis). In this chapter we will restrict ourselves to the use of MRI, and criteria by which to judge what is an abnormal MRI scan. We will therefore first have to look closer at the pathology of MS, to understand how this translates into MRI abnormalities.

A short description of the pathology of MS

MS is primarily a demyelinating disease: that is to say, destruction of the myelin sheath takes place with relative preservation of axons. This type of discontinuous demyelination is in contrast to the type of secondary demyelination seen in Wallerian degeneration, where damage of the axon is the primary event. The acute plaque[11] is not well demarcated, is oedematous, and contains many lymphocytes, myelin fragments and lipid-laden macrophages. Moreover, perivenular lymphocytic cuffs are found in the vicinity of active plaques. The chronic plaque[11] is sharply demarcated and shrunken. In the chronic plaque one finds naked axons (without myelin sheaths), hypertrophic astrocytes, microglia (macrophages), plasma cells, and expanded extracellular space. At the edge of the plaque T-lymphocytes can be found. If a plaque is still somewhat active, foam cells can be observed, with marked glial reaction, consisting of astrocytic activation, oligodendrocyte proliferation and microglial phagocytosis. Shadow plaques represent areas of partial demyelination, and are nowadays considered to be the result of remyelination, and contain numerous proliferating oligodendrocytes.

As the cause of MS remains obscure, the exact sequence of events in the evolution of MS lesions can only be hinted at. Prineas summarizes the following concepts: (1) both myelin and oligodendrocytes are targets of (2) macrophages and their proteolytic enzymes (3) after being recognized by oligoclonal IgG antigens or T-lymphocytes, and (4) remyelination occurs in acute and chronic plaques.[12] Why remyelination eventually fails in MS is an important question. In between plaques, in macroscopically normal brain tissue, numerous perivenular infiltrates can be found in what is called the Virchow–Robin spaces; it is of particular interest that these infiltrates can also be found in the retina[13] and in the meninges.[14] The perivenular distribution of infiltrates and plaques is noticed by many observers, and accounts for the finger-like extension of lesions along venules, often referred to as Dawson fingers.[15]

Since the venules of the white matter drain into the lateral ventricle, MS plaques have a predilection for the ventricular lining. Periventricular lesions are found in more than 90 per cent of cases; the anterior (Steiner's 'Wetterwinkel') and posterior and inferior horns of the lateral ventricles are often involved, as are the subcallosal surface, the peri-aqueductal region and the floor of the fourth ventricle. The shrinkage of chronic lesions accounts for the ventricular dilatation found in long-standing cases. Cortical lesions are found in the majority of cases and are usually small and often only seen on microscopy.[16] Although the lesions of MS do not follow a specific pattern, in most cases the number of lesions in both hemispheres is roughly equal and the distribution is, by and large, symmetrical. In a series of 10 cases with a total of 482 plaques,[16] 58 per cent were cortical, 13 per cent in the centrum semiovale and corpus callosum, 9 per cent in the basal ganglia, 4 per cent in the midbrain, 6 per cent pontine, 6 per cent cerebellar, and 3 per cent medullary. Plaques are usually not larger than 1.5 cm, although plaques up to 4.5 cm have been reported; most chronic gliotic plaques, however, are smaller than 3 mm.

How does MRI reflect the pathology of MS?

The major lessons which can be learned from the pathology of MS are: (1) the dynamic evolution with early inflammation; and (2) the remarkable topographical distribution of lesions. Both of these cardinal features should be considered in the execution and interpretation of MRI in suspected MS. Any alteration in the brain tissue will increase T_2 relaxation times. The signal on T_2-weighted images will therefore be hyperintense from the earliest stage of inflammation until the chronic stages

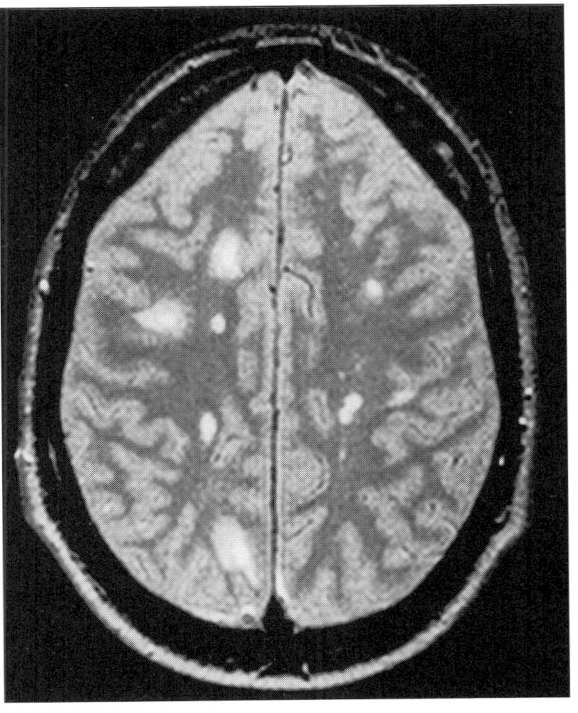

(a)

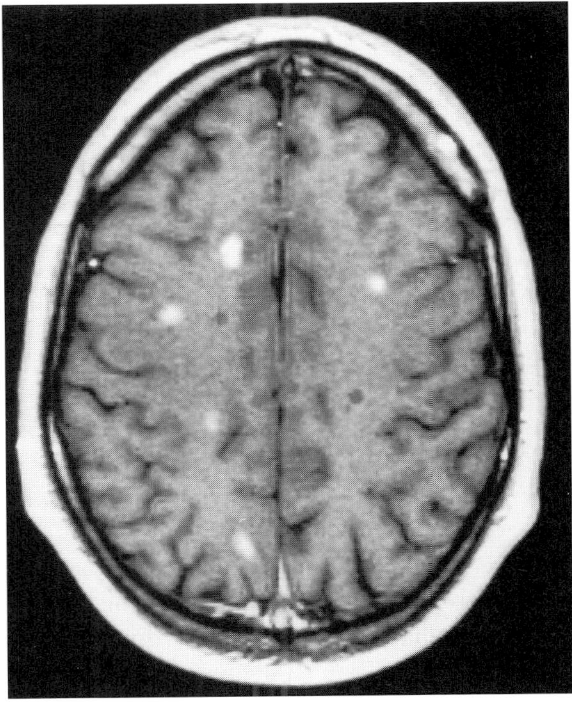

(b)

Fig. 4.2
Dissociation in time. *Multiple lesions are seen on the mildly T_2-weighted image (a), only some of which are enhancing with gadolinium on the T_1-weighted image (b), demonstrating dissociation of the disease in time. Note that the area of enhancement in (b) frequently is smaller than the corresponding T_2 abnormality in (a), the fuzzy border of which is determined by a halo of oedema. Also note that some lesions have hypointense signal on T_1 (b); these so-called black holes represent severely demyelinated, gliotic lesions. The T_2-weighted image (a) displays all these aspects of acute and chronic lesions with high signal, explaining the high sensitivity (and poor specificity) of increased signal* per se.

(*Fig. 4.2*); even remyelinated lesions will probably still have abnormal signal, since remyelinated axons have thinner myelin sheaths. Signal increase on T_2-weighted images therefore is a very sensitive but completely non-specific finding, and occurs in the vast majority of white matter diseases. Early lesions can be surrounded by a vague halo of less markedly increased signal, representing oedema (*Fig. 4.2*), which resolves over time. Many lesions shrink substantially in the first month, but only rarely does a lesion disappear completely (beyond the scanner resolution).

One of the earliest features in the acute inflammatory lesion is disruption of the blood–brain barrier, which can be demonstrated with gadolinium enhancement.[17] Evidence from animal work[18] and biopsy studies[19,20] indicate that gadolinium enhancement correlates in time with the acute inflammatory phase, which coincides with acute demyelination (*Fig. 4.2*). It should be noted that treatment with corticosteroids strongly suppresses gadolinium enhancement, and this suppression correlates with clinical improvement and reduction in myelin breakdown products.[21] Without treatment, enhancement subsides after about one month, leaving a T_2 abnormality in virtually every case. Further differentiation of those residual lesions is now possible with the use of magnetization transfer imaging and hypointensity on T_1-weighted SE images (*Fig. 4.2*).

The morphology of lesions is informative; based on their centring along venules, MS lesions typically have an ovoid shape (*Fig. 4.1*). The periventricular location, with early involvement of the corpus callosum, the characteristic extensions into the adjacent white matter (Dawson fingers), are dictated by the perivenular distribution of MS plaques. All these features can elegantly be demonstrated by MRI. MR images frequently display corti-

cal lesions in MS patients, which is in agreement with histopathological observations (*Fig. 4.3*). The presence of cortical lesions probably accounts for the increased prevalence of epilepsy among MS patients.[22]

Choosing the best MR technique

Although the first report on MR detection of MS lesions used an inversion recovery technique,[1] T_2-weighted spin–echo sequences are more sensitive than inversion recovery, T_1-weighted spin–echo,[23] and gradient-echo techniques[24] in detecting MS lesions. Fast or turbo spin–echo sequences are quicker than conventional ones (several phase encoding steps per excitation) and probably detect roughly the same number of lesions.[25] One should bear in mind that fast–turbo SE is technically more complicated; image quality is easily compromised and the sensitivity of this technique to detect MS lesions shows regional variation within the brain.[25] For example, in the posterior fossa, fast–turbo SE sequences have limited sensitivity, which is unfortunate, since posterior fossa lesions especially are quite specific for MS.

Axial dual echo long repetition time spin–echo images provide the most relevant information in standard brain scans. The short echo time provides a proton density type of image, which is the most useful image (*Figs 4.1–4.3*). The longer echo time provides stronger T_2-weighting, and can be used to verify the presence of a lesion. More sophisticated techniques, such as fluid attenuated inversion recovery (FLAIR) and sagittal imaging planes, can further improve the diagnostic possibilities. The FLAIR sequence provides strong T_2-weighting and cerebro-spinal fluid (CSF) suppression at the same time, and improves the detection of cortical lesions. Sagittal

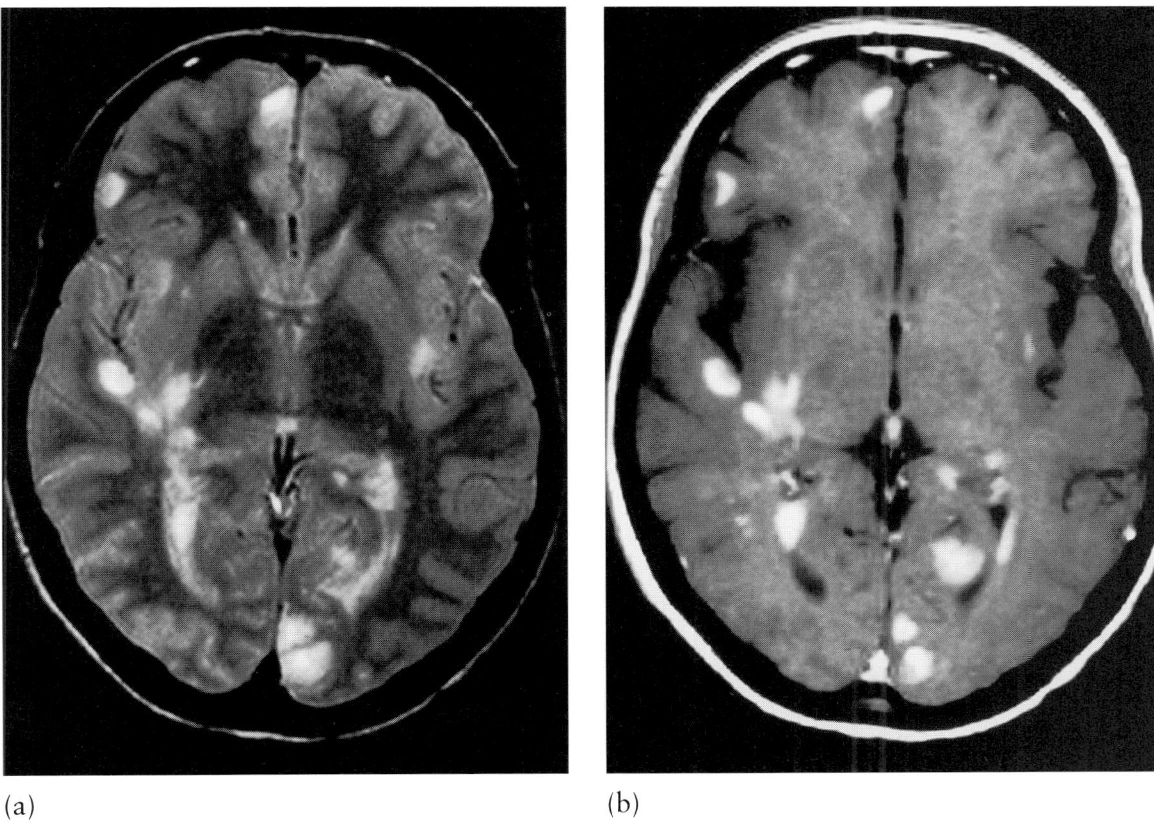

(a)

(b)

Fig. 4.3
*Cortical lesions. Patient with very active MS,
showing multiple lesions on the mildly T$_2$-
weighted image, with enhancement in the vast
majority (b). Note that many lesions are located
in the cortex or immediately adjacent to it, which
is very uncommon for white matter lesions in
small vessel arteriosclerotic disease.*

images elegantly depict the corpus callosum,
the infratentorial region and medulla oblon-
gata, regions typically involved in MS.[26–28]

Gadolinium enhancement can best be
demonstrated using T$_1$-weighted spin–echo
sequences (*Figs 4.2 and 4.3*). Gradient echo
images are less well suited, although recent
observations with thin-section inversion-
prepared 3D gradient–echo techniques are
promising. Enhancement with gadolinium is
dose- and time-dependent. Triple dose detects
more enhancing lesions,[29] but in a diagnostic
setting conventional single dose (0.1 mmol/kg)
will usually suffice. Whenever possible, scanning

should be postponed until 15–30 minutes after injection to increase the conspicuity of enhancing lesions.

With advances in technique of spinal cord imaging (3 mm slices obtained with a phased array coil) MS lesions can also be demonstrated in the spinal cord (*Fig. 4.4*) in the vast majority of patients.[30] This is of considerable interest, since incidental lesions are not seen in the cord with normal ageing,[31] offering a potential place for spinal MRI to increase the specificity of MRI in the diagnosis of MS. Furthermore, spinal imaging also rules out a compressive lesion, and might be necessary in case of symptomatology restricted to the spinal cord. Lesions in the optic nerve can be demonstrated using coronal images, either T_2-weighted spin–echo with frequency selective fat-saturation or using a short T_1 inversion recovery (STIR) technique[32] (*Fig. 4.5*).

Differential diagnosis of MR white matter lesions: pattern recognition

Many other types of tissue change, such as infarction, gliosis, dilatation of Virchow–Robin spaces, and others, will also increase the magnetic resonance (MR) signal intensity. This accounts for the low specificity of MR signal changes *per se*. Acquired white matter diseases can be classified according to their causative mechanism as hypoxic–ischaemic, inflammatory, infectious, toxic–metabolic, or traumatic, while hereditary white matter diseases are classified according to the subcellular organelle which is abnormal.[33] Although many investigators have tried to classify different types of pathology based on their relaxation characteristics, such attempts have been frustrated by a biological overlap. A rather

extensive differential diagnosis of MR abnormalities, of the type seen in MS, exists and is summarized in *Table 4.2*.

Notwithstanding this extensive differential diagnosis, there are certain specific features on brain MR images which can make a diagnosis of MS more probable, especially in relation to hypoxic–ischaemic disease, by far the most common other type of lesion. Diagnostic clues include the presence of irregular and confluent periventricular lesions, especially around the frontal, occipital and temporal horn. It has been suggested[34] that the finding of lesions greater than 6 mm abutting the bodies of the ventricles is specific for MS; the same authors state that the presence of lesions in the infratentorial region is specific as well. The presence of ovoid lesions (which relates to the finding of Dawson fingers in pathology) is found in 86 per cent of MS patients.[35] Cortical lesions are very rare in, for example, normal ageing but are frequently seen in MS.[16] On the other hand, there are certain features which make a diagnosis of MS less probable. These include symmetrical abnormalities and extensive involvement of the basal ganglia.

One of the most typical brain MRI signs for MS is probably an abnormal corpus callosum. Callosal atrophy can be encountered relatively early in the disease, in the absence of clinical disability. Callosal and subcallosal periventricular lesions are frequently found in MS.[36] It has been shown that callosal lesions and medial temporal lobe lesions (which are rare in vascular disease) are related to cognitive and psychiatric disturbances.[37,38] Callosal lesions and atrophy can best be demonstrated on coronal or sagittal MR images. A recent study showed that abnormalities at the junction of the corpus callosum and the septum pellucidum (callosal–septal interface) can be found in 93 per cent of MS patients, and have a high specificity.[27] The differences between

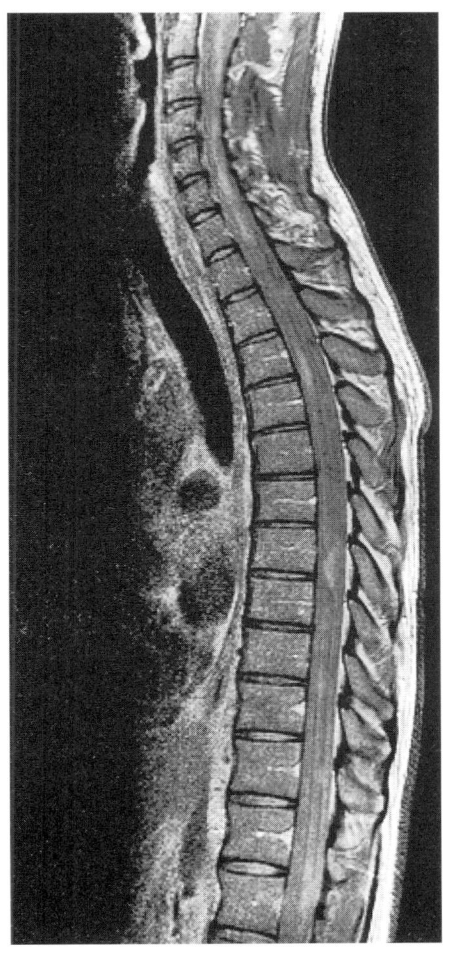

(a)

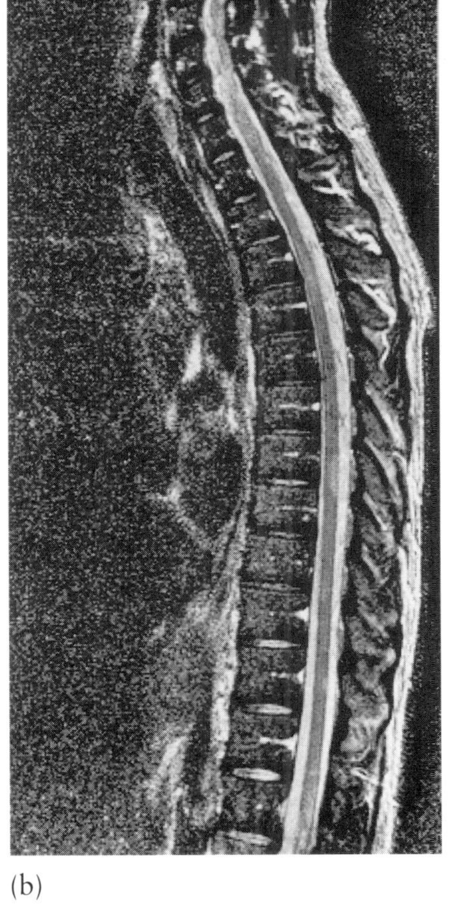

(b)

Fig. 4.4
Spinal lesions. *Dual echo images with 3 mm slice thickness, 1 mm in-plane resolution obtained with a phased array coil and cardiac gating. Multiple spinal lesions are visualized, with best contrast on the mildly T_2-weighted image (a), while the location of the cord and CSF spaces are best appreciated on the corresponding heavily T_2-weighted image (b).*

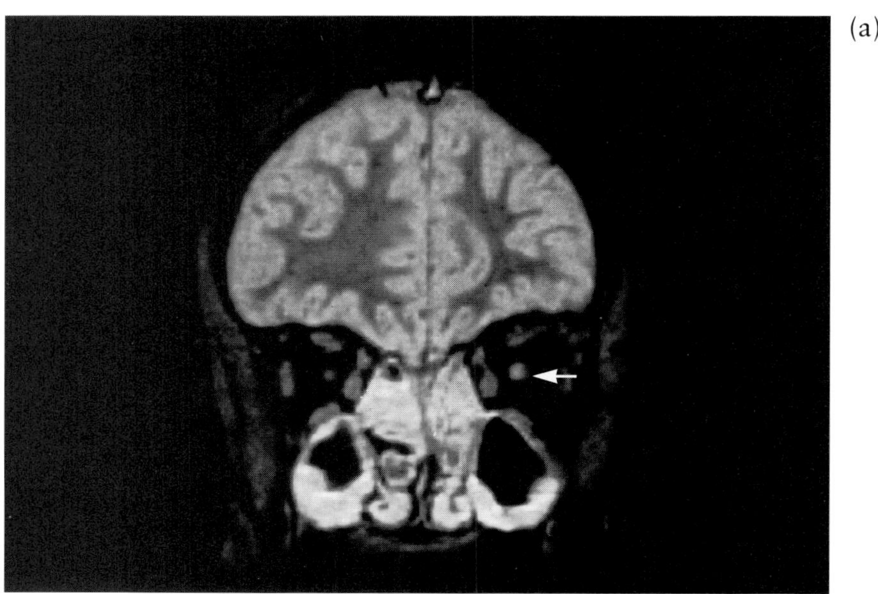

(a)

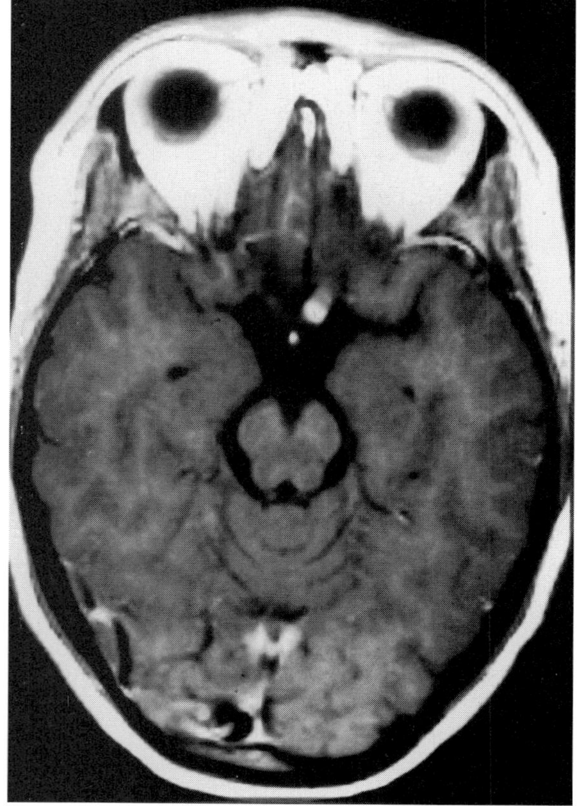

(b)

Fig. 4.5
Optic neuritis. *The lesion in the left optic nerve is seen with high signal on the coronal fat-suppressed STIR image (compare normal low signal in right nerve (a)) and displays gadolinium enhancement on the transverse T_1-weighted image (b).*

Hypoxic/ischaemic

- Hypertension: macroangiopathy, microangiopathy
- Hypotension: borderzone infarcts, Binswanger's disease
- Atherosclerosis: ideopathic, diabetes mellitus (DM)
- Unknown origin: Alzheimer's disease, major depression, normal pressure hydrocephalus, migraine
- Embolic: cardiac, atheromatous, peri-operative
- Wallerian degeneration

Inflammatory

- MS and variants: Charcot type (classic), Marburg type (fulminant), Balo type (concentric sclerosis), Schilder type (diffuse sclerosis), Devic type (neuromyelitis optica)
- Peripheral inflammatory demyelinating diseases: Fisher's syndrome, chronic inflammatory demyelinating polyneuropathy (CIDP)
- Vasculitis: lupus erythematodes, Behçet disease, giant cell arteritis, Sjögern's disease, polyarteritis nodosa
- Sarcoid
- Inflammatory bowel disease

Infectious

- Protozoal: cryptococcus, toxoplasmosis, cysticercosis
- Fungal: candida, aspergillus
- Spirochetal: syphilis, neuroborreliosis (Lyme's disease)
- Bacterial: tuberculosis, brucellosis
- Viral: herpes simplex, HIV, progressive multifocal leucencephalopathy (PML), HTLV-I (TSP)

Post-infectious

- Acute demyelinating encephalomyelopathy (ADEM), subacute sclerosing postinfectious encephalitis (SSPE)

Toxic-metabolic

- Central pontine myelinolysis (CPM), carbonmonoxide (CO) intoxication, methotrexate (MTX) treatment, Marchiafavi-Bignami, funicular myelinolysis (B_{12} deficiency)

Traumatic

- Radiation, contusion

Table 4.2
Differential diagnosis of incidental MR white matter lesions.

Criteria	MS	Hypoxic/ischaemic disease
Corpus callosum lesions	+ +	−
U-fibre involvement	+ +	−
Basal ganglia lesions	±	+ +
Infratentorial lesions	+	−
Gadolinium enhancement	+	−
Temporal lobe lesions	+ +	−
Arterial territory	−	±
Ovoid shape	+ +	−
Periventricular location	+ +	−

Table 4.3
*MR criteria to distinguish MS from
hypoxic/ischaemic disease.*

hypoxic–ischaemic and MS lesions are summarized in *Table 4.3*.

Variants of MS, mass lesions and acute disseminated encephalomyelitis (ADEM)

In the typical form of MS (sometimes referred to as 'Charcot type') lesions are usually small to medium in size, homogeneous and multiple. This is especially true for relapsing–remitting and secondary progressive MS patients. There are some specific subtypes of MS which produce a different picture. Patients with primary progressive MS have fewer and smaller lesions, which only rarely enhance with gadolinium.[39] In Balò's concentric sclerosis large multilaminated lesions are found with alternating zones of demyelination and normal myelin, which can be appreciated as bands with low and high signal on MR.[40] In Schilder's disease, only one or two huge lesions are found which can extend from the ventricles into the cortex. In Devic's neuromyelitis optica (frequently occurring in Japan) lesions are found only in the optic nerve and spinal cord.[41]

In some patients with Charcot type MS huge lesions can be observed with irregular incomplete enhancement (*Fig. 4.6*). Such lesions can easily be misinterpreted as tumours, and indeed they sometimes have frightening appearances. In cases of established MS one should not of course be too aggressive, biopsy should be postponed for at least several weeks, by which time a follow-up MRI will show partial resolution of the lesion, thus excluding the possibility of a neoplasm. Nevertheless, large series of biopsies in MS patients have been published,[20] all of which were probably performed to rule out neoplasm.

In ADEM, MR abnormalities can be indistinguishable from MS, showing multiple

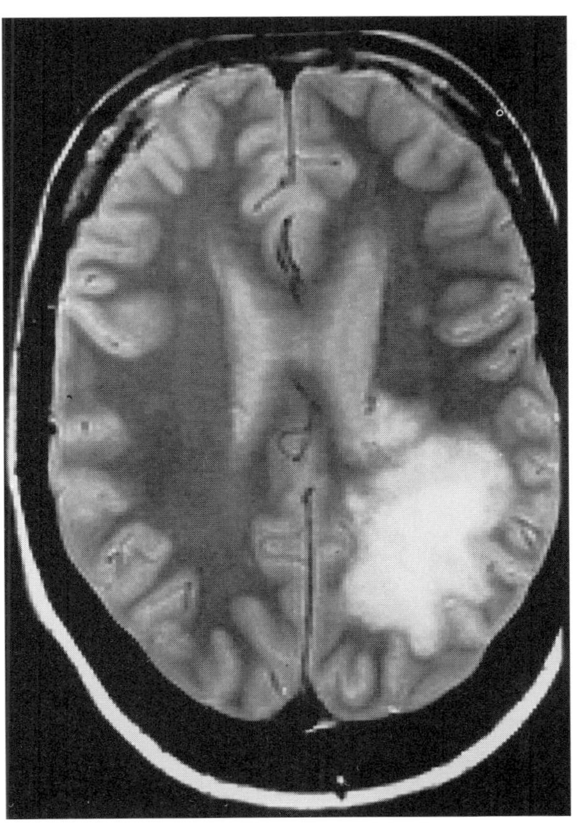

(a)

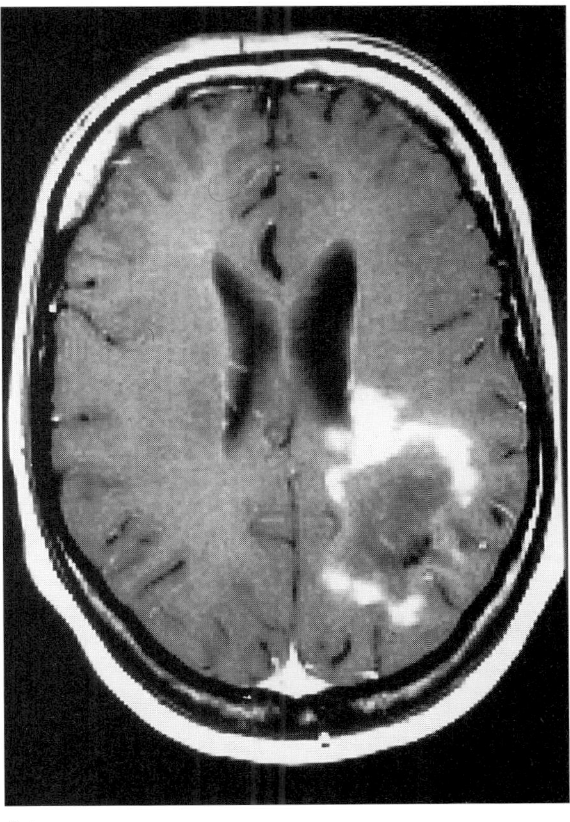

(b)

Fig. 4.6
Tumour-like MS. *Mildly T$_2$-weighted image displays huge lesion in the left parietal lobe (a), which displays irregular, ring-like, enhancement with gadolinium on the corresponding T$_1$-weighted image (b). This frightening appearing lesion might easily be confused with a neoplasm, but the presence of other white matter lesions (a) should suggest the correct diagnosis, obviating biopsy.*

lesions around the ventricles. In contrast to the clinical monophasic course, both enhancing and non-enhancing lesions can be found.[42,43] More in keeping with the monophasic course is the fact that new MR lesions are rarely found at follow-up.[44] ADEM occurs most commonly in children and young adults. As in childhood MS, lesions can be very large[45] and show a tendency to resolve almost completely over time.

Criteria	Description
Paty's[7]	Either 4 lesions or 3 lesions, one of which is periventricular
Fazekas'[51]	3 lesions, fulfilling 2 of the following criteria • a lesion larger than 6 mm • a lesion abutting the ventricles • an infratentorial lesion

Table 4.4
Commonly used diagnostic MR criteria for MS.

Classical diagnostic MR criteria focus on sensitivity

Most of the pathological processes involved in MS will increase the signal intensity of T_2-weighted images because they increase proton density and/or T_2 (*Fig. 4.2*). This accounts for the high sensitivity of MR for MS lesions. Classically, MR diagnostic criteria for MS relied on the presence of more than three lesions larger than 3 mm, sometimes reinforced by the presence of a 'lumpy-bumpy' periventricular border. Those features are incorporated into the commonly used MR criteria by Paty *et al.*[7] (*Table 4.4*): more than 95 per cent of the patients with clinically definite MS will show abnormalities strongly suggestive of MS on T_2-weighted images. In addition, in a follow-up study of the same patients after three years, 85 per cent of the patients who developed clinically definite MS had MR scans strongly suggestive of MS initially, while only 6 per cent had a completely normal MR scan.[46]

As MRI is very sensitive in detecting the lesions of MS, one could speculate that, with the advent of MRI and a widespread use of this tool, clinically silent cases would be revealed. This has proved to be the case in a study of twins, discordant for MS, where white matter abnormalities on MRI were found in roughly 10 per cent of clinically unaffected twins,[47] and in a study of familial MS, where white matter abnormalities were found in clinically unaffected family members.[48] On the other hand, in a large epidemiological study,[49] only 3 of the 69 new MS cases would have been missed without MRI. In addition 18 out of 50 cases changed from possible to probable MS.

As with any medical test showing a high sensitivity, the specificity of MRI for MS is usually considerably lower, reaching 57 per cent after a follow-up of two years.[46] Likewise, the positive predictive value of an abnormal brain MR scan (minimum four lesions) in patients presenting with isolated syndromes suspected of MS is 65 per cent, while the negative predictive value of a normal brain MRI scan at presentation is 97 per cent.[50] These figures illustrate that probably too much emphasis is placed on sensitivity, while specificity lags behind. This is somewhat unfortunate, as the prevalence of MS in a group of patients suspected of MS is usually lower than 50 per cent; in such situations, it is more important to be specific.

Towards more specific diagnostic MR criteria

Paty's criteria have been evaluated prospectively in patients presenting with isolated syndromes suggestive of MS, showing high sensitivity but relatively low specificity.[7] The most extensively used alternative criteria are those by Fazekas *et al.*[51] (*Table 4.4*); in a retrospective study of patients with established MS, these criteria showed both high sensitivity and specificity, but the criteria of Fazekas[52] perform less well in a prospective fashion when applied to patients presenting with an isolated syndrome suggestive of MS.

Given the typical pathology of MS, it is not surprising that both Paty's and Fazekas' criteria incorporate periventricular lesions, and that ovoid and callosal–subcallosal MRI abnormalities are a frequent finding. Moreover, MS lesions typically are located in the occipital and temporal lobes, regions which are usually spared in small vessel vascular disease (*Fig. 4.1*). The same holds true for the basal ganglia, where MS lesions centre on the internal capsule, but relatively spare the basal nuclei itself. Even in subjects under 50 years old, incidental white matter lesions are a frequent finding. Therefore, in most criteria a minimum number of lesions is required (e.g. three or four). By increasing the minimum number of T_2 lesions required for a scan to be abnormal to nine, the specificity of MS can be increased.[53] Actually, one could simply count the number of lesions, and provide the chance of developing MS rather then being forced to a yes-or-no answer. The relationship between the number of lesions at presentation and the risk of developing MS is shown in *Fig. 4.7*.

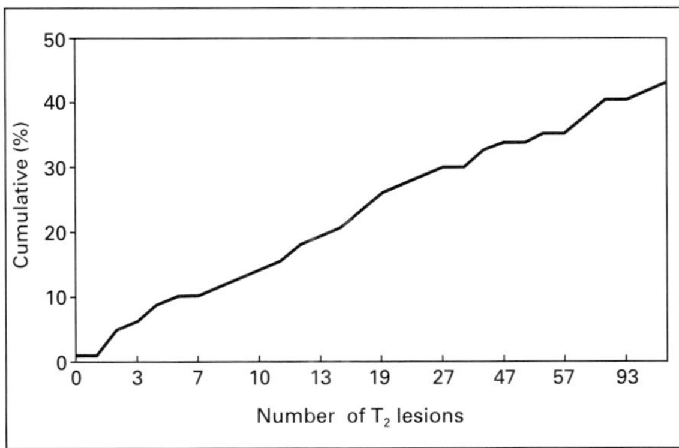

Fig. 4.7
Predictive value of number of lesions. *Plot of the cumulative chance of developing MS within three years plotted against the number of lesions at presentation. Note the almost linear relationship, indicating that the number of lesions at presentation is an important prognostic factor.*

In agreement with pathological findings,[16] MR quite frequently depicts lesions in the direct subcortical U-fibres. These areas tend to be spared in vascular disease,[33] since they have a different (cortical) blood supply. On the other hand, so-called juxta-cortical lesions are a frequent finding in MS (*Fig. 4.3*).[54] Intuitively many people disregard this feature, as MS is considered to be a white matter disease. However, one should realize that myelinated axons arise within all layers of the cortex, and that the cortex contains a considerable amount of myelin.

A crucial difference between small vessel disease and MS is that, in the latter, there is an acute onset of lesion development with inflammation (*Figs 4.2 and 4.3*). Since this phase can be visualized with gadolinium, it has been speculated that the presence of both enhancing and non-enhancing MRI lesions is the radiological counterpart of dissociation in space and time.[55] One study[52] indeed showed that gadolinium enhancement was more specific for diagnosing MS than abnormalities on T_2-weighted imaging. The alternative MR findings which can be used to increase specificity are summarized in *Table 4.5*.

What is the role of spinal MRI?

Using phased array coils, spinal MRI has become feasible within a limited time frame (*Fig. 4.4*). The most robust technique is dual echo cardiac triggered spin echo. Short echo-time inversion recovery is a good alternative, while FLAIR is disappointing, notwithstanding initial favourable reports. Spinal lesions can be found in the vast majority of patients (90 per cent), while they are not found in controls, even with ageing. The prevalence of spinal lesions in other neurological diseases is largely unknown, but spinal lesions in lupus erythemathodes, for example, can be found.

Spinal imaging in a diagnostic setting can perform two roles. The first is in patients with typical spinal cord symptomatology (e.g. transverse myelitis or bladder symptoms),

where a spinal MR is needed to rule out a compressive lesion. The finding of multiple focal lesions confirms the diagnosis of MS. The other role is in patients with few brain lesions, or with cerebrovascular risk factors, in whom the presence of spinal lesions increases the specificity of the examination. In patients with a negative brain scan (approximately 5 per cent of patients), spinal MR reveals lesions in the majority.[30,56,57] Interestingly, spinal lesions can also be found in patients with no clinical cord symptomatology. Clinically silent lesions are found, for example, in patients with a first attack of optic neuritis. Most MS lesions are focal and circumscribed, spindle shaped, eccentrically located and extend one vertebral segment. Diffuse signal increase throughout the cord is found in progressive patients, notably primary progressive ones.[30] Whether this feature is also diagnostically useful remains to be evaluated.

A tailored approach to the use of MR in diagnosis

The major role of MR is to demonstrate clinically silent dissociation in space which, in the most recent diagnostic criteria, can be used to make a diagnosis of laboratory-supported definite MS.[3] Standard T_2-weighted MRI has a high sensitivity (95 per cent), and hence a negative brain scan has high negative predictive power. In addition, MRI is capable of showing clinically relevant lesions in places which are not accessible to other imaging techniques, such as the optic nerve, the posterior fossa and the spinal cord. One should always keep in mind the poor specificity of T_2-weighted MR using classical criteria; although the positive predictive value will therefore inherently be poor, it will increasingly become so with a lower *a priori* chance of MS (i.e. lower prevalence). One should realize that while MS in

- Minimum of 9 lesions
- Infratentorial lesions
- Gadolinium enhancement (part of lesions)
- Occipital and temporal lesions
- Juxta-cortical lesions

Table 4.5
MR imaging findings with higher specificity.

high prevalence areas occurs in 1 per 1000 inhabitants at the maximum (0.1 per cent), small vessel white matter disease probably occurs in 5 per cent of the population! If white matter lesions are an incidental discovery, they are vascular in nature until proven otherwise. Suggesting MS in the absence of any clinical suspicion based on the finding of white matter lesions alone is one of the most common mistakes in this field.

In the past decade, emphasis has been placed on excluding MS, since the diagnosis of MS itself offered no therapeutic opportunities. This is starting to change with the introduction of effective drugs, such as interferon-β and copolymer-1, and many other drugs are on the verge of obtaining approval. Therefore,

the emphasis is shifting from excluding MS, towards ascertaining the presence of MS. Were a fully effective treatment to become available, one would of course like to start that treatment as early as possible. In other words, we increasingly need to be specific, since early treatment might be given encompassing serious side effects. Therefore, there now is a need for more specific criteria (*Table 4.5*)

In order to be specific we can look for infratentorial, juxtacortical and enhancing lesions. It will of course strongly depend on the clinical situation whether sensitivity or specificity should prevail, and the frequently asked question, whether gadolinium should be routinely used, cannot be simply answered

Clinical setting	Type of MR scan	Finding	Interpretation
No suspicion	Brain T$_2$	WM lesions	no MS
Exclude MS (atypical symptom)	Brain T$_2$	(a) no lesions (b) ≥4 lesions	(a) no MS (b) MS not ruled out
Diagnose MS (typical symptoms)	Brain T$_2$ ±spine/optic nerve	≥4 WM lesions or ≥1 spinal lesion	probably MS (laboratory-supported definite MS)
Certify MS (consider treatment)	Brain T$_2$ & Gd* ±spine/optic nerve	>7 WM lesions or ≥1 spinal lesion or Gd enhancement	MS extremely likely (risk of side-effects outweighed by chance of appropriate treatment)

*Gd = gadolinium; in case of contrast administration not all lesions should be enhancing.

Table 4.6
Diagnostic MR strategy in the diagnosing of MS.

with yes or no. *Table 4.6* provides rough directions. Indications for the use of spinal imaging have been provided in the previous paragraph, and should not be performed routinely. An integrated flow chart for the use of various MR parameters in the diagnostic work-up of suspected MS, depending on the *a priori* classification, is presented in *Fig. 4.8*.

Acknowledgements

The Dutch MR centre for MS research is supported by the 'Stichting Vrienden MS Research', the 'Academisch Ziekenhuis der Vrije Universiteit' and the Medical Faculty of the 'Vrije Universiteit'. Professor CH Polman for his useful comments on the manuscript.

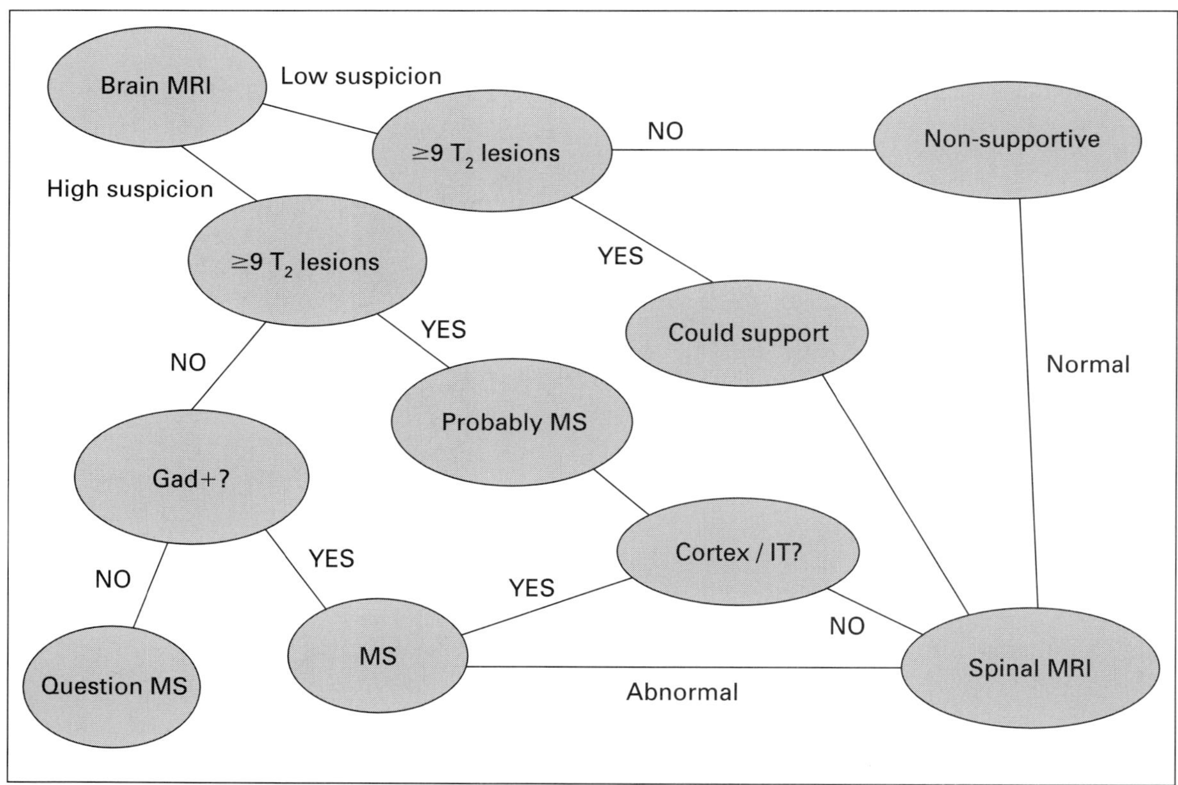

Fig. 4.8
Diagnostic flow diagram for MR imaging. *The choice of the MR examination, method of analysis, and interpretation should be guided by the clinical setting. Note: Gad + means presence of gadolinium enhancement in part of the lesions; cortex/IT means presence of cortical and infratentorial lesions.*

References

1. Young IR, Hall AS, Pallis CA *et al*. Nuclear magnetic resonance imaging of the brain in multiple sclerosis. *Lancet* 1981; **ii**: 1063–1066.

2. Schumacher GA, Beebe G, Kibler RE *et al*. Problems of experimental trials of therapy in multiple sclerosis: report by the panel on evaluation of experimental trials of therapy in multiple sclerosis. *Ann N Y Acad Sci* 1965; **122**: 552–568.

3. Poser CM, Paty DW, Scheinberg L *et al*. New diagnostic criteria for multiple sclerosis: guidelines for research protocols. *Ann Neurol* 1983; **13**: 227–231.

4. Herndon RM, Brooks B. Misdiagnosis of multiple sclerosis. *Semin Neurol* 1985; **5**: 94–98.

5. Gilbert JJ, Sadler M. Unsuspected multiple sclerosis. *Arch Neurol* 1983; **40**: 533–536.

6. Georgi VW. Multiple Sklerose: Pathologisch-Anatomische Befunde multipler Sklerose bei klinisch nicht diagnostizierten Krankheiten. *Schweiz Med Wochenschr* 1966; **20**: 605–607.

7. Paty DW, Oger JJF, Kastrukoff LF *et al*. MRI in the diagnosis of MS: a prospective study with comparison of clinical evaluation, evoked potentials, oligoclonal banding and CT. *Neurology* 1988; **38**: 180–185.

8. Scotti G, Scialfa G, Biondi A *et al*. Magnetic resonance in multiple sclerosis. *Neuroradiology* 1986; **28**: 319–323.

9. Appel B, Moens E, Rinck P *et al*. Abord de la sclérose en plaque par l'IRM. *J Neuroradiol* 1988; **15**: 108–136.

10. Uhlenbrock D, Seidel D, Gehlen W *et al*. MR imaging in multiple sclerosis: comparison with clinical, CSF and visual evoked potential findings. *Am J Neuroradiol* 1988; **9**: 59–67.

11. Adams CW. The general pathology of multiple sclerosis: morphological and chemical aspects of the lesions. In: Hallpike JF, Adams CWM, Toutelotte WW, eds. *Multiple Sclerosis. Pathology, Diagnosis and Management*, London: Chapman and Hall 1983; 203–240.

12. Prineas JW. The neuropathology of multiple sclerosis. In: Koetsier JC, ed. *Handbook of Clinical Neurology*, Vol. 47: *Demyelinating Diseases*. Amsterdam: Elsevier Science Publishers 1985; 213–257.

13. Lightman S, McDonald WI, Bird AC *et al*. Retinal venous sheathing in optic neuritis. Its significance for the pathogenesis of multiple sclerosis. *Brain* 1987; **110**: 405–414.

14. Guseo A, Jellinger K. The significance of perivascular infiltrations in multiple sclerosis. *J Neurol* 1975; **211**: 51–60.

15. Dawson JW. The histology of disseminated sclerosis. *Trans Roy Soc Edinb* 1916; **50**: 517–740.

16. Lumsden CE. The neuropathology of multiple sclerosis. In: Vinken PJ, Bruyn GW, eds. *Handbook of Clinical Neurology*, Vol. 9. Amsterdam: North-Holland Publishing Company 1970; 217–309.

17. Grossman RI, Gonzalez-Scarano F, Atlas SW *et al*. Multiple sclerosis: gadolinium enhancement in MR imaging. *Radiology* 1986; **161**: 721–725.

18. Hawkins CP, Munro PMG, MacKenzie F *et al*. Duration and selectivity of blood–brain barrier breakdown in chronic relapsing experimental allergic encephalomyelitis studied by gadolinium-DTPA and protein markers. *Brain* 1990; **113**: 365–378.

19. Katz D, Taubenberger J, Raine C *et al*. Gadolinium-enhancing lesions on magnetic resonance imaging: neuropathological findings. *Ann Neurol* 1990; **28**: 243.

20. Nesbit GM, Forbes GS, Scheithauer BW *et al*. Multiple sclerosis: histopathologic and MR and/or CT correlation in 37 cases at biopsy and 3 cases at autopsy. *Radiology* 1991; **180**: 467–474.

21. Barkhof F, Frequin STFM, Hommes OR *et al*. A correlative triad of gadolinium-DTPA MRI, EDSS, and CSF-MBP in relapsing/remitting multiple sclerosis patients treated with high-dose intravenous methylprednisolone. *Neurology* 1992; **42**: 63–67.

22. Truyen L, Barkhof F, Frequin STFM *et al*. Magnetic resonance imaging of epilepsy in multiple sclerosis: a case control study. Impli-

cations for treatment trials with 4-aminopyridine. *Multiple Sclerosis* 1996; **1**: 213–217.

23. Uhlenbrock D, Sehlen S. The value of T1-weighted images in the differentiation between MS, white matter lesions, and subcortical arteriosclerotic encephalopathy (SAE). *Neuroradiology* 1989; **31**: 203–212.

24. Shah M, Ross JS, Van Dyke C *et al.* Three-dimensional T1-weighted MP Rage versus T2-weighted spin–echo imaging in the detection of multiple sclerosis plaques. *Radiology* 1991; **181**(P): 210–211.

25. Thorpe JW, Halpin SF, MacManus DG *et al.* A comparison between fast and conventional spin–echo in the detection of multiple sclerosis lesions. *Neuroradiology* 1994; **36**: 388–392.

26. Hashemi RH, Bradley WG, Chen DY *et al.* Suspected multiple sclerosis: MR imaging with a thin-section fast FLAIR pulse sequence. *Radiology* 1995; **196**: 505–510.

27. Gean-Marton AD, Vezina LG, Marton KI *et al.* Abnormal corpus callosum: a sensitive and specific indicator of multiple sclerosis. *Radiology* 1991; **180**: 215–221.

28. Truyen L, Gheuens J, van de Vyver FL *et al.* Improved correlation of magnetic resonance imaging (MRI) with clinical status in multiple sclerosis (MS) by use of an extensive standardized imaging protocol. *J Neurol Sci* 1990; **96**: 173–182.

29. Filippi M, Yousry T, Campi A *et al.* Comparison of triple dose versus standard dose gadolinium-DTPA for the detection of MRI enhancing lesions in patients with MS. *Neurology* 1996; **46**: 379–384.

30. Lycklama à Nijeholt GL, Barkhof F, Scheltens P *et al.* MR of the spinal cord in multiple sclerosis: relations to clinical subtype and disability. *J Neuroradiol* 1997; **18**: 1041–1048.

31. Thorpe JW, Kidd D, Miller DH *et al.* Spinal cord MRI using multi-array coils and fast spin–echo. I. Findings in normal controls. *Neurology* 1993; **43**: 2625–2631.

32. Miller DH, Newton MR, van der Poel JC *et al.* Magnetic resonance imaging of the optic nerve in optic neuritis. *Neurology* 1988; **38**: 175–179.

33. van der Knaap MS, Valk J. *Magnetic Resonance of Myelin, Myelination and Myelin Disorders*, 2nd edn. Berlin: Springer Verlag 1995.

34. Fazekas F, Offenbacher H, Fuchs S *et al.* Criteria for an increased specificity of MRI interpretation in elderly subjects with suspected multiple sclerosis. *Neurology* 1988; **38**: 1822–1825.

35. Horowitz AL, Kaplan RD, Grewe G *et al.* The ovoid lesion: a new MR observation in patients with multiple sclerosis. *Am J Neuroradiol* 1989; **10**: 303–305.

36. Simon JH, Holtås SL, Schiffer RB *et al.* Corpus callosum and subcallosal-periventricular lesions in multiple sclerosis: detection with MR. *Radiology* 1986; **160**: 363–367.

37. Simon JH, Schiffer RB, Rudick RA *et al.* Quantitative determination of MS-induced corpus callosum atrophy in vivo using MR imaging. *Am J Neuroradiol* 1987; **8**: 599–604.

38. Honer WG, Hurwitz T, Li DKB *et al.* Temporal lobe involvement in multiple sclerosis patients with psychiatric disorders. *Arch Neurol* 1987; **44**: 187–190.

39. Thompson AJ, Kermode AG, MacManus DG *et al.* Patterns of disease activity in multiple sclerosis: clinical and magnetic resonance imaging study. *Br Med J* 1990; **300**: 631–634.

40. Chen CJ, Ro LS, Chang CN *et al* Serial MRI studies in pathologically verified Balò's concentric sclerosis. *J Comput Assist Tomogr* 1996; **20**: 732–735.

41. Barkhof F, Scheltens P, Valk J *et al.* Serial quantitative MR assessment of optic neuritis in a case of neuromyelitis optica, using gadolinium-"enhanced" STIR imaging. *Neuroradiology* 1991; **33**: 70–71.

42. Mader I, Stock KW, Ettlin T *et al.* Acute disseminated encephalomyelitis: MR and CT features. *Am J Neurorad* 1996; **17**: 104–109.

43. Caldemeyer KS, Smith RR, Harris TM *et al.* MRI in acute disseminated encephalomyelitis. *Neuroradiology* 1994; **36**: 216–220.

44. Kesselring J, Miller DH, Robb S *et al.* Acute disseminated encephalomyelitis. MRI findings and the distinction from multiple sclerosis. *Brain* 1990; **113**: 291–320.

45. van der Meyden CH, de Villiers JFK, Middlecote BD *et al.* Gadolinium ring enhancement and mass effect in acute disseminated encephalomyelitis. *Neuroradiology* 1994; **36**: 221–223.

46. Lee KH, Hashimoto S, Hooge JP *et al*. Magnetic resonance imaging of the head in the diagnosis of multiple sclerosis: a prospective 2-year follow-up with comparison of clinical evaluation, evoked potential, oligoclonal banding, and CT. *Neurology* 1991; **41**: 657–660.

47. Thorpe JW, Mumford CJ, Compston DAS *et al*. British Isles survey of multiple sclerosis twins: MRI. *J Neurol Neurosurg Psychiatry* 1994; **57**: 491–496.

48. Lynch SG, Rose JW, Smoker W *et al*. MRI in familial multiple sclerosis. *Neurology* 1990; **40**: 900–903.

49. Poser S, Scheidt P, Kitze B *et al*. Impact of magnetic resonance imaging (MRI) on the epidemiology of MS. *Acta Neurol Scand* 1991; **83**: 172–175.

50. Morissey SP, Miller DH, Kendall BE *et al*. Prognostic significance of brain MRI at presentation in patients with a clinically isolated syndrome suggestive of MS – a five year follow-up study. *Brain* 1993; **116**: 115–146.

51. Offenbacher H, Fazekas F, Schmidt R *et al*. Assessment of MRI criteria for diagnosis of MS. *Neurology* 1993; **43**: 905–909.

52. Tas MW, Barkhof F, van Walderveen MAA *et al*. The effect of gadolinium on the sensitivity and specificity of MR imaging in the initial diagnosis of multiple sclerosis. *Am J Neuroradiol* 1995; **16**: 259–264.

53. Barkhof F, Filippi M, Losseff N *et al*. Towards specific magnetic resonance imaging criteria in the early diagnosis of multiple sclerosis (abstract). *Neurology* 1995; **45** (suppl 4): A398.

54. Filippi M, Mammi S, Yousry T *et al*. Comparison of fast-FLAIR vs conventional SE sequences for measurement of brain MRI lesion load in patients with multiple sclerosis. *J Neuroimmunol* 1995; **62** (suppl 1): 62.

55. Heun R, Kappos L, Bittkau S *et al*. Magnetic resonance imaging and early diagnosis of multiple sclerosis. *Lancet* 1988; **ii**: 1202–1203.

56. Kidd D, Thorpe JW, Thompson AJ *et al*. Spinal cord MRI using multi-array coils and fast spin–echo. II. Findings in multiple sclerosis. *Neurology* 1993; **43**: 2632–2637.

57 Thorpe JW, Kidd D, Moseley IF *et al*. Spinal MRI in patients with suspected multiple sclerosis and negative brain MRI. *Brain* 1996; **119**: 709–714.

5

Differential diagnosis in multiple sclerosis

Cesare Fieschi, Claudio Gasperini and Giovanni Ristori

Introduction

Multiple sclerosis (MS) is an inflammatory demyelinating disorder and is the most common cause of neurological disability in young adults. Classically it begins with a relapsing–remitting course and the most usual initial clinical manifestations are sensory (40 per cent) and visual (35 per cent), followed by motor (21 per cent), brain stem (16 per cent), cerebellar (15 per cent) and bladder (4 per cent) symptoms. In time, the remissions tend to be less than complete and many patients subsequently pass into a progressive phase (secondary progression) with gradually worsening irreversible disability. However, up to one-third of patients do not develop progressive disability and remain unimpaired many years after the onset of the illness (benign MS). A smaller number of patients (<10 per cent) develop progressive disability from the onset without relapses and remissions (primary progressive MS).

The diagnosis of MS is fundamentally clinical. The essential diagnostic criteria are the signs of lesions disseminated in time and space and the exclusion of other conditions which may produce the same clinical picture. A number of clinically based diagnostic classifications have been used (see Barkhof, Chapter 4). The criteria by Schumaker *et al.*[1] require that symptoms and signs be attributable to more than one central nervous system (CNS) lesion (dissociation in place) and the occurrence of more than one individual period of signs or symptoms, or progression over more than half a year (dissociation in time).

In clinical practice, difficulties arise when trying to diagnose patients at onset of MS or with recurrent episodes of neurological deficit which may be attributable to a single lesion, and patients with a variety of recurring symptoms but with signs of damage at only one site. For these reasons, Schumaker's criteria have been superseded by an agreed classification which incorporates evidence of subclinical involvement, as demonstrated by abnormalities in evoked responses and on magnetic resonance imaging (MRI). In addition, the ability to detect immunological abnormalities of cerebrospinal fluid (CSF), such as oligoclonal bands or increased intrathecal immunoglobulin G (IgG) synthesis, has introduced a new category of laboratory-supported definite MS (*Table 5.1*).[2]

Modern immunochemical techniques have made it possible to show intrathecal synthesis of oligoclonal IgG in around 95 per cent of patients with clinically definite MS.[3] Nevertheless, the oligoclonal bands are also present in a wide range of inflammatory and immunological disorders, many of which form part of the differential diagnosis of MS (see *Table 5.2*). Furthermore, a few patients with 'clinically definite' MS have no evidence of intrathecal IgG synthesis, the absence of which has been

Category	Attacks	Clinical evidence		Paraclinical evidence	Cerebrospinal fluid OB/IgG
Clinically definite MS	2	2			
	2	1	and	1	
Laboratory-supported definite MS	2	1	or	1	+
	1	2			+
	1	1	and	1	+
Clinically probable MS	2	1			
	1	2			
	1	1	and	1	
Laboratory-supported probable MS	2				+

OB, oligoclonal band

Table 5.1
Poser diagnostic criteria for MS.[2]

Inflammatory disorders
  MS
  Systemic lupus erythematosus
  Primary Sjögren's syndrome
  Behçet's disease
  Polyarteritis nodosa

Infectious diseases
  Viral encephalitis
  Neuroborreliosis
  Chronic fungal meningitis
  Neurosyphilis
  Subacute sclerosing panencephalitis
  Progressive rubella panencephalitis

Sarcoidosis

Cerebrovascular disorders

Guillain–Barré syndrome

Table 5.2
Common diseases cause oligoclonal bands in the CSF.

identified as one of the most important factors which should cast doubt on the diagnosis.[4–6]

Recently, diagnosis has been facilitated by use of MRI which has proved to be very sensitive[7] (see Barkhof, Chapter 4). Areas of high signal on T_2-weighted MRI are seen in approximately 95 per cent of patients with clinically definite MS. Magnetic resonance documentation of new lesions occurring over time may meet the criteria for 'dissociation in time and space'. However, despite the high sensitivity of MRI for the diagnosis of MS, the typical pattern of discrete multifocal white matter areas of increased signal on T_2-weighted scans is not specific solely to MS: a number of diseases exhibit typical MS lesions on MRI (*Table 5.3*).

Particular care is needed in those patients who have a clinical picture compatible with MS and multiple white matter abnormalities, but who have normal CSF; in a consecutive series of 405 patients, we found 18 such cases.[5] After extensive investigations, we reached a new diagnosis in six patients, comprising vasculitis (two cases), one case of mitochondrial encephalomyopathy with lactic acidosis and stroke-like episodes (MELAS), multiple ischaemic lesions caused by atrial septum aneurysm (one case), oligopontocerebellar atrophy (one case) and one case of Lyme disease. A further disease which shows this clinical, MRI and immunological pattern is the CADASIL syndrome which should always be considered in patients presenting these characteristics.

MRI specificity is increased by diagnostic criteria based on the number, size and location of lesions. Kuroda *et al.*[8] evaluated the MRI criteria for MS previously proposed[7,9] in 36 MS patients and 36 control patients with HTLV-I associated myelopathy/tropical spastic paraparesis. The primary criterion (at least three MRI lesions >3 mm) was fulfilled in 31 MS patients and in 2 controls, yielding 93 per cent specificity and 86 per cent sensitivity. However, another study showed that about 30 per cent of patients with cerebral systemic lupus erythematosus have lesions >6 mm.[10]

MS variants
    Charcot type, Devic type, Schilder type, Marburg type, isolated syndromes
Normal aging
Alzheimer's disease
Migraine
Subcortical arteriosclerotic encephalopathy or Binswanger's disease
Multiple metastases
Vasculitis
    Sjögren's syndrome, polyarteritis nodosa, systemic lupus erythematosus, Behçet's disease,
    giant cell arteritis
Sarcoidosis
Leucodystrophies
Encephalitides
    Viral:
    HTLV-1 myelopathy, subacute sclerosing panencephalitis, progressive multifocal
    leucoencephalopathy (papova), acute disseminated encephalomyelitis (ADEM)
    Mycoplasmal:
    Tuberculosis
    Spirochaetal:
    Syphilis, neuroborreliosis or Lyme disease
Chronic demyelinating inflammatory polyneuropathy
Subacute combined degeneration of the spinal cord (B_{12} deficiency)

Table 5.3
Diseases which mimic MS on MRI.

Furthermore, although MRI detects the white matter lesions of MS within the brain with high sensitivity, a minority of patients have normal brain MRI. Several series report occasional patients, some of whom fulfil the criteria of definite MS, in whom MRI reveals lesions typical of MS only in the spinal cord and not in the brain.[11–13] Recently it has been suggested that the finding of a normal brain MRI, although rare, is nevertheless quite compatible with a diagnosis of MS. Spinal cord MRI in such patients frequently displays intrinsic cord lesions, the presence of which is of considerable diagnostic value.[14]

Thus, there is no single laboratory test which is pathognomonic for MS. Many conditions can produce a multifocal central nervous system (CNS) syndrome with a relapsing–remitting course in young adults.[15] The rate of misdiagnosis is around 5 per cent, indicating that 1 in 20 patients thought to have MS have, instead, a condition resembling MS. Such conditions, which should always be investigated, can be classified approximately into those which are commonly mistaken for MS and those which are less like MS (see *Tables 5.4–5.6*). Recently some authors reported 'red flags' to alert the neurologist to an incorrect diagnosis. They found that four red flags were strongly correlated with alternative diagnoses: normal cerebrospinal fluid, absent eye findings, normal brain MRI, and absent bowel or bladder symptoms. Each had a predictive value for an alternative diagnosis of more than 90 per cent, which increased to 98 per cent when three or more red flags were present.[16]

Other demyelinating diseases have been regarded as a variant of MS. Devic's neuromyelitis optica is characterized by an acute–subacute onset of blindness of one or both eyes preceded or followed within days or weeks by a transverse or ascending myelitis. Recently the following diagnostic criteria have been proposed to distinguish strict Devic's neuromyelitis optica from MS:[17]

- Clinical – acute involvement of spinal cord and optic nerves, either coincidental or separated by months or years, independent of its subsequent progression, but without the development of brainstem cerebellar, or cortical features at any time in the disease course
- Imaging – normal appearing brain MRI; enlargement and cavitation on spinal cord MRI
- Cerebrospinal fluid – decreased serum/CSF albumin ratio with normal CNS, daily IgG synthesis and usually an absence of oligoclonal bands.

Marburg's disease is described as a fulminant, monophasic, malignant form of MS. A combination of cerebral, brain stem and spinal manifestations evolve over a few weeks, rendering the patient stuporous or comatose, or decerebrate with prominent cranial nerve and corticospinal abnormalities.[18,19] Death may end the illness within a few weeks to months without any remission having occurred.

Wegener's granulomatosis
Whipple's disease
Arnold–Chiari malformation

Isolated spinal cord syndromes:
Extrinsic or intrinsic compressive lesions
Vitamin B_{12} deficiency
Intracranial tumour

Table 5.4
Diseases mimicking MS clinically but with a clearly different diagnosis on MRI.

Disease	Differential diagnosis by
AIDS	Antibodies to HIV in serum
Prothrombotic states	EGC – extracranial Doppler of the carotid arteries and echocardiography. Coagulopathy: determination of protein S, protein C, antithrombin III, detection of the lupus anticoagulant, tissue plasminogen activator concentrations, plasminogen activator inhibitor activities
Spinocerebellar degeneration	Clinical course and normality of other laboratory tests
Mitochondrial encephalopathies:	Estimation of lactate and pyruvate in plasma and CSF. Analysis for mitochondrial DNA mutation, skeletal muscle biopsy to detect a mitochondrial disorder
CADASIL:	Clinical course, genetic linkage analysis, arteriopathic alterations

Table 5.5
*Diseases mimicking MS clinically and on MRI
(CSF normal or not available).*

MS in Asians may present with disseminated signs, similar to MS in white populations, or with a distinctive predilection for severe optic–spinal involvement.[20,21] Recently a comparison between Western and Asian types of MS has been reported: patients with Asian-type MS had fewer brain lesions on MRI, but more gadolinium-enhanced spinal cord lesions than did patients with Western-type MS. Furthermore, the DR2-associated DRB1 1501 allele and DRB5 0101 allele were associated with Western-type MS, but not with either Asian-type MS or healthy control subjects. The presence of heterogeneity in the immuno-genetic background and in the MRI features between the two subtypes of MS thus suggests the presence of an aetiologically distinct disease in Asians.[22]

Monosymptomatic MS

The first manifestation of MS is in many cases an acute, clinically isolated syndrome involving the optic nerves (36 per cent) or the spinal cord (33 per cent). Follow-up studies show a risk of progression to MS after an episode of acute unilateral optic neuritis (ON) or acute partial myelopathy which ranges from 12 to 85 per cent.[23,24] Brain MRI demonstrates multifocal white matter abnormalities indistinguishable from those seen in MS in 50 to 70 per cent of patients with such clinically isolated syndrome.[25,26] Several prospective studies have shown that the presence of these MRI abnormalities markedly increases the risk of developing MS within the first 1 to 3 years[24,26,27] and has a greater prognostic value

Disease	Differential diagnosis by
Vasculitis: Sjögren's syndrome, polyarteritis nodosa, systemic lupus erythematosus	Estimation of anticardiolipin antibodies, detection of antinuclear antibodies, determination of antibodies to native. DNA against Ro SS-A and La SS-B. If necessary, cerebral angiography, retinal fluoroangiography, slit lamp examination and biopsy
Behçet's disease	Clinical course (mucocutaneous ulcerations)
Lyme disease	Measurements of antibodies to *B. burgdorferi* in serum and CSF. Positive reactions confirmed by a Lues TPHA test
Sarcoidosis	Kveim test, estimation of the level of angiotensin-converting enzyme in serum and CSF, biopsy of any possible accessible lesion
Adrenoleucodystrophy	Determination of very long fatty acids
HTLV-I	Test for HTLV-I antibodies
Leber's optic atrophy	Mitochondrial DNA analysis to exclude a mutation at position 11778
ADEM	Serial MRI examinations and clinical course

Table 5.6
Disease clinically mimicking MS with both MRI and CSF criteria.

than the presence of oligoclonal IgG in CSF or evoked potential abnormalities.[28,29] Finally, Filippi *et al.*[30] demonstrated that the risk of developing MS increases and the time to development of MS decreases with increasing lesion load at presentation.

Optic Neuritis

There is wide belief that monosymptomatic ON is usually a first manifestation of MS. ON is usually characterized by rapid deterioration of vision in one or both eyes. Retrobulbar pain, exaggerated by eye movements, is common. Other symptoms are loss of brightness, disturbed colour vision and altered depth perception. Central scotomas can be present. The recovery phase of ON begins within a few weeks of onset. The best visual outcome usually occurs 3–6 months after onset, but may occur within a few weeks.

Short-term follow-up studies indicated that patients presenting with ON who had lesions on MRI frequently developed a clinically definite MS, whereas patients with normal MRI had a better prognosis and may never develop clinically definite MS. The relative risk of developing MS after a median of one year was 5.4 ($p < 0.05$) in unilateral monosymptomatic acute ON with abnormal MRI at onset.[31]

By reviewing previous studies, increased leucocyte count in the CSF has been found in 13–60 per cent and oligoclonal bands (OB) in 24–61 per cent of patients with acute monosymptomatic ON.

Although visual loss is more usually caused by primary demyelination of the optic nerve, it has to be distinguished from secondary demyelination in optic neuropathies mimicking ON, such as those caused by compression, ischaemia or toxic aetiology.[32] Moreover, bacterial, viral, parasitic and fungal infections producing an inflammatory process within the optic nerve are encountered. Post-viral and post-vaccination ON have also been described and in rare cases ON has been associated with collagenoses.

The form most difficult to distinguish from that in MS is Leber's hereditary optic atrophy which will be described in a following paragraph.

Myelopathy

Another difficult clinical problem is an isolated spinal cord syndrome, particularly when the patient presents with progressive spastic paraplegia in middle life. In this case the first step is to exclude extrinsic or intrinsic compressive lesions. The onset of spinal cord compression by extramedullary masses is usually of gradual progression. There may be pain in a radicular distribution or tenderness over the spine. Pain may be increased on coughing. Bowel or bladder dysfunction usually occurs late with extramedullary lesions (the exceptions being sacral and lower thoracic masses), and early sphincter dysfunction should increase the index of suspicion for disease intrinsic to the spinal cord. Cervical spondylosis generally has its onset in the fifth or later decades, whereas MS occurs in younger age groups. Moreover, the deep tendon reflexes in cervical spondylosis may be focally depressed in a segmental pattern due to root compression. Although depressed deep tendon reflexes occasionally occur in MS, hyperactive tendon reflexes are much more common.

The majority of patients with isolated noncompressive spinal cord lesions at MRI are found to have MS, particularly if there are multiple lesions on cerebral scans.[2c]

If patients are of Caribbean or Japanese origin, tropical spastic paraparesis resulting from HTLV-I infection must be considered.

Diseases mimicking MS
Clinically

We can include diseases mimicking MS clinically but with a clearly differential diagnosis on MRI.

Wegener's granulomatosis

This is a rare disease of unknown aetiology which usually affects adults rather than children, and has a male:female predominance of 2:1. It is characterized by necrotizing vasculitis and granulomatous inflammation and primarily affects the lungs and kidneys. However, small vessels anywhere in the body can be involved. Neurological complications occur in approximately 50 per cent of cases and take either the form of a peripheral neuropathy or multiple cranial neuropathies resulting from extension of nasal and sinus granulomas to the upper cranial nerves, and pharyngeal lesions to the lower nerves. In rare cases, this latter form may present as clinical manifestations which mimic MS.[33] The diagnosis is confirmed by demonstrating the presence of both granulomas and vasculitis.

Whipple's disease

This is a rare disorder predominantly of middle-aged men, which may give rise to a number of neurological syndromes; cognitive problems, visual impairment, ophthalmoplegia and myoclonus have been reported. Frederikson[34] described a male patient who presented after having multiple neurological episodes for two months. His MRI scan showed enhancement of the dura over one convexity. Many periodic acid Schiff's stain (PAS)-positive macrophages were found in a biopsy of his dura and cortex, indicating the presence of certain bacterial polysaccharides. Whipple's disease was diagnosed and he was treated with penicillin and streptomycin and recovered within ten days. Diagnostic guidelines in central nervous system Whipple's disease have recently been suggested.[35]

Arnold Chiari malformation

The form of Chiari malformation which appears in adult life may also cause some diagnostic difficulty. The symptoms may be those of increased intracranial pressure, progressive cerebellar ataxia, syringomyelia, or a combination of disorders of the lower cranial nerves, cerebellum, medulla and spinal cord. The condition occasionally appears to have a relapsing–remitting course, with gradual onset of spastic paraparesis and little involvement until many years later.[36] The diagnosis is facilitated by the use of MRI and laboratory tests.

The CSF total protein may be moderately increased while the OB are usually absent. Definitive diagnosis depends on the MRI picture which shows abnormalities of the cranio-

cervical regions but with no lesions located in the white matter.[37]

Isolated spinal cord syndrome

Extrinsic or intrinsic compressive lesions The first step is to exclude extrinsic or intrinsic compressive lesions. MRI has a unique role in this situation, particularly in the diagnosis of intraspinal tumours. Most patients with isolated non-compressive spinal cord lesions are found to have MS, particularly if there are multiple lesions on cerebral MRI scans.[24,38]

Vitamin B_{12} deficiency In clinical practice the distinction between MS and 'subacute combined degeneration' due to vitamin B_{12} deficiency occasionally leads to difficulty with diagnosis. Demyelination in the spinal cord is a prominent feature of the neuropathology of vitamin B_{12} deficiency and is characterized by the symmetrical involvement of the posterior and lateral columns. There are some reports of patients in whom a diagnosis of MS has been made or suspected, only for the diagnosis to be changed to subacute combined degeneration following the discovery of an abnormality of vitamin B_{12} metabolism.[39,40]

Although the presence of gastric achlorhydria, megaloblastic anaemia and macrocytic anaemia should be considered, the diagnosis of vitamin B_{12} deficiency has, until recently, been very dependent on serum vitamin B_{12} assay. However, since significant lowering of serum vitamin B_{12} and elevation of plasma unsaturated R-binder capacity has also been reported in relapsing–remitting MS, it cannot be relied upon to diagnose tissue vitamin B_{12} deficiency. New evidence suggests that total plasma homocysteine may be a useful guide to functional vitamin B_{12} deficiency.[41]

Intracranial tumour

The clinical pattern of tumours is occasionally indistinguishable from that observed in relapsing–remitting MS. Arteriovenous malformations and other forms of angioma involving the brain stem can create particular diagnostic difficulties.

Bickerstaff *et al.*[42] described unilateral visual loss, with a central scotoma occurring during pregnancy, with subsequent complete recovery, caused by a meningioma pressing on the optic nerve. A relapsing–remitting condition caused by a glioma located in the brain stem[43] and an epidermoid of the fourth ventricle have also been reported.[44] A patient with cerebellar ataxia which remitted repeatedly on treatment with adrenocorticotrophic hormone, and who had for several years been diagnosed as having MS, was later found to have a primary cerebral lymphoma.[45]

Lehaman and Fieger[46] described a patient who, between the ages of 9 and 22 years, had suffered remitting–relapsing symptoms characterized by repeated episodes of weakness of the right arm. This was then followed by a left hemiparesis and diplopia. Eventually arachnoid cysts in the cisterna magna were diagnosed.

Clinical and MRI criteria (CSF normal or not available)

In these diseases the CSF finding is not sufficient for the differential diagnosis and a detailed diagnostic battery of laboratory tests for the most likely alternative diagnoses have to be performed.

AIDS

Involvement of the CNS is frequent in human immunodeficiency virus (HIV)-infected patients. It usually occurs in the later stages of the disease[47] but in 10 per cent of cases it may be the initial manifestation of HIV infection.[48] Berger *et al.*[49] described seven men suffering from neurological disease clinically indistinguishable from MS which occurred in association with seropositivity for HIV. In four patients the neurological disease preceded the demonstration of HIV seropositivity by several years, suggesting a concurrence of the two illnesses, but in three cases HIV seropositivity occurred in close chronological association with the onset of the neurological disease, making an aetiological association more likely.

The clinical evidence of multiple lesions may be supported by cerebral white matter lesions, displayed by MRI, indistinguishable from those of MS.[47]

In AIDS patients, the total protein concentration and cell count in the CSF are usually increased to within the range still acceptable for MS, but oligoclonal bands are uncommon.[47]

Mitochondrial encephalopathies

'Mitochondrial encephalopathies' refer to mitochondrial diseases in which both muscle and the CNS are involved but, in contrast to the mitochondrial myopathies, CNS dysfunction dominates the clinical picture. Patients with mitochondrial encephalopathies can be divided into two groups. In the first group, the child is either seriously ill from birth or deteriorates rapidly shortly thereafter. In the second group, the child appears normal at birth and only later is the presence of a progressive neurological disorder recognized. This group, which should be included in the differential diagnosis of MS, includes MELAS and myoclonic epilepsy with ragged-red fibres (MERRF). In most cases they are hereditary disorders characterized by the presence of external opthalmoplegia, progressive ptosis, proximal weakness and generalized tonic–clonic seizures. It has been reported that MRI can be extremely useful in the diagnosis of these disorders; MRI abnormalities considered specific to mitochondrial encephalopathy have been described in three patients with complete or partial MELAS syndromes.[50] In this study, all patients showed a T_2-weighted MRI pattern of multifocal areas of hyperintense signal confined to the cortex of the cerebrum, cerebellum, and white matter immediately adjacent. In contrast, we made a diagnosis of MELAS in one patient with 'clinically definite' MS who, on MRI, had white matter abnormalities considered fully compatible with MS, and normal CSF examination.[4]

It is important to note that the compilation of MS-like genetic disorders described in this review may not be exhaustive. Based on the disorders and metabolic pathways already discussed, it is reasonable to predict other possible mimics of MS.[51] It has been suggested that if one or more first-degree relatives of a patient with MS also has MS, the diagnosis of MS should be viewed cautiously and a search for monogenic genocopies of MS undertaken. Alternatively, if one or more first-degree relatives of a patient with MS has an unexplained CNS disorder, the diagnosis of MS should also be cautiously considered, especially in view of the intrafamilial variability of some genetic conditions, such as the mitochondrial cytopathies. In these instances it is important to evaluate critically the medical records of affected family members and, in certain instances, to directly examine them. Finally, the presence of any unexplained non-CNS disease in a patient with known or suspected MS, such as an unexplained anaemia, skin angiokeratoma, cardiomyopathy, proteinuria or metabolic acidosis, should alert the physician to another, possibly genetic, diagnosis.[51]

When the diagnosis of mitochondrial encephalopathy is suspected, based on clinical and MRI features or family history, lactic and pyruvic acid levels should be measured in both blood and CSF and the lactate:pyruvate ratio calculated. If no other reason for the secondary elevation of lactate can be found, the diagnosis should be pursued with a muscle biopsy.

Cerebrovascular disease

Cerebrovascular disease rarely causes diagnostic difficulty, although the possibility of subacute bacterial endocarditis and prothrombotic states must be considered. In these cases, rarely the presence of several clinical attacks, multiple MRI abnormalities mimicking MS and OB of IgG in the CSF, can create some difficulty in making a correct diagnosis. We reported a case of multiple ischaemic lesions caused by atrial septal aneurysm, initially considered as clinically definite MS.[4] Previously, a patient in whom emboli from a tumour of the left ventricle (classified as cavernous angiectasia) was diagnosed as having MS.[52]

Spinocerebellar degeneration

The differential diagnosis between MS and classical Friedreich's ataxia does not usually create problems. Much greater difficulty is presented by atypical cases of hereditary or sporadic cerebellar ataxia and, in particular, by hereditary spastic paraplegia. Of course, if it is possible to examine several members of a family, all of whom show a similar clinical syndrome, the diagnosis may be quite easy, but this is not usually possible in practice.

Visual evoked potentials are of limited value in diagnosis because they are often abnormal in both conditions. Magnetic resonance imaging may show periventricular and, rarely, discrete white matter abnormalities in both sporadic and hereditary cerebellar degeneration.[53] The CSF is normal in patients with hereditary spastic paraplegia and oligoclonal bands have not been described.

CADASIL

This syndrome is a 'cerebral autosomal dominant arteriopathy with subcortical infarcts and leukoencephalopathy' linked to chromosome *19q12*.

The neurological manifestations are characteristic: the age of onset of first symptoms ranges between 30 and 50. The key features consist of recurrent stroke-like episodes. The progressive development of a subcortical dementia after a history of recurrent stroke-like episodes has been found in most of the reported cases.

Brain MRI shows multiple well-delineated subcortical white matter lesions and diffuse leukoencephalopathy often mimicking the MS MRI pattern.

Examination of CSF usually gives normal results for cell count, protein and glucose; CSF immunoglobulins are normal by isoelectric focusing.

The diagnosis is established by the typical clinical course, the neuroradiological findings, the arteriopathic alterations, and the results of the genetic linkage analysis.

Clinical and both MRI and CSF criteria

In this section, the risk of a misdiagnosis is possible in some patients. In such cases a detailed diagnostic battery of laboratory tests should be performed in order to exclude less frequent alternative diseases.

Inflammatory disorders
Systemic lupus erythematosus In some cases the clinical picture of systemic lupus erythematosus (SLE) is indistinguishable from that of MS.[55] The most common presentation which can be confused with MS is that of varying combinations of ON and myelopathy.[55,56] Moreover, bilateral internuclear ophthalmoplegia[57] has also been described in SLE.

In SLE, the CSF may be normal, or the cell count and total protein may be within the MS range. The proportion of IgG has been found to be increased in 69 per cent of cases.[58] Oligoclonal IgG bands may be found[59] but their presence may be a strong factor against

the diagnosis of SLE. Cranial MRI in SLE patients shows white matter lesions mimicking those seen in MS[60] and about 30 per cent of patients with cerebral SLE have lesions >6 mm,[61] which is one of the diagnostic criteria proposed for MS to increase MRI specificity.[9]

The diagnosis of SLE can be obtained by laboratory tests of immune function. These, however, must be interpreted with caution as antinuclear factor has been found in the serum of 25 per cent of patients with MS[62] and low titre in 81 per cent.[63]

Primary Sjögren's syndrome Sjögren's syndrome is a chronic inflammatory and autoimmune disease in which the salivary and lacrimal glands undergo progressive destruction, resulting in decreased production of saliva and tears (sicca syndrome). Focal CNS disease occurs in at least 25 per cent of patients with the syndrome.[64]

Characteristically the neurological dysfunction has been described as multifocal, recurrent and progressive, and involving both the brain and spinal cord.[65] Alexander *et al.*[66] drew attention to the occurrence of central nervous system disease in primary Sjögren's syndrome and emphasized a remarkable resemblance between Sjögren's syndrome and MS. They described 20 patients, all of whom had been regarded as having MS. In these patients sicca syndrome, which is the symptom which can help to differentiate MS from Sjögren's syndrome, had been diagnosed before the onset of neurological disease in only four cases. The clinical features included a relapsing–remitting course in the majority, signs of spinal cord and cerebellar disease, internuclear ophthalmoplegia in three cases and visual loss. Oligoclonal IgG was present in the CSF in nearly all cases examined. On MRI, multiple small lesions, predominantly in the white matter, were seen in periventricular and subcortical locations. Such lesions were often not distinguishable from demyelinating lesions seen in patients with MS.

Because of the similarity in the clinical presentations and laboratory findings of patients with MS and Sjögren's syndrome, we recommend that Sjögren's syndrome be added to the differential diagnosis of patients presenting with a syndrome which resembles MS. We suggest that such patients should be evaluated for evidence of Sjögren's syndrome, including an ocular examination and minor salivary gland biopsy. Furthermore, such patients should be carefully examined for evidence of cutaneous and systemic vasculopathy, peripheral neuropathy, inflammatory myositis, and serological abnormalities.

Polyarteritis nodosa Polyarteritis nodosa is an inflammatory disease of arteries and arterioles throughout the body. Involvement of the CNS is unusual and takes the form of widespread microinfarcts. Brain stem syndromes resembling MS have also been described. Cranial MRI reveals multiple white matter lesions not immediately distinguishable from those of MS, and IgG OB have also been seen.[67] However, neurological dysfunctions occur often relatively later in the disease so that, even if they are present, evidence of systemic disease is usually well recognized and a diagnosis of MS is not likely to be considered.

Behçet's disease Behçet's disease is a multisystem, mainly inflammatory, disorder of unknown cause in which the nervous system is often affected.[68] Although the characteristic mucocutaneous ulceration of the mouth and perineum usually precedes or accompanies the neurological symptoms, they may occasionally occur later.[68] It is the involvement of the optic nerve and spinal cord which is most likely to cause confusion with MS. Retrobulbar neuritis has been described as the initial neurological symptom. Paraplegia has been reported in about 17 per cent of cases.[69]

On examination of the CSF, the total protein and cell count may be within the range found in MS,[70] but there are sometimes very high protein levels. Oligoclonal bands can be present as observed by McLean *et al.* in 2 of the 12 patients studied retrospectively using CSF and serum analysis.[59] Multifocal brain lesions may be demonstrated by MRI, the white matter abnormalities resembling those of MS; however, the presence of leptomeningeal enhancement, previously reported in two patients with neuro-Behçet's disease,[71] can help in the differential diagnosis of MS.

Lyme disease

Neuroborreliosis is a frequent and serious manifestation of Lyme disease caused by the tick-borne spirochaete *Borrelia burgdorferi*.[72] The neurological presentation of Lyme disease is extremely variable and it may mimic MS very closely. Meningitis, cranial neuritis and painful radiculoneuritis have been reported as the most common forms of CNS involvement.[73] However, myelopathy,[74] encephalitis,[75] psychiatric disorders,[76] and an 'MS-like disease',[77] have also been reported. Facial palsy, often bilateral, recurrent cranial nerve palsies and hemiparesis,[73] spastic paraparesis,[78] transverse myelitis,[74] and cerebellar ataxia[79] are the most frequent symptoms which could raise difficulties in the differential diagnosis of MS. On MRI, white matter and periventricular lesions mimicking MS may be seen.[77]

In patients with Lyme disease, CSF findings of high cell counts, inflammatory lymphocytosis, intrathecal synthesis of IgG and OB on isoelectric focusing have been reported.[80] In view of this, the diagnostic differentiation of neuroborreliosis from MS using laboratory methods may be difficult. Serological tests for antibodies can be useful[81] but, even when these are positive, some doubts should persist since

B. burgdorferi antibodies can be found in several inflammatory diseases of the CNS, including MS.[82] Therefore, the primary diagnosis of neuroborreliosis is based on antibodies synthesized within the CNS against *B. burgdorferi*.[80]

Sarcoidosis

Sarcoidosis involves the CNS in approximately 5 per cent of cases.[83] The neurological presentation makes the differential diagnosis from MS very difficult, particularly if the neurological symptoms are the first sign of the disease, as happens in about 6 per cent of the patients.[84] The onset may occasionally be rapid or sudden, followed by complete or partial spontaneous remission. Of particular importance is the involvement of the optic nerve characterized by blurred vision and pain in one or both eyes which can be the only neurological manifestation.[85] Relapsing–remitting cranial nerve palsies, particularly of the facial nerve but also including bulbar palsy, may occur over a period of several weeks or months. Moreover, a progressive spastic paraparesis caused by compression, ischaemia or parenchymal disease of the spinal cord has been described.[86] In this case, the course of the disease is indistinguishable on clinical grounds from that of progressive MS.

Examination of the CSF in patients with sarcoidosis can reveal a local synthesis of oligoclonal IgG.[87]

Periventricular and discrete white matter abnormalities may be seen on MRI which are not easily distinguishable from those seen in MS. However, gadolinium enhancement can be particularly useful in differentiating MS from neurosarcoidosis. In a study of 24 neurosarcoidosis patients with stringent clinical criteria for the diagnosis, the presence of enhancing structures in the CNS seen in 17 patients on MRI (leptomeningeal enhancement, parenchymal enhancing mass, periventricular enhancement, enhancing cord masses, enhancing nerve roots and chiasmal enhancement) was a useful clue to the diagnosis in 88 per cent of the cases, while in about 46 per cent of the cases the T_2 scans revealed abnormalities identical to those of MS.[88]

Adrenoleucodystrophy

Adrenoleucodystrophy (ALD) is a genetically determined disorder which is associated with the accumulation of very long-chain fatty acids (VLFA). If it is in the form which predominantly affects the brain and adrenal glands, it mainly occurs in children and is unlikely to be mistaken for MS. However, the X-linked type may manifest in adult life as adrenomyeloneuropathy (AMN), with progressive spinal cord disease combined with some clinical evidence of peripheral neuropathy. In these cases, the absence of a family history indicating sex-linked inheritance might create diagnostic difficulty with MS. Differential diagnosis is particularly difficult in female heterozygotes who may also present with spastic paraparesis[89] or with mild remitting neurological symptoms and oligoclonal bands seen on CSF examination.[90] In some cases, the resemblance to MS is even closer on MRI, when diffuse white matter abnormalities predominantly located in the parietal–occipital lobes are characteristically seen.[91] The diagnosis can be established in both homozygous cases and in carriers by estimation of VLFA in the plasma.

Human lymphotropic virus type I (HTLV-I)

Tropical spastic paraparesis is associated with HTLV-I. Although this syndrome does not mimic the relapsing–remitting form of MS, it is not immediately distinguishable from the onset of the progressive form. Tropical spastic paraparesis usually begins in patients in their mid-40s. The disease runs a slowly progressive course, usually with back pain, bladder disturbance and, invariably, sensory symptoms. There are no ocular symptoms, but visual and other evoked potentials have been often reported as being abnormal.[92,93] Intrathecal production of IgG and the presence of OB have also been described.[93] MRI, which may show periventricular lesions similar to those in MS, must be interpreted with care. Recently, Kuroda *et al.*[8] found that 2 of 36 patients with HTLV-I-associated myelopathy/tropical spastic paraparesis, fulfilled the MRI criteria for MS which were previously proposed by Paty *et al.*[7] and by Fazekas *et al.*[9]

Therefore, if chronic myelopathy is present, particularly in a patient of Caribbean or Japanese origin, a test for HTLV-I antibodies must be considered.

Leber's optic atrophy

This rare condition is characterized by the relatively rapid development of bilateral blindness with optic atrophy, beginning in early adult life. Leber's hereditary optic neuropathy is exclusively maternally transmitted; in contrast to X-linked disease, the descendants of male patients are not affected. In most patients the visual loss begins between 18 and 25 years, with an insidious onset and a subacute or slow evolution, but it may begin so abruptly as to suggest a retrobulbar neuritis. Usually both eyes are affected simultaneously – although in some patients, one eye is affected first, followed by the other after an interval of several weeks or months. Optic atrophy may occur in combination with degeneration in many other parts of the nervous system such as corticospinal tract and cerebellum. MS may sometimes resemble these symptoms, but without a definitive hereditary background and with a much better outlook for improvement of vision. This pattern of inheritance is consistent with an underlying mutation of mitochondrial DNA and three

such mutations, exclusively found in affected families, have been described.[94–96] The most common is a point mutation at position 11778 of mtDNA. From the clinical point of view, mtDNA analysis is indicated in women who present with simultaneous or sequential bilateral optic neuropathy, even if there is no family history of subacute visual failure or other neurological features develop later.[97]

Acute disseminated encephalomyelitis

Acute disseminated encephalomyelitis (ADEM) and MS are both inflammatory demyelinating diseases of the CNS. Whereas ADEM is usually a monophasic illness frequently preceded or accompanied by a viral infection, MS is by definition a multiphasic disease which usually results in stepwise or steadily progressive deterioration in neurological function. Problems in diagnosis may arise when there is a polysymptomatic presentation in the absence of a preceding infection, and in patients presenting with an isolated clinical deficit of a type common to both diseases, such as optic neuritis.

Certain clinical features may help to differentiate the two conditions. Acute disseminated encephalomyelitis often produces a widespread CNS disturbance with coma or drowsiness, seizures and multifocal neurological signs involving the brain, spinal cord and optic nerves. In contrast, MS usually presents with one symptom such as ON or a subacute myelopathy. Although acute disseminated encephalomyelitis may also present in this way, the ON which occurs in ADEM is usually simultaneously bilateral whereas in MS it is more often unilateral; in addition, the myelopathy in MS patients is frequently partial but in ADEM it is often complete and associated with areflexia. Nevertheless, no clinical feature is exclusive to one or other disorder.

Examination of the CSF cannot be relied

upon to differentiate the two conditions. While a moderate CSF pleocytosis is usual in ADEM, high cell counts may occasionally be seen in MS. Likewise, although oligoclonal IgG bands are a characteristic feature of MS, they may also occur in ADEM.[94] However, in MS OB almost always persist, so their disappearance is a useful distinguishing feature of ADEM.[98]

MRI may reveal multifocal asymmetric white matter lesions in the brain, which are indistinguishable from those seen in MS.[99]

In these patients, the differential diagnosis of MS and ADEM from a single scan could be possible if there was a reliable method of determining the age of lesions. Studies in MS patients using gadolinium enhanced MRI show a mixture of enhancing and non-enhancing lesions,[100] while in ADEM, which is usually a monophasic disease, it might be expected that all lesions would be enhanced in the acute phase, while none would be in the chronic phase. Serial MRI offers help in differentiating monophasic from multiphasic disease. Using unenhanced serial MRI in ADEM, many lesions resolve and new lesions do not develop,[99] whereas in MS, although some lesions resolve, new lesions develop. In addition, it has been demonstrated that the combination of gadolinium-enhancing lesions and non-enhancing T_2 lesions, rather than the presence of non-enhancing lesions alone, increases the likelihood of early progression from a clinically isolated syndrome to clinically definite MS.[101]

Unusual symptoms

Although white matter in any area of the CNS system may be involved in MS, there are a number of favoured sites, notably the optic nerve, periventricular region, and cervical cord. Thus, ON and sensory or motor disturbance of the limbs are common initial presen-

tations, as are syndromes referable to the brain stem and cerebellum. However, other less frequent symptoms are also described:

Extrapyramidal movement disorders

Although extrapyramidal movement disorders are rare in MS, numerous case reports have been published and clearly document the occurrence of a wide range of these disorders. They include hemiballismus, resulting from a lesion involving the contralateral subthalmic nucleus,[102] spasmodic torticollis associated with a midbrain lesion,[103] chorea, and parkinsonism.[104]

Recently, Trachant *et al.*[105] reported 14 new cases of movement disorders other than tremor, associated with MS; 9 had dystonia, 3 had parkinsonism and 2 had myoclonus. They also reviewed 135 such cases from the literature, concluding that paroxysmal dystonias (tonic spasm), ballism–chorea and palatal myoclonus can be caused by demyelinating lesions.

Paroxysmal symptoms

In addition to paroxysmal pain which occurs in up to 50 per cent of MS patients, such paroxysmal symptoms as tonic seizure, paroxysmal dysarthria and ataxia, and paroxysmal sensory disturbance, although relatively uncommon, can be observed in MS and rarely occur in other conditions.[106]

Seizure

Approximately 5 per cent of patients with MS develop focal Jacksonian or generalized seizures at some time during the course of their disease.[106]

This association may seem surprising in a white matter disease, but pathological and MRI studies using new sequences, such as FLAIR, have implicated cortical and subcortical lesions in the pathogenesis.[107]

Aphasia

Remitting aphasia is uncommon in MS, but rare cases have been described, associated with lesions located in the left hemisphere.[108]

Psychosis

Rarely, cases of MS presenting as acute or chronic psychosis without abnormal neurological signs, have been reported.[109,110]

Conclusion

MS can usually be diagnosed from a patient history, clinical examination, CSF studies and MRI scan. However, rarely, the classical clinical criteria, even when supported by MRI findings or by the presence of abnormalities on CSF, may not be sufficiently specific. The need to reach diagnostic certainty is particularly important given the availability of therapeutic modalities which may potentially prevent the progression of the disease. Therefore the search for new methodological approaches which increase the sensitivity and specificity of the diagnosis should be encouraged.

While waiting for further development of new techniques which could facilitate an early and correct diagnosis, we suggest that several steps should be followed by a neurologist when he is first confronted by a patient suspected of having MS. These include:

- extremely accurate clinical and familiar history
- expertise in performing and interpreting MRI examinations combined with
- a CSF study early in the diagnostic process of all patients with suspected MS which sometimes may reveal unsuspected pathology or raise doubts which leads to
- a detailed diagnostic battery of laboratory tests for alternative, less frequent diagnoses.

Cerebral biopsy is advised in very selected clinical cases with serious worsening of the clinical condition in the absence of any other diagnostic clue.

References

1. Schumaker GA, Beebe G, Kibler RE *et al.* Problems of experimental trials of therapy in multiple sclerosis. *Ann NY Acad Sci* 1965; **122**: 552–568.
2. Poser CM, Paty DW, Scheinberg L *et al.* New diagnostic criteria for multiple sclerosis: guidelines for research protocols. *Ann Neurol* 1983; **13**: 227–231.
3. Matteson EL, Flager DG, Mesara BW. IgG synthesis rate in evaluation of multiple sclerosis in a community hospital. *Neurology* 1987; **37**: 847–849.
4. Fieschi C, Gasperini C, Ristori G *et al.* Diagnostic problems in 'clinically definite' multiple sclerosis patients with normal CSF and multiple MRI abnormalities. *Europ J Neurol* 1994; **1**: 127–133.
5. Fieschi C, Gasperini C, Ristori G *et al.* Patients with clinically definite multiple sclerosis, white matter abnormalities on MRI, and normal CSF: if not multiple sclerosis, what is it? *J Neurol Neurosurg Psychiatry* 1995; **58**(2): 255–256.
6. Zeman AZJ, Kidd D, McLean BN *et al.* A study of oligoclonal band negative multiple sclerosis. *Neurol Neurosurg Psychiatry* 1996; **60**: 27–30.
7. Paty DW, Oger JJF, Kastrukoff LF *et al.* MRI in the diagnosis of MS: a prospective study with comparison of clinical evaluation, evoked potentials, oligoclonal banding and CT. *Neurology* 1988; **38**: 180–185.
8. Kuroda Y, Matsui M, Yukitake M *et al.* Assessment of MRI criteria for MS in Japanese MS and HAM/TSP. *Neurology* 1995; **45**: 30–33.
9. Fazekas F, Offenbacher H, Fuchs S *et al.* Criteria for an increased specificity of MRI interpretation in elderly subjects with suspected multiple sclerosis. *Neurology* 1988; **38**: 1822–1825.
10. Taccari E, Sili Scavalli A, Spadaro A *et al.* Magnetic resonance imaging (MRI) of the brain in SLE: ECLAM and SLEDAI correlations. *Clin Exp Rheumatol* 1994; **12**: 23–28.
11. De Lapaz RL, Floris R, Norman D *et al.* High field MRI of the spinal cord in multiple sclerosis [abstract]. *Proceedings of the Society of Magnetic Resonance in Medicine, 6th Annual Meeting* 1986; 45.
12. Honig LS, Sheremata Wa. Magnetic resonance imaging of spinal cord lesions in multiple sclerosis. *J Neurol Neurosurg Psychiatry* 1989; **52**: 459–466.
13. Kidd D, Thorpe JW, Thompscn AJ *et al.* Spinal cord MRI using multi-array coils and fast spin echo. Findings in multiple sclerosis. *Neurology* 1993; **43**: 2632–2637.
14. Thorpe JW, Kidd D, Moseley F *et al.* Spinal MRI in patients with suspected multiple sclerosis and negative brain MRI. *Brain* 1996; **119**: 709–714.
15. Paty DW, McFarlin De, McDonald WI. Magnetic resonance imaging and laboratory aids in the diagnosis of multiple sclerosis. *Ann Neurol* 1991; **13**: 227–231.
16. Katzan I, Rudick R. Guidelines to avoid errors in the diagnosis of multiple sclerosis. *Ann Neurol* 1996; **40** (suppl 3): 554.
17. Mandler RN, Davis LE, Jeffrey DR *et al.* Devic's neuromyelitis optica: a clinicopathological study of 8 patients. *Ann Neurol* 1993; **34**: 162–168.
18. Johnson MD, Lavin P, Whetsell WO Jr. Fulminant monophasic multiple sclerosis, Marburg's type. *J Neurol Neurosurg Psychiatry* 1990; **53**: 918–921.
19. Mendez MF, Pogacar S. Malignant monophasic multiple sclerosis or Marburg's disease. *Neurology* 1988; **38**: 1153–1155.
20. Shibasaki H, McDonald WI, Kuroiwa Y. Racial modification of clinical picture of multiple sclerosis: comparison between British and Japanese patients. *J Neurol Sci* 1981; **49**: 253–271.
21. Kira J, Tobimatsu S, Goto I *et al.* Primary progressive versus relapsing remitting multiple sclerosis in Japanese patients: a combined

clinical, magnetic resonance imaging and multimodality evoked potential study. *J Neurol Sci* 1993; **117**: 179–185.

22. Kira J, Kanai T, Nishimura Y *et al.* Western versus Asian types of multiple sclerosis: immunogenetically and clinically distinct disorders. *Ann Neurol* 1996; **40**: 569–574.

23. Morrissey SP, Miller DH, Kendall BE *et al.* Prognostic significance of brain MRI at presentation with a clinically isolated syndrome suggestive of MS – a five-year follow-up study. *Brain* 1993; **116**: 135–146.

24. Miller DH, Ormerod IEC, Rudge P *et al.* The early risk of multiple sclerosis following acute syndromes of the brainstem and spinal cord. *Ann Neurol* 1989; **26**: 635–639.

25. Jacobs L, Kinkel PR, Kinkel WR. Silent brain lesions in patients with isolated optic neuritis. A clinical and nuclear magnetic resonance study. *Arch Neurol* 1986; **43**: 452–455.

26. Miller DH, McDonald WI, Blumhardt LD *et al.* Magnetic resonance imaging in isolated non-compressive spinal cord syndromes. *Ann Neurol* 1987; **22**: 714–723.

27. Ford B, Tampieri D, Francis G. Long-term follow-up of acute partial transverse myelopathy. *Neurology* 1992; **42**: 250–252.

28. Frederiksen JL, Larsson HBW, Olesen J *et al.* MRI, VEP, SEP and biothesiometry suggest monosymptomatic acute optic neuritis to be a first manifestation of multiple sclerosis. *Acta Neurol Scand* 1991; **83**: 343–350.

29. Lee KH, Hashimoto SA, Hooge JP *et al.* Magnetic resonance imaging of the head in the diagnosis of multiple sclerosis: a prospective 2-year follow-up with comparison of clinical evaluation, evoked potentials, oligoclonal banding, and CT. *Neurology* 1991; **41**: 657–660.

30. Filippi M, Horsfield MA, Morrissey SP *et al.* Quantitative brain MRI lesion load predicts the course of clinically isolated syndromes suggested of multiple sclerosis. *Neurology* 1994; **44**: 635–641.

31. Miller DH, Ormerod IEC, McDonald WI. The early risk of multiple sclerosis after optic neuritis. *J Neurol Neurosurg Psychiatry* 1988; **51**: 1569–1571.

32. Burde RM, Savino PJ, Trobe JD (eds). *Clinical Decisions in Neuro-ophthalmology*, 2nd edn. Mosby, St. Louis: 1992; 41–73.

33. Adams RD, Victor M. *Principles of Neurology*, New York: McGraw-Hill 1985; 628.

34. Frederikson S. *Proceedings of the MS Forum, Modern Management Workshop, Berlin December 1993*; 24 (personal communication).

35. Louis ED, Lynch T, Kaufmann P *et al.* Diagnostic guidelines in central nervous system Whipple's disease. *Ann Neurol* 1996; **40**: 561–568.

36. Mohr PD, Strang FA, Sambook MA *et al.* The clinical and surgical features in 40 patients with primary ectopia (adult Chiari malformation). *Q J Med* 1977; **46**: 85–96.

37. Wolpert SM, Anderson M, Scott RM *et al.* Chiari malformation: MR imaging evaluation. *Am J Roentgenol* 1987; **149**: 1033–1042.

38. Kempster PA, Iansek R, Ball JI *et al.* Value of visual evoked response and oligoclonal bands in cerebrospinal fluid in diagnosis of spinal multiple sclerosis. *Lancet* 1987; **1**: 769–771.

39. Carmel R, Watkins D, Goodman SI *et al.* Hereditary deficit of cobalamin metabolism (cbl/G mutation) presenting as a neurological disorder in adulthood. *N Engl J Med* 1988; **318**: 1738–1741.

40. Ransohoff RM, Jacobsen DW, Green R. Vitamin B12 deficiency and multiple sclerosis. *Lancet* 1990; **335**: 1286–1296.

41. Allen RH, Stabler SP, Savage DG. Lindembaum J. Diagnosis of cobalamin deficiency I: Usefulness of serum methylmalonic acid and total homocysteine concentrations. *Am J Hematol* 1990; **34**: 90–98.

42. Bickerstaff ER, Small JM, Guest IA. The relapsing remitting course of certain meningiomas in relation to pregnancy and menstruation. *J Neurol Neurosurg Psychiatry* 1958; **21**: 89–91.

43. Sarkari NBS, Bickerstaff ER. Relapses and remission in brain stem tumours. *Br Med J* 1969; **2**: 21–23.

44. Rosenbluth PR, Lichtenstein BW. Pearly tumor (epidermoid cholesteatoma) of the brain. Clinicopathology study of two cases. *J Neurosurg* 1960; **17**: 35–42.

45. Ruff RL, Petito CK, Rawlinson DG. Primary cerebral lymphoma mimicking multiple scle-

rosis. *Arch Neurol* 1979; **36**: 598.

46. Lehaman RAW, Fieger HG. Arachnoid cyst producing recurrent neurological disturbances. *Surg Neurol* 1978; **10**: 134–136.

47. McArthur JC. Neurological complications of AIDS. *Medicine (Baltimore)* 1987; **66**: 407–437.

48. Levy RM, Breseden DE. Central nervous system dysfunction in acquired immunodeficiency syndrome. *J Acquir Immune Defic Syndr Hum Retrovirol* 1988; **1**: 41–64.

49. Berger JR, Sheretema WA, Resnick L *et al.* Multiple sclerosis-like illness occurring with human immunodeficiency virus infection. *Neurology* 1989; **39**: 324–329.

50. Matthews PM, Tampieri D, Berkovic SF *et al.* Magnetic resonance imaging shows specific abnormalities in the MELAS syndrome. *Neurology* 1991; **41**: 1043–1046.

51. Natowicz MR, Bejjani Bassem. Genetic disorders that masquerade as multiple sclerosis. *Am J Med Genet* 1994; **49**: 149–169.

52. Albers GW, Avalos SM, Weinrich M. Left ventricular tumor masquerading as multiple sclerosis. *Arch Neurology* 1987; **44**: 779–780.

53. Ormerod IEC, Miller DH, McDonald WI *et al.* The role of NMR imaging in the assessment of multiple sclerosis and isolated neurological lesions. A quantitative study. *Brain* 1987; **110**: 1579–1616.

54. Hutchinson M, Bresnihan B. Neurological lupus erythematosus with tonic seizures simulating multiple sclerosis. *J Neurol Neurosurg Psychiatry* 1983; **9**: 336–337.

55. Hackett ER, Martinez RD, Larson PF *et al.* Optic neuritis in systemic lupus erythematosus. *Arch Neurol* 1974; **31**: 9–11.

56. Yamamoto M. Recurrent transverse myelitis associated with collagen disease. *J Neurol* 1986; **233**: 185–187.

57. Cogen MS, Kline LB, Duvall ER. Bilateral internuclear ophthalmoplegia in systemic lupus erythematosus. *J Clin Neuro-Ophthalmol* 1987; **7**: 69–73.

58. Small P, Mass MF, Kohler PF *et al.* Central nervous system involvement in SLE. *Arthritis Rheum* 1977; **20**: 869–878.

59. McLean BN, Miller D, Thompson EJ. Oligoclonal banding of IgG in CSF, blood–brain barrier function, and MRI findings in patients with sarcoidosis, systemic lupus erythematosus, and Behçet's disease involving the nervous system. *J Neurol Neurosurg Psychiatry* 1995; **58**: 548–554.

60. Ormerod IEC, Miller DH, MacDonald WI *et al.* The role of NMR imaging in the assessment of multiple sclerosis and isclated neurological lesions. A quantitative study. *Brain* 1987; **110**: 1579–1616.

61. Taccari E, Sili Scavalli A, Spadaro A *et al.* Magnetic resonance imaging (MRI) of the brain in SLE: ECLAM and SLEDAI correlations. *Clin Exp Rheumatol* 1994; **12**: 23–28.

62. Singh VK. Detection of antinuclear antibodies in the serum of patients with multiple sclerosis. *Immunol Lett* 1962; **4**: 317–319.

63. Dore-Duffy P, Donaldson JO, Rothman BL *et al.* Antinuclear antibodies in multiple sclerosis. *Arch Neurol* 1982; **39**: 504–506.

64. Alexander EL, Provost TT, Stevens MB *et al.* Sjögren's syndrome: central nervous system manifestations. *Neurology* 1981; **31**: 1391–1396.

65. Alexander EL, Provost TT, Stevens MB *et al.* Neurologic complications of primary Sjögren's syndrome. *Medicine (Baltimore)* 1982; **61**: 247–257.

66. Alexander EL, Malinow K, Lejewski JE *et al.* Primary Sjögren's syndrome with central nervous system disease mimicking multiple sclerosis. *Ann Intern Med* 1986; **104**: 323–330.

67. Miller JR, Burke A, Bever CT. Occurrence of oligoclonal bands in multiple sclerosis and other CNS diseases. *Ann Neurol* 1983; **13**: 53–58.

68. Chajek T, Fainaru M. Behçet's disease. Report of 41 cases and review of literature. *Medicine (Baltimore)* 1975; **54**: 179–186.

69. Motomura S, Tabira T, Kuroiwa Y. A clinical comparative study of multiple sclerosis and neuro-Behçet's syndrome. *J Neurol Neurosurg Psychiatry* 1980; **43**: 210–213.

70. Schotland DL, Wolf SM, White HH *et al.* Neurologic aspects of Behçet's disease. *Am J Med* 1963; **34**: 544–553.

71. Devlin T, Gray L, Allen NB *et al.* Neuro-Behçet's disease: factors hampering proper diagnosis. *Neurology* 1995; **45**: 1754–1757.

72. Burgdorfer W, Barbours AG, Hayes SF *et al.*

Lyme disease – a tick-borne spirochetosis? *Science* 1982; **216**: 1317–1319.

73. Pachner AR, Steere AC. The triad of neurologic manifestations of Lyme disease: meningitis, cranial neuritis and radiculoneuritis. *Neurology* 1985; **35**: 47–53.

74. Reik L, Burgdorfer W, Donaldson JO. Neurologic abnormalities in Lyme disease without erythema chronicum migrans. *Am J Med* 1986; **81**: 73–78.

75. Ackerman R, Rehse-Kupper B, Gollmer E *et al.* Chronic neurologic manifestations of erythema migrans borreliosis. *Ann NY Acad Sci* 1988; **539**: 16–23.

76. Pachner A. Spirochetal diseases of the CNS. *Neurol Clin* 1986; **4**: 207–222.

77. Kohler J, Kern U, Kasper J *et al.* Chronic central nervous system involvement in Lyme borreliosis. *Neurology* 1988; **38**: 863–867.

78. Kohler J, Kasper J, Kern U *et al.* Borrelia encephalomyelitis. *Lancet* 1986; **2**: 35.

79. Benoit P, Douron E, Destel A *et al.* Spirochaetes and Lyme disease. *Lancet* 1986; **2**: 1223.

80. Heller J, Holzer G, Schimrigk K. Immunological differentiation between neuroborreliosis and multiple sclerosis. *J Neurol* 1990; **237**: 465–470.

81. Muhulemann MF, Wright DJ. The emerging pattern of Lyme disease in the United Kingdom and Irish Republic. *Lancet* 1987; **1**: 260–262.

82. Coyle PK. *Brorrelia burgdorferi* antibodies in multiple sclerosis. *Neurology* 1989; **39**: 760–761.

83. Delaney P. Neurologic manifestations of sarcoidosis. *Ann Intern Med* 1977; **87**: 336–345.

84. Stern BJ, Krumholz A, Johns C *et al.* Sarcoidosis and its neurological manifestations. *Arch Neurol* 1985; **42**: 909–917.

85. Graham EM, Ellis CJK, Sanders MD *et al.* Optic neuropathy in sarcoidosis. *J Neurol Neurosurg Psychiatry* 1986; **49**: 756–763.

86. Day AL, Sypert GW. Spinal cord sarcoidosis. *Ann Neurol* 1976; **1**: 79–85.

87. Kinnman J, Link H. Intrathecal production of oligoclonal IgM and IgG in CNS sarcoid. *Acta Neurol Scand* 1984; **69**: 97–106.

88. Lexa JF, Grossman RI. MR sarcoidosis in the head and spine: spectrum of manifestations and radiographic response to steroid therapy. *Am J Neuroradiol* 1994; **15**: 973–982.

89. Noetzel MJ, Landau WM, Moser HW. Andrenoleukodystrophy carrier state presenting as a chronic nonprogressive spinal cord disorder. *Arch Neurol* 1987; **44**: 566–567.

90. Dooley JM, Wright BA. Adrenoleukodystrophy mimicking multiple sclerosis. *Can J Neurol Sci* 1985; **12**: 73–74.

91. Bewermeyer H, Bamborshke S, Ebhardt G *et al.* MR imaging in adrenoleukomyeloneuropathy. *J Comput Assist Tomogr* 1985; **9**: 793–796.

92. Bhagavati S, Ehrlich G, Kula R *et al.* Detection of human T-cell lymphoma/leukaemia virus type 1 DNA and antigen in spinal fluid and blood of patients with chronic progressive myelopathy. *N Engl J Med* 1988; **318**: 1141–1147.

93. Newton M, Cruikshank KK, Miller D *et al.* Antibody to human virus type I in West-Indian-born UK residents with spastic paraparesis. *Lancet* 1987; **1**: 415–416.

94. Wallace DC, Singh G, Lott MT *et al.* Mitochondrial DNA mutation associated with Leber's hereditary optic neuropathy. *Science* 1988; **242**: 1427–1430.

95. Howell N, Kubacka I, Xu M *et al.* Leber hereditary optic neuropathy: involvement of the mitochondrial NDI gene and evidence for an intragenic suppressor mutation. *Am J Hum Genet* 1991; **48**: 935–942.

96. Huoponen K, Vilkki J, Aula P *et al.* A new mtDNA mutation associated with Leber hereditary optic neuroretinopathy. *Am J Hum Genet* 1991; **48**: 1147–1153.

97. Harding AE, Sweeney MG, Miller DH *et al.* Occurrence of a multiple sclerosis-like illness in women who have a Leber's hereditary optic neuropathy mitochondrial DNA mutation. *Brain* 1992; **115**: 979–989.

98. Kesserling J, Miller DH, Robb SA *et al.* Acute disseminated encephalomyelitis. MRI findings and the distinction from multiple sclerosis. *Brain* 1990; **113**: 291–302.

99. Kesserling J, Atlas SW, Grosman RI *et al.* MR diagnosis of acute disseminated encephalomyelitis. *J Comput Assist Tomogr* 1986; **10**: 798–801.

100. Miller DH, Rudge P, Johnson G *et al*. Serial gadolinium enhanced magnetic resonance imaging in multiple sclerosis. *Brain* 1988; **111**: 927–939.

101. Tas MW, Barkhof F, van Walderveen MAA *et al*. The effect of gadolinium on the sensitivity and specificity of MR in the initial diagnosis of multiple sclerosis. *Am J Neuroradiol* 1995; **16**: 259–264.

102. Riley D, Lang AE. Hemiballismus in multiple sclerosis. *Mov Disord* 1988; **1**: 88–94.

103. Plant GT, Kermode AG, Du Boulay EPGH *et al*. Spasmodic torticollis due to a midbrain lesion in a case of multiple sclerosis. *Mov Discord* 1989; **4**: 359–362.

104. Mao CC, Gancher ST, Herdon RM. Movement disorders in multiple sclerosis. *Mov Disord* 1988; **2**: 109–116.

105. Trachant C, Bhatia KP, Marsden CD. Movement disorders in multiple sclerosis. *Mov Disord* 1995; **10**: 418–423.

106. Matthews WB. Clinical aspect. In: Matthews WB, ed. *McAlpine's Multiple Sclerosis*, 2nd edn., Edinburgh: Churchill Livingstone 1991; 43–105.

107. Thompson AJ, Kermode AG, Moseley IF *et al*. Seizures due to multiple sclerosis: seven patients with MRI correlations. *J Neurol Neurosurg Psychiatry* 1993; **56**: 1317–1320.

108. Hunter SB, Ballinger WE, Rubin JJ *et al*. Multiple sclerosis mimicking primary brain tumour. *Arch Path Lab Med* 1987; **111**: 464–468.

109. Kohler J, Heildeyer H, Volk B. Multiple sclerosis presenting as chronic atypical psychosis. *J Neurol Neurosurg Psychiat* 1988; **51**: 281–284.

110. Ron MA, Feinstein A. Multiple sclerosis and the mind [editorial]. *J Neurol Neurosurg Psychiatry* 1992; **55**: 1–3.

6

The role of T cells and cytokines in the pathogenesis of multiple sclerosis

Norbert Sommer and Roland Martin

Introduction

The exact pathogenesis of multiple sclerosis (MS) is not known. However, it is now widely accepted that MS is an autoimmune disease, which is (*a*) at least in part caused by T cellular mechanisms, (*b*) can be triggered by environmental factors, and (*c*) is related to the immunogenetic background of an individual and associated with multiple genes. Major arguments for the autoimmune origin of the disease are the inflammatory histopathological changes in the central nervous system (CNS), the (relative) response to immunomodulatory drugs, and the similarities to experimental autoimmune encephalomyelitis (EAE), the animal model of MS.

The role of T cells and cytokines in the pathogenesis of MS has been investigated extensively during the past ten years. Analysis of the immune response in MS patients is difficult, because a single target autoantigen has not been defined. Mainly for practical reasons most studies originally concentrated on myelin basic protein (MBP) which is readily isolated from CNS white matter. In the meantime a considerable number of other CNS target antigens have also been investigated. This will be outlined in the first part of this chapter. EAE can be produced in susceptible animal strains by immunization with myelin components or transfer of myelin-specific T cells. Although it is not possible to transfer EAE findings directly to MS, most of the current pathogenetic concepts rely on findings in the animal models. The second part of this section deals with the immune response in EAE and its relevance to the human disease. Finally, cytokines have attracted great attention as immune mediators and potential targets for therapeutic intervention. Their role in MS and EAE is outlined in the third part of this chapter.

T-cell responses in MS

With the currently available methods, studies in MS patients can only provide circumstantial evidence for the relevant immunopathogenetic mechanisms involved. During the past decade an enormous pool of data was created in order to investigate the specificity and function of myelin-reactive T cells. Some of the key questions asked were:

- How frequent are myelin-reactive T cells in MS patients and unaffected individuals?
- What is their fine specificity and HLA-restriction?
- Is there a restricted T cell receptor (TCR) repertoire in these T cells?
- Are there any quantitative or functional differences in the T cell response between MS patients and controls?

Myelin basic protein as a major target antigen

MBP was most thoroughly investigated as a candidate target antigen, because it makes up 30 per cent of the CNS myelin protein and is easy to purify.[1,2] Initially, the most striking finding was that MBP-reactive T cells could be isolated from MS patients, as well as from unaffected controls, with considerable heterogeneity of epitope specificity and T cell receptor usage.[3–7] Frequency estimations of MBP-reactive T cells depended on the methods used. The highest frequencies were reported by Olsson and colleagues using an ELISPOT protocol for detection of interferon-γ (IFN-γ)-secreting cells.[8,9] They found MBP-reactive T cells at a frequency of $10–20/10^5$ in peripheral blood, which was at least ten times higher than in their controls. Even higher frequencies $(185/10^5)$ were found in the cerebrospinal fluid (CSF) of MS patients, some 40 times higher than in the control group.[9] For reasons not fully understood, significantly lower frequencies were reported in proliferation assays measuring the uptake of tritiated thymidine (i.e. between 0.7 in 10^5 and 0.5 in 10^7).[10,11] In some of the studies somewhat higher frequencies were found in MS patients compared with controls, but could not be confirmed by others.[12] The fact that the patient and control groups were heterogeneous and not HLA-matched in these studies might explain some of the negative results.

The overwhelming majority of T cell lines investigated were restricted by HLA-DR, and only a small minority by HLA-DQ or -DP.[4,10] In the context of certain HLA-types, immuno-dominant regions were identified in various parts, i.e. the N-terminal, middle, and the C-terminal regions of the MBP molecule.[5–7,10,12,13] Altogether, there is promiscuous HLA-binding of various MBP-epitopes,[14] and most epitopes

can be presented by several different HLA-DR molecules,[4,5] explaining the heterogeneity of the T cell response in terms of HLA restriction.

A number of studies investigated the TCR usage of MBP-specific T cells. This approach was initiated by findings in some commonly used EAE models which showed the preferential usage of certain TCR genes by encephalitogenic T cells, most often Vβ8. The hypothesized TCR predominance in MS patients would have greatly increased the chances for an immunospecific therapy. Indeed, initial reports raised the hope of a restricted usage of Vβ17 and Vβ12, or Vβ5.2 and Vβ6.1 in MBP-specific T cells.[15,16] However, these studies were contradictory and investigated only a small number of patients. Further studies analysing larger numbers of T cells with different fine specificity from a greater pool of patients, or even clones with the same peptide specificity, then made a strong TCR-limitation unlikely.[17,18] It was generally agreed that MBP-specific T cells have a high degree of heterogeneity in their TCR usage; however, new observations indicate that the heterogeneity or restriction of the TCR repertoire is influenced by a number of factors. These data indicate that the TCR usage is heterogeneous in situations where a peptide binds with high affinity to the HLA-molecule, i.e. the immunodominant MBP peptide (83–99) to DR2 molecules (Vergelli, Martin *et al.*, unpublished results), allowing for low affinity TCR-MHC–peptide interactions and consequently also TCR heterogeneity. The opposite is seen in peptides which bind with low affinity to the HLA molecule, i.e. MBP (111–129) to DR4 Dw4 (Muraro *et al.*, unpublished results). Here, the unstable HLA–peptide complex requires high affinity TCR molecules to allow for recognition. This is similar to the situation in PL/J mice and recognition of MBP (Ac1-11) which binds very poorly to I-A[u,19] and where one there-fore observed a strikingly uniform TCR repertoire.[19]

Interesting and valuable information was obtained from family and twin studies which circumvented the selection bias in otherwise heterogeneous patient populations. Martin *et al.* studied six sets of monozygotic twins, three concordant and three discordant for MS.[20] There were similar frequencies of MBP-specific T cells, with a slightly higher percentage of cytotoxic lines in the affected twins. In some of the twin pairs, but not in others, there were differences in fine specificity. Joshi *et al.* found similar frequencies of MBP-reactive T cells in peripheral blood from MS patients and their unaffected siblings.[21] Even HLA-identical sibling pairs discordant for MS had similar frequencies. Moreover, there was great heterogeneity in the recognized epitopes even in HLA-identical siblings. Therefore, the data of both studies are clearly not sufficient to prove the involvement of MBP-specific T cells in the pathogenesis of MS.

Utz *et al.* analysed the role of TCR genes in MS by comparing TCR usage in discordant versus concordant twin pairs.[22] Concordant twin sets select similar Vα chains, whereas discordant twins select different TCR after antigen stimulation. Interestingly and importantly, these findings apply to the T cell response against MBP, but also to the foreign recall antigen tetanus toxoid. This is the first study that provides unequivocal *in vitro* evidence for the involvement of T cell responses in the pathogenesis in MS. The data also suggest that exogenous factors might shape the T cell repertoire in MS patients and so skew the response towards a pathogenic phenotype.[22] In a subsequent study the complementarity determining region (CDR) 3 of Vα8-positive cells was analysed in the same set of twins.[23]

Marked amino acid sequence heterogeneity was found in MBP-reactive cells from all individuals with severe MS. By contrast, CDR3 regions were more restricted in MBP cells from healthy controls and individuals with only mild MS. Moreover, tetanus toxoid-specific cells bearing the Vα8-TCR were also relatively homogeneous within individuals regardless of disease activity.[23] These findings provide evidence for the hypothesis that increasing disease duration and severity is associated with an increased variety and diversity of MBP-reactive T cells. This probably reflects an impaired ability of regulatory mechanisms to control the anti-self responses.[23]

Other candidate CNS antigens

Among the remaining myelin proteins, proteolipid protein (PLP) and myelin–oligodendrocyte glycoprotein (MOG) were studied to a considerable extent (*Table 6.1*). PLP is an extremely hydrophobic protein and therefore difficult to isolate. Consequently most studies showing T cell reactivity to PLP were done by using synthetic peptides derived from the hydrophilic loops of the protein. Two peptides (40–60 and 89–106) were recognized by large numbers of T cell lines from patients and controls.[24,25] These peptides proved to bind well to MS-associated major histocompatibility complex (MHC) class II alleles (DR2a and -b). Also, some of the heterogeneous functional features typical of MBP-lines were found in PLP-lines.[26–28] In a longitudinal study, Correale *et al.*[29] established T cell clones against PLP during different clinical stages. They found that, during clinical exacerbations, T helper-1-like clones prevail, whereas interleukin (IL-4) and IL-10 producing clones dominate during remission. Also, this group has recently shown that PLP-specific T cell clones from patients with chronic progressive MS, which express co-stimulatory molecules, are resistant to inhibitory regulation, including the induction of anergy and sensitivity to transforming growth factor (TGH)-β-induced growth inhibition. This might be one of several possible mechanisms for driving the disease into a chronic progressive phase. As seen for MBP-T cells, using an ELISPOT assay PLP-specific cells were more frequent in blood and CSF from MS patients than in controls.[9]

The T cell response against MOG has been investigated by two groups.[30,31] Both studies found strong T cell responses to MOG. In one study 50 per cent of the patients, but only 1 out of 16 controls, showed *in vitro* T cell responses to MOG.[31] If this can be confirmed, it would strongly argue in favour of MOG being a relevant autoantigen in MS.

2',3'-cyclic nucleotide 3'-phosphodiesterase (CNP) is the third most frequent myelin antigen (*Table 6.1*), but has only recently been studied as a target antigen in MS. The protein is difficult to isolate and tends to copurify with MBP. First studies with purified CNP, recombinant protein and synthetic peptides have shown T cell reactivity in patients as well as controls.[32]

Myelin-associated glycoprotein (MAG) was also shown to elicit T cell reactivity in MS patients, but only a few studies with conflicting results have been performed.[35,36] MAG is also present in the peripheral nervous system, and – unrelated to MS – in a subgroup of patients with inflammatory polyneuropathy, monoclonal antibodies against MAG probably play a key role in the mechanism of demyelination.[37,38]

Transaldolase-H is an enzyme expressed in oligodendrocytes and important for myelination and cellular integrity. Searching for endogenous retroviral sequences in MS, Perl and colleagues found sequence homology and cross reactivity between transaldolase and epitopes of the HTLV-I and HIV-1 retroviruses.[37]

Subsequently, they found serum antibodies as well as evidence for T cell reactivity against transaldolase in a number of MS patients, but rarely in controls.[37]

A different approach to identify key antigens in MS was chosen by van Noort *et al.*[38] They examined proliferative responses of blood lymphocytes to an HPLC-fractionated whole myelin protein. Myelin proteins isolated from MS brains contained a single fraction to which T cells from MS patients and controls responded. This protein was identified as αB-crystallin, a small heat shock protein, which is present in oligodendrocytes and astrocytes from MS lesions, but not in unaffected myelin.[38]

In summary, T cell reactivity to a considerable number of CNS proteins has been documented in MS patients and regularly also in healthy individuals. The response to MBP is particularly well documented, but T cells to PLP and other much less abundant proteins are being examined thoroughly at the moment. Most of the myelin-reactive T cells investigated are CD4-positive, T helper-1-like (secreting interferon-γ (IFN-γ) and lymphotoxin (LT)), cytotoxic, and restricted by HLA-DR. So far they resemble the autoreactive encephalitogenic T cells in EAE. However, it is not possible to analyse their pathogenic potential *in vivo*.

The detection of *in vivo* pre-activated T cells with myelin-specificity would support their pathogenetic role and different experimental methods were chosen for this approach. Allegretta *et al.*[39] used somatic mutations in a commonly expressed gene (hypoxanthine guanine phosphoribosyltransferase, HPRT) as an index for T cell amplification *in vivo*. This method is based on the observation that gene mutations in human T lymphocytes occur preferentially in dividing cells. It could be shown that HPRT-mutated

Protein	Mol. weight	Rel. per cent of myelin	T-cell responses in humans		Induction of EAE
Proteolipid protein (PLP)	26,30 kDa	50%	Yes	(Pelfrey et al.;[25] Correale et al.;[28] Kondo et al.;[27])	Yes (Numerous refs.)
Myelin basic protein (MBP)	14–21.5 kDa (several isoforms)	30%	Yes	(Numerous refs.)	Yes (Numerous refs.)
2',3'-cyclic nucleotide 3'-phosphodiesterase (CNPase, CNP)	46,48 kDa	4%	Yes	(Rösener et al.[32])	?
Myelin-oligodendrocyte glycoprotein (MOG)	26,28 kDa	<1%	Yes	(Sun et al.;[30] Kerlero de Rosbo et al.[31])	Massive infiltrates with little clinical disability (Linington et al.[71])
Myelin-associated glycoprotein (MAG)	67,72 kDa	1%	Yes	(Johnson et al.;[33] Zhang et al.[34])	?
Transaldolase-H	38 kDa	<1%	Yes	(Banki et al.[37])	?
S-100β	11 kDa	Non-myelin protein	?		Panencephalitis with cellular infiltrates in CNS, retina, and uvea (Kojima et al.[73])
αβ-crystallin	23 kDa	Heat-shock protein (inducible in glial cells)	Yes	(van Noort et al.[38])	?

Table 6.1

CNS proteins as potential autoantigens. Listed are antigens which elicit T-cell responses in MS patients, and usually also controls, or induce EAE (with selected references) cells with reactivity to MBP were found in MS patients but not in healthy individuals.[40] Similarly, Zhang *et al.*[41] investigated pre-activated myelin-reactive T cells in MS patients and controls. While there were no differences in the frequency of autoreactive T cells after primary antigen stimulation, the frequency of MBP or PLP but not tetanus-toxoid-reactive T cells generated after primary IL-2 stimulation was significantly elevated in MS patients.

CD8-positive T cells have also been established specific for MBP, PLP, and MAG; however, considering the elusive role of this cell type in EAE, their role in MS is still uncertain.[42] Moreover, γδ-T-cells were detected in demyelinated CNS plaques in MS patients.[43,44] Their biological role is unclear, but some of them might respond against heat shock proteins (HSP). HSP are a group of proteins with important functions during stress responses, highly conserved in phylogeny, and T cells against bacterial HSP might cross-react with human HSP in inflammatory lesions.[43,44]

Animal models and T-cell responses

The immunological pathogenesis of EAE is much better analysed than that of MS. In fact, many theories and experimental treatment approaches are based on findings in EAE, although most of them have never been formally proven in MS. A basic problem, therefore, lies in the applicability of these experimental animal findings to the human disease.

EAE can be induced in susceptible animal strains and a large number of different models have been used since the first description in the 1930s.[45] Inbred rodent strains have been studied most thoroughly.[46–50] The Lewis rat model is probably the easiest of all to induce by active immunization with MBP or transfer of MBP-specific T cell. However, the disease is monophasic and demyelination in the CNS is atypical.[48] Among the mouse models, EAE in the SJL-strain resembles closest the human disease.[50] These mice show (*a*) clinical remissions and spontaneous relapses, (*b*) histological evidence of demyelination, and (*c*) a relatively broad immunological T cell response against various myelin antigens. All these features make it probably the most valuable and practical animal model of MS to date. Furthermore, the TCR-gene repertoire of this strain is deleted by approximately 50 per cent (without gross immunological deficiency) including the otherwise very dominant Vβ8 gene family.[51] This results in a greater heterogeneity in the TCR repertoire of MBP-specific T cells,[52,53] again making the model more similar to MS.

Two recently developed EAE models are also briefly described here, because they demonstrate how technical and experimental effort might eventually bridge the gap between animal studies and human disease. Hauser and colleagues established an innovative EAE model in the non-human primate Callithrix jacchus.[54,55] These marmosets are unique in that they are born as naturally occurring bone marrow chimeras, despite being genetically distinct. The individual animals arise from separate ova which are fertilized independently, but have a fused placenta resulting in cross-circulation and mutual tolerance of each other's bone marrow-derived cells. In this model it could clearly be shown that MBP-specific T cells raised from a healthy monkey, cultured *in vitro* and injected into another sibling can successfully induce EAE.[54] Also, MRI studies are relatively easy in this model, but have obvious technical limits in rodents.[56]

Severe combined immunodeficient (SCID)-mice might also be valuable tools for studying autoreactivity. These mice have a combined T- and B-cell defect and are not able to reject foreign tissue.[57] The transfer of EAE from another mouse strain to SCID-mice has been achieved after transfer of myelin-reactive T cells plus co-transfer of haematopoietic tissue.[58] It is therefore conceivable that human autoreactive T cells could be transferred into these mice, thus allowing a better characterization of their pathogenetic potential.

EAE is mediated by CD4+ positive T cells which are class II-restricted and secrete IFN-γ and tumour necrosis factor (TNF).[47,59] As there is no spontaneous animal model of encephalomyelitis (as in autoimmune diabetes) active immunization or adoptive T cell transfer are the only ways of initiating the autodestructive process. It is now believed by many researchers that the activation of autoreactive T cells as a trigger event, occurs in the periphery and not in the CNS, although this is not definitely proven.[60] After activation of T cells these are able to adhere to cerebral endothelial cells and subsequently enter the CNS parenchyma. Certain adhesion molecules seem to be particularly important in this process. Baron *et al.*[61] showed that only T cells expressing VLA-4 (very late antigen-4, also α4β1-integrin or CD49d/CD29) can penetrate into the CNS. Accordingly, blocking of VLA-4 by monoclonal antibodies can suppress EAE.[62]

MBP and PLP have been studied thoroughly as encephalitogenic antigens in various inbred rodent strains. The T cell epitopes of both molecules in several different models have been characterized.[63–66] In most strains there is one dominant epitope in each myelin protein which, after immunization with the whole protein, elicits the strongest immune response as defined by using synthetic peptides. However, immunization with some of the synthetic peptides might elicit T cell responses which were not detected after whole protein immu-

nization.[67] These so-called 'subdominant' epitopes are thought to be relevant for the stimulation of T cells in CNS lesions in EAE and MS, and could considerably broaden the T cell specificities involved in the autoimmune attack. Another, probably related, phenomenon of 'epitope spreading' has been observed in EAE experiments studying the time course of T cell responses. Several weeks after immunization with an MBP or PLP peptide significant systemic T cell responses to other peptides of the same protein as well as to other myelin proteins could be detected.[68–70] This observation suggests the *in vivo* priming of autoreactive T cells; moreover the successive recruitment of T cells with new anti-myelin specificities has been interpreted as one possible mechanism responsible for the induction of relapse and perpetuation of disease.

Besides PLP and MBP the role of less common CNS proteins in EAE is also increasingly being investigated. MOG-specific T cells mediate an intense inflammatory response in the CNS which, however, does not lead to significant neurological deficit.[71] This phenomenon seemed to correlate with the relative paucity of macrophages in the infiltrates, whereas the number and function of T cells in the lesions were unchanged. By contrast, antibodies against MOG enhance demyelination EAE in the Lewis rat after adoptive T cell transfer.[72] Thus, an anti-MOG immune response can induce both inflammation and demyelination, depending on the experimental setting used.

S100β is a small non-myelin calcium-binding protein which is present in astrocytes, and also in the peripheral nervous system and the retina.[73] Adoptive transfer of S100β-specific T cells leads to a severe inflammatory response in the nervous system with only minimal neurological deficit. Interestingly, inflammation was also found in the uvea and retina.[73] This finding is of clinical relevance in MS, as uveitis and periphlebitis retinae are not uncommon in patients with MS.[74,75]

The role of cytokines

Cytokines take part in multiple effector mechanisms of the immune system and also other tissues, and their role in autoimmune demyelinating diseases has been addressed by countless studies. Nevertheless, it has been difficult and sometimes even controversial to define the pathogenetic contribution of each cytokine precisely. In general, pro-inflammatory cytokines, such as tumour necrosis factor-α (TNF-α), LT, IFN-γ, and IL-2 have been accused of contributing to the autodestructive process, whereas cytokines with immunosuppressive properties, such as IL-4 or transforming growth factor-β (TGF-β), have been ascribed a counter-regulatory, disease-limiting role. Nevertheless, it should be noted that cytokines have principally short-range action and their effect (as discussed below for IFN-γ) depends on their presence *in situ* and the form of application in the respective experimental setting.

TNF-α and LT*

TNF-α is a principal cytokine in the immune response against bacteria and other micro-organisms. It is mainly produced by mononuclear phagocytes (macrophages) and also by T cells, and thought to be a link between specific immune responses and acute inflammation. LT is closely related to TNF-α and binds to the same cell surface receptor. LT has similar biological actions as TNF, but is produced

**TNF (in contrast to TNFα or LT) was used either as a common term for both cytokines or (usually in earlier studies) when the specific cytokine was not defined.*

exclusively by activated T cells. The genes for human TNF-α, LT (and a recently described third family member, lymphotoxin-β) are located within the MHC-complex on chromosome 6.[76] A considerable number of studies have assigned a role for these cytokines in the pathogenesis of autoimmune demyelination (*Table 6.2*).

Immunocytochemistry

TNF-α and LT are probably among the most important cytokines involved in local tissue damage in MS and EAE. First of all, TNF-positive cells could be identified by immunohistological techniques in brains from patients with MS.[77] In MS lesions, TNF-staining is associated with both astrocytes and macrophages mostly located at the lesion edge. Astrocytes and macrophages–microglia have some common functional properties, such as class II expression, IL-1 secretion and antigen presentation, the latter probably being mediated primarily by microglia. Since astrocytes can be induced to produce TNF-α *in vitro*, they are likely to be an important source of TNF-α production.[77] Selmaj and colleagues[78] identified TNF-α as well as LT in acute and chronic active MS lesions. LT was found to be associated with T lymphocytes and microglial cells, whereas TNF-α was located with astrocytes and foamy macrophages in active lesions, and infrequently with endothelial cells at the lesion edge in acute lesions.[78] Enhanced CNS expression of TNF-α and LT is not specific for MS. The cytokines were also found in other inflammatory conditions such as subacute sclerosing panencephalitis (SSPE),[77] and adrenoleucodystrophy,[78] but not in Alzheimer's or Parkinson's disease brain tissue, nor non-inflammatory CNS disease.[79]

Supporting results were found in various EAE models. In Lewis rat EAE, a study using *in situ* hybridization shows that TNF-α

Condition	Finding	Reference
MS	Detection of TNF-α and LT in lesions by immunocytochemistry	Hofman *et al.*[77] Selmaj *et al.*[78]
	Enhanced serum and/or CSF levels of TNF-α	Spuler *et al.*[85]
	Increased TNF production before clinical exacerbation in a whole blood mitogen stimulation assay	Beck *et al.*[83]
	Enhanced levels of TNF-α and LT mRNA in blood mononuclear cells before exacerbation	Rieckmann *et al.*[86]
Tissue culture	Recombinant human TNF-α mediates myelin and oligodendrocyte damage	Selmaj and Raine[87]
EAE	Detection of TNF-α in CNS lesions by *in situ* hybridization	Held *et al.*[80]
	EAE susceptibility in different rat strains correlates with TNF-α expression by their astrocytes	Chung *et al.*[91]
	Encephalitogenicity of T-cell clones requires TNF-α/LT-expression	Powell *et al.*[89] Kuchroo *et al.*[50]

	Various anti-TNF therapies ameliorate neurological signs
	    monoclonal antibody to TNF-α/LT
	    polyclonal anti-TNF-α antibody
	    soluble TNF-receptor I
	    pentoxifylline
	    selective phosphodiesterase 4-inhibitors
		Ruddle *et al.*[93] Selmaj *et al.*[94] Selmaj *et al.*[95]
		
		Rott *et al.*[96] Sommer *et al.*[100] Genain *et al.*[98]

Table 6.2
The pathogenetic role of TNF-α/LT in MS and EAE. The table summarizes experimental evidence with selected references.

expressing cells appear with the signs of paralysis and are markedly reduced during recovery, despite the presence of mononuclear cells in the CNS.[80] In chronic-relapsing EAE of the SJL mouse, reverse transcriptase-PCR was used to detect cytokine gene expression in the CNS. Apart from IL-2 and IFN-γ, detectable in infiltrating CD4-positive T cells, TNF-α was predominantly produced by CNS-resident microglia and also infiltrating macrophages.[81]

Serum and CSF TNF-levels in MS patients

A number of studies have described elevated cytokine levels in MS patients. It should be noted that normal serum levels of TNF-α and other cytokines are very low and initially the results between, and even within, laboratories differed significantly.[82] High titres were mainly found in severe conditions such as septic shock and cerebral malaria.[82] In MS, serum levels of TNF-α and IFN-γ were reported to be increased before exacerbations.[83] In another study CSF TNF-α levels were increased in chronic progressive, but not in stable, MS.[84] In a prospective, serial study of nine MS patients who were followed monthly for one year, TNF-α values were correlated to clinical symptoms and MRI activity.[85] High serum TNF-α-levels (>50 pg/ml) and detectable CSF levels were always associated with contrast-enhancing MRI lesions, although an overall correlation between serum cytokine levels and MRI activity did not reach statistical significance. After steroid treatment TNF-α levels were suppressed for several months, while new contrast-enhancing MRI lesions appeared.[85]

Measuring TNF-α-mRNA levels in circulating blood cells offers a more sensitive way of determining cytokine expression, although this does not necessarily reflect the absolute protein levels. Rieckmann *et al.*[86] showed, by using a semiquantitative polymerase chain reaction (PCR), that significant increases in TNF-α and LT expression preceded clinical relapse. In parallel, the expression of the counter-regulatory cytokines TFG-β and IL-10 mRNA declined.[86] On the basis of this study it seems reasonable to use semiquantitative PCR for patient monitoring in clinical trials.

In vitro *toxicity*

Further evidence for the pathogenic role of TNF-α came from *in vitro* studies showing a direct toxicity for oligodendrocytes. TNF-α induced oligodendrocyte necrosis and irreversible myelin dilatation in myelinated cultures of mouse spinal cord tissue.[87] This effect was peculiar to TNF-α, and not observed with

the pro-inflammatory cytokines IFN-γ or IL-2.[87] In another *in vitro* study it could be shown that microglial cells, when activated with IFN-γ, expressed TNF which was subsequently capable of killing oligodendrocytes.[88]

TNF-α/LT *expression of encephalitogenic T cell clones*

As outlined above, encephalitogenic T cells in EAE carry the Th1 phenotype. The two relevant investigations concerning cytokine patterns of T cells conclude that TNF-α/LT production, and also the expression of the adhesion molecule VLA-4 (α4β1-integrin, CD49d/CD29), are important properties of encephalitogenic T cell clones.[89,90] Powell *et al.* describe seven T-cell clones reactive against the encephalitogenic peptide MBP-Ac1-11 in PL/J mice. Following adoptive transfer, one of the clones induced severe EAE, three others mild EAE, and the remaining three were not pathogenic. The most prominent feature of the strongly pathogenic clone was its massive production of TNF; however, the weakly encephalitogenic clones were very heterogeneous in their TNF production.[89] Kuchroo *et al.* describe another two encephalitogenic T-cell clones reactive for the immunodominant PLP peptide (amino acids 139–151) in SJL-mice. At least one of these two clones produced more TNF compared with five sister clones; clearly non-encephalitogenic clones were low TNF-producers.[90] Both these studies show that TNF production was among the most consistent features of encephalitogenic T-cell clones, compared with other cytokines and most surface markers (except for VLA-4, see above). However, a direct correlation to the level of TNF-production could not be drawn and it is likely that a number of other factors are involved to render a certain myelin-reactive T cell pathogenic.

Genetic variability of TNF expression

EAE-sensitive and -resistant rat strains can be distinguished by the capacity of their astrocytes to secrete TNF-α. Astrocytes from Brown-Norway (BN) rats, which are EAE-resistant, produce much lower amounts of TNF, compared with astrocytes from the highly susceptible Lewis rats.[91] Astrocytes from BN rats express TNF-α mRNA and protein in response to lipopolysaccharide (LPS) alone, yet IFN-γ does not significantly enhance LPS-induced TNF-α expression, nor do they express appreciable TNF-α in response to the combined stimuli of IFN-γ/IL-1β. By contrast, astrocytes from Lewis rats express low levels of TNF-α mRNA and protein in response to LPS, and are extremely responsive to the priming effect of IFN-γ for subsequent TNF-α gene expression. Also, Lewis rat astrocytes produce TNF in response to IFN-γ/IL-1β. Therefore, the capacity for TNF-α production by Lewis astrocytes is likely to contribute to their susceptibility for EAE.[91]

Investigations of the role of TNF-genes have also been performed in humans, but were equivocal. The production of TNF-α and LT is controlled by inherited alleles (for TNF-α: TNFA 1 or 2; for LT: TNFB 1, 2.1 or 2.2). For some autoimmune diseases (lupus erythematosus and autoimmune diabetes), in which TNF is also considered pathogenetically relevant, an association of high TNF-α production with HLA-DR3 (lupus) and HLA-DR3 and DR4 (diabetes) was found. In these studies HLA-DR2 patients usually were low TNF-α producers. These results were partly controversial, and not obtained with T-cell lines, but with unselected mononuclear cells from peripheral blood. By contrast, more recent data show that antigen-specific T-cell lines from HLA-DR2 donors (MS patients as well as controls) produced significantly more TNF-α and LT than lines from donors with other HLA-haplotypes.[92] Such a difference was not found for the production of IFN-γ (gene located on chromosome 12). Nevertheless the amount of the cytokine production was not correlated with the known TNF-α and LT alleles. These data show that the MS-susceptible HLA-haplotype DR2 correlates with increased production of TNF-α and LT and further supports the assumed pathogenetic roles of these cytokines.[92]

Anti-TNF treatment in EAE

Direct functional evidence for the role of the cytokines stems from EAE-treatment studies. A number of different anti-TNF treatment approaches have been investigated and practically all of them suppress the neurological signs in EAE animals. Monoclonal antibodies against TNF-α/LT largely suppress the clinical and histological signs of EAE.[93,94] EAE can also be prevented by the administration of soluble tumour necrosis factor receptor I.[95] A number of pharmacological compounds have been investigated as potential TNF-suppressing agents. Pentoxifylline is an unspecific phosphodiesterase inhibitor and has been described as a suppressor of Th1-associated lymphokine production[96] and of EAE. The specific phosphodiesterase type 4 inhibitor rolipram, an antidepressant, is an even more potent inhibitor of TNF-α[97] and has been shown to suppress EAE in three different models including the relapsing SJL-mouse and the Callithrix jacchus-marmoset model in which the treatment also reduced MRI abnormalities.[98–100] Although the actual *in vivo* mechanism of this effect has not been fully elucidated, it is likely that suppression of TNF is at least partially responsible for the therapeutic effect.[99] A number of newly developed phosphodiesterase type 4 inhibitors similarly suppress EAE and make this group of compounds attractive candidates for treatment studies in MS (N Sommer, A Bittner, P-A Löschmann, R Martin, unpublished).

In summary, there is considerable evidence that the tumour necrosis factors are important effector molecules in EAE and MS. An interesting clinical observation related to cytokine actions was reported by Compston and colleagues.[101] They treated MS patients with a monoclonal antibody (CAMPATH-1H) which targets the CD52 antigen mainly present on T cells. A pilot study had shown that treatment with this lymphocyte-depleting antibody reduced disease activity in MS patients. However, in some patients the first antibody infusion was followed by an exacerbation or reactivation of MS symptoms for several hours. It was found that these neurological symptoms correlated with a rapid transient increase in TNF-α, IFN-γ and IL-6 serum levels and could be prevented by corticosteroids. Although the mechanism of cytokine release has not been fully characterized, this study provides an impressive example of the *in vivo* action of cytokines.[101]

IFN-γ

IFN-γ is produced by T-helper cells, particularly Th1 cells, which also produce LT, and often TNF-α and IL-2, but also by CD8+ cytotoxic T cells and NK-cells. It is a central immunoregulatory cytokine and its primary effect on target cells is activation and enhanced expression of MHC-molecules. Although IFN-γ is generally believed to play a pivotal role in MS and EAE the mechanism of its potential action in the pathogenesis is far from clear. Moreover, experimental evidence in EAE was controversial regarding the disease-enhancing or -suppressing effects of IFN-γ.

One clinical trial with IFN-γ in MS was discontinued, because an unacceptably high relapse rate was attributed to the cytokine.[102] In this trial 18 patients with relapsing–remitting MS were treated with different doses (1–1000 µg) of recombinant IFN-γ twice a week for four weeks. Seven of the 18 patients had exacerbations of MS during the treatment period, and the average exacerbation rate per patient per year increased from 1.42 before the trial to 4.67 during the trial, with prompt reduction to 1.05 after stopping IFN-γ.[102] The causal relationship between exacerbations and administrations of IFN-γ was further supported by the findings of a dose-dependent induction of HLA-DR surface antigens on peripheral blood cells.[102] The trial was originally based on the hypothesis that IFN-γ production is deficient in MS patients.[103–105] Moreover, it had been shown that intraventricular administration of IFN-γ in rats may inhibit EAE.[106] More recent findings show that the abrogation of IFN-γ expression in mice on a genetic background known to be resistant to the induction of EAE (BALB/c) converted them to a susceptible phenotype.[107] In addition, IFN-γ was not necessary for the induction of EAE using genetic knockout mice, in which the IFN-γ gene was disrupted and backcrossed to an EAE-susceptible strain.[108]

By contrast, a number of the EAE findings point towards a disease-enhancing role of IFN-γ. EAE-inducing T cells produce IFN-γ besides TNF-α and other proinflammatory cytokines (see above).[89,90] IFN-γ is localized in inflammatory lesions,[109] and cooperates with TNF-α in many actions, such as upregulating class II and adhesion molecules.[76] Furthermore, adoptive transfer of encephalitogenic T cells after incubation with IFN-γ enhances EAE, and direct injection of IFN-γ into the spinal cord causes EAE-like inflammation.[110]

It is hard to summarize the action of IFN-γ in MS and EAE. It seems that in most experimental settings IFN-γ is essential for amplification of an inflammatory response. In addition, however, there is clear evidence that in some special situations its action is redundant or even antagonistic, although this is mostly observed in somewhat artificial experimental animal models.

IL-2 and IL-2R

IL-2 is a major autocrine growth factor for T cells. It stimulates other T-cell derived cytokines, such as IFN-γ and LT, and lack of IL-2 may be a cause of T-cell anergy. IL-2 has such a central role in T-cell activation that it is difficult to delineate a more specific function in the pathogenesis of MS and EAE. Like other proinflammatory cytokines IL-2,[79] as well as IL-2R,[111] were detected in MS lesions. Levels of IL-2 and soluble IL-2R were measured in patients' sera and CSF and were found to be elevated in most, but not all, studies.[112–117] In any case, the clinical usefulness of these markers is probably low.[118]

In EAE, the possibility of direct CNS tissue analysis has made the picture clearer. The levels of IL-2 mRNA (and IFN-γ in parallel) are increased in EAE mice with active disease,[119] whereas they are low in controls and in spontaneous remission of EAE.[81] In addition, a decrease of IL-2 mRNA (in parallel with TNF-α) in the CNS accompanies clinical improvement of EAE in treatment studies with compounds, such as IL-4, retinoid, and phosphodiesterase inhibitor.[99,120,121]

IL-4

IL-4 is produced by T cells and mast cells and acts as a regulator of allergic reactions and growth and differentiation factor for T cells. It also increases expression of MHC class II molecules and stimulates the proliferation of B cells. IL-4 has been shown to regulate T lymphocytes towards a Th2-profile, which was hypothesized to be favourable in a Th1-mediated disease such as EAE. Indeed, therapeutic application of IL-4 resulted in amelioration of clinical disease, the induction of MBP-specific Th2-cells, reduction of demyelination, and inhibition of the inflammatory cytokines TNF-α and IL-2 in the CNS.[120] These data support the model that production of IL-4, and other related cytokines such as IL-10, modulates disease activity by antagonizing the effect of pathogenic Th1 cytokines.

TGF-β

TGF-β is a family of closely related cytokines with pleiotropic actions including stimulation and/or inhibition of various cell types. TGF-β also seems to have a major role in immunoregulation, and suppresses T-cell and macrophage activation. Therefore, in MS and EAE it has mainly been studied as an antagonist of proinflammatory cytokines.

A number of studies show that EAE can be suppressed by TGF-β1.[122–124] Accordingly, the administration of anti-TGF-β antibodies led to a worsening of the neurological signs of EAE. Also, TGF-β was detected by immunohistology in CNS areas and was ascribed an endogenous immunoregulatory function.[125]

There are a number of mechanisms by which TGF-β might exert these effects. TGF-β inhibits antigen-specific proliferation of myelin-reactive T cells and their capacity to transfer EAE.[122,126] It has also been shown that TGF-β downregulates MHC class II expression *in vitro*,[127] which may be a relevant immunosuppressive mechanism *in vivo*. Moreover, oral administration of MBP as a method of suppressing EAE ('oral tolerance') has been shown to be mediated by TGF-β-secreting T cells which are induced in Peyer's patches.[128]

A time course study in MS patients showed that decreased production of TGF-β by blood lymphocytes correlated directly with disease activity. Patients with active MS produced less TGF-β than those with stable disease.[129] These and other findings would suggest that the balance of pro-inflammatory cytokines and anti-inflammatory cytokines, such as TGF-β, are an important mechanism for the manifestation of MS.

Other cytokines

A number of other cytokines have been investigated in MS and EAE and, although their role may be less prominent, they add to the complex picture and some of them have been targeted in EAE-treatment studies.

IL-1 is mainly produced by mononuclear phagocytes and acts in many ways synergistic to TNF.[76] IL-1 stimulates various cell types, but its effect on T cells, stimulation of IL-2 production and enhancement of adhesion and T-cell extravasation are probably most important in MS.[130] IL-1 reactivity was found in MS plaques.[111]

IL-6 is also a major inflammatory cytokine. Elevated IL-6 levels in the CNS were found in mice suffering from a severe form of EAE, suggesting a possible pathogenic role of IL-6 in demyelinating diseases.[131]

IL-12 is a cytokine which promotes the development of Th1 cells and induces IFN-γ and also TNF-α production. *In vitro* preincubation of encephalitogenic T cells with IL-12 leads to more severe and prolonged EAE after adoptive transfer. Accordingly, treatment of mice with an anti-IL-12 antibody completely prevented neurological signs.[132]

IL-10 inhibits T-cell proliferation and production of pro-inflammatory cytokines. IL-10 mRNA is greatly increased in the CNS during the recovery phase of EAE, complementary to the decrease of IL-2 expression.[133]

IL-13 is a potent mediator of macrophage functions, such as the production of the inhibition of IL-1 and TNF production. The application of an IL-13-producing treatment regime (by injection of a cell line transfected with IL-13 cDNA) EAE was markedly suppressed.[134]

What is, after all, certain in the pathogenesis of MS?

Despite the enormous amount of neurological and immunological research over the past 20 years, remarkably little is known about the pathogenesis of MS. Still the most consistent indicator for an immune-mediated pathogenesis is the detection of oligoclonal banding and intrathecal immunoglobulin G (IgG) synthesis in the patients' CSF.[135] Nevertheless this is not specific for MS and is also found in other inflammatory and immune-mediated conditions.

Numerous T-cell studies have increased our knowledge of how T cells recognize, and can be activated by, myelin autoantigens. However, a consistent picture of the underlying abnormalities in MS has not emerged. Further investigations with advanced techniques, e.g. the transfer of human T cells into SCID mice, are underway. Studies in monozygotic twins have, for the first time, provided evidence that the T-cell response in general is different in MS patients as compared with unaffected controls.[22]

A highly reproducible finding in MS epidemiology is the relatively strong hereditary component. All attempts to identify the genes involved in disease susceptibility have not solved the problem of MS genetics, but recent studies have shown interesting results (see Sawcer, Robertson, and Compston, Chapter 2). Three groups performed genome screens of multiplex families in Canada, the UK and the USA, using sets of polymorphic markers which span the whole genome. There was consistently at least a weak association of MS and the MHC-locus on chromosome 6.[136–138] This supports the hypothesis that a cellular immune abnormality is involved in the pathogenesis, but does not exclude the involvement of other non-immune genes in this region (including the TNF genes).

Animal studies have greatly improved the understanding of CNS autoimmunity. Critics of EAE studies argue that the various models are always induced by strong artificial stimuli and never completely reflect all aspects of the human disease. Nevertheless, recently developed models do reproduce the relapsing clinical course and the demyelinating histopathological changes after a single induction step. EAE is a T-cell dependent disease and the most straightforward way to induce EAE is by intravenous injection of activated myelin-specific T cells. It remains elusive, however, why some induction protocols are less reliable than others and what properties are required to render T cells encephalitogenic. First important insights as to the role of T- and B-cell interaction in the pathogenesis of demyelination were provided by studies showing a significant enhancement of EAE by antibodies against MOG.[72]

Future research will have to find better read-out systems for human T-cell function in humans. Also, animal studies will have to improve the artificial and still relatively variable induction steps (in many models) towards more transparent and 'physiologic' mechanisms. Beyond these pathophysiological issues, the current knowledge will nevertheless enable the development of clinically attractive new therapies for MS, e.g. the blocking of cytokine action in the CNS.

References

1. Williams KA, Deber CM. The structure and function of central nervous system myelin. *Crit Rev Clin Lab Sci* 1993; **30**: 29–64.
2. Martin R, McFarland HF, McFarlin DE. Immunological aspects of demyelinating diseases. *Annu Rev Immunol* 1992; **10**: 153–187.
3. Burns J, Rosenzweig A, Zweiman B *et al.* Isolation of myelin basic protein-reactive T-cell lines from normal human blood. *Cell Immunol* 1983; **81**: 435–440.
4. Chou YK, Vainiene M, Whitham R *et al.* Response of human T lymphocyte lines to myelin basic protein: association of dominant epitopes with HLA-class II restriction molecules. *J Neurol Sci* 1989; **23**: 207–216.
5. Martin R, Jaraquemada D, Flerlage M *et al.* Fine specificity and HLA restriction of myelin basic protein-specific cytotoxic T cell lines from multiple sclerosis patients and healthy individuals. *J Immunol* 1990; **145**: 540–548.
6. Pette M, Fujita K, Kitze B *et al.* Myelin basic protein-specific T lymphocyte lines from MS patients and healthy individuals. *Neurology* 1990; **40**: 1770–1776.
7. Meinl E, Weber F, Drexler K *et al.* Myelin basic protein-specific T lymphocyte repertoire in multiple sclerosis. Complexitity of the response and dominance of nested epitopes due to recruitment of multiple T cell clones. *J Clin Invest* 1993; **92**: 2633–2643.
8. Olsson T, Sun J, Hillert J *et al.* Increased numbers of T cells recognizing multiple myelin basic protein epitopes in multiple sclerosis. *Eur J Immunol* 1992; **22**: 1083–1087.
9. Olsson T, Wei Zhi W, Höjeberg B *et al.* Autoreactive T lymphocytes in multiple sclerosis determined by antigen-induced secretion of interferon-γ. *J Clin Invest* 1990; **86**: 981–985.
10. Ota K, Matsui M, Milford EL *et al.* T-cell recognition of an immunodominant myelin basic protein epitope in multiple sclerosis. *Nature* 1990; **346**: 183–187.
11. Chou YK, Bourdette DN, Offner H *et al.* Frequency of T cells specific for myelin basic protein and myelin proteolipid protein in blood and cerebrospinal fluid in multiple sclerosis. *J Neuroimmunol* 1992; **38**: 105–113.
12. Jingwu Z, Medaer R, Hashim GA *et al.* Myelin basic protein-specific T lymphocytes in multiple sclerosis and controls: precursor frequency, fine specificity, and cytotoxicity. *Ann Neurol* 1992; **32**: 330–338.
13. Martin R, Howell MD, Jaraquemada D *et al.* A myelin basic protein peptide is recognized by cytotoxic T cells in the context of four HLA-DR types associated with multiple sclerosis. *J Exp Med* 1991; **173**: 19–24.
14. Valli A, Sette A, Kappos L *et al.* Binding of myelin basic protein peptides to human histocompatibility leukocyte antigen class II molecules and their recognition by T cells from multiple sclerosis patients. *J Clin Invest* 1993; **91**: 616–628.
15. Wucherpfennig KW, Ota K, Endo N *et al.* Shared human T cell receptor V beta usage to immunodominant regions of myelin basic protein. *Science* 1990; **248**: 1016–1019.
16. Kotzin BL, Karuturi S, Chou YK *et al.* Preferential T-cell receptor Vβ-chain variable gene use in myelin basic protein-reactive T-cell clones from patients with multiple sclerosis. *Proc Natl Acad Sci USA* 1991; **88**: 9161–9165.
17. Martin R, Utz U, Coligan JE *et al.* Diversity in fine specificity and T cell receptor usage of the human CD4+ cytotoxic T cell response specific for the immunodominant myelin basic protein peptide 87–106. *J Immunol* 1992; **148**: 1359–1366.
18. Giegerich G, Pette M, Meinl E *et al.* Diversity of T cell receptor alpha and beta chain genes expressed by human T cells specific for similar myelin basic protein peptide/major histocompatibility complexes. *Eur J Immunol* 1992; **22**: 753–758.
19. Acha-Orbea H, Steinman L, McDevitt, HO.

T-cell receptors in murine autoimmune diseases. *Annu Rev Immunol* 1989; **7**: 371–406.

20. Martin R, Voskuhl R, Flerlage M *et al*. Myelin basic protein-specific T-cell responses in identical twins discordant or concordant for multiple sclerosis. *Ann Neurol* 1993; **34**: 524–535.

21. Joshi N, Usuku K, Hauser SL. The T-cell response to myelin basic protein in familial multiple sclerosis: Diversity of fine specificity, restricting elements, and T-cell receptor usage. *Ann Neurol* 1993; **34**: 385–393.

22. Utz U, Biddison WE, McFarland HF *et al*. Skewed T cell receptor repertoire in genetically identical twins with multiple sclerosis correlates with disease. *Nature* 1993; **364**: 243–247.

23. Utz U, Brooks JA, McFarland HF *et al*. Heterogeneity of T-cell receptor α-chain complementarity-determining region 3 in myelin basic protein-specific T cells increases with severity of multiple sclerosis. *Proc Natl Acad Sci USA* 1994; **91**: 5567–5571.

24. Pelfrey CM, Trotter JL, Tranquill LR *et al*. Identification of a novel T cell epitope of human proteolipid protein (residues 40–60) recognized by proliferative and cytolytic CD4+ T cells from multiple sclerosis. *J Neuroimmunol* 1993; **46**: 33–42.

25. Pelfrey CM, Trotter JL, Tranquill LR *et al*. Identification of a second T cell epitope of human proteolipid protein (residues 89–106) recognized by proliferative and cytolytic CD4+ T cells from multiple patients. *J Neuroimmunol* 1994; **53**: 153–161.

26. Ohashi T, Yamamura T, Inobe J-I *et al*. Analysis of PLP-specific T cells in multiple sclerosis: identification of PLP 95–116 as an HLA-DR2,w15-associated determinant. *Int Immunol* 1995; **7**: 1771–1778.

27. Kondo T, Yamamura T, Inobe J-I *et al*. TCR repertoire to proteolipid protein (PLP) in multiple sclerosis (MS): homologies between PLP-specific T cells and MS-associated T cells in TCR junctional sequences. *Int Immunol* 1996; **8**: 123–130.

28. Correale J, McMillan M, McCarthy K *et al*. Isolation and characterization of autoreactive proteolipid protein-peptide specific T-cell clones from multiple sclerosis patients. *Neu-rology* 1995; **45**: 1370–1378.

29. Correale J, Gilmore W, McMillan M *et al*. Patterns of cytokine secretion by autoreactive proteolipid protein-specific T cell clones during the course of multiple sclerosis. *J Immunol* 1995; **154**: 2959–2968.

30. Sun J, Link H, Olsson T *et al*. T and B cell responses to myelin-oligodendrocyte glycoprotein in multiple sclerosis. *J Immunol* 1991; **146**: 1490–1495.

31. Kerlero de Rosbo N, Milo R, Lees MB *et al*. Reactivity to myelin antigens in multiple sclerosis. Peripheral blood lymphocytes respond predominantly to myelin oligodendrocyte glycoprotein. *J Clin Invest* 1993; **92**: 2602–2608.

32. Rösener M, Muraro P, Riethmüller A *et al*. 2',3'-cyclic nucleotide 3'-phosphodiesterase: a novel target antigen in demyeliniting diseases. *J Neuroimmunol* 1997 **75**: 28–34.

33. Johnson D, Hafler DA, Fallis RJ *et al*. Cell-mediated immunity to myelin-associated glycoprotein, proteolipid protein, and myelin basic protein in multiple sclerosis. *J Neuroimmunol* 1986; **13**: 99–108.

34. Zhang YD, Burger D, Saruhan M *et al*. The T-lymphocyte response against myelin-associated glycoprotein and myelin basic protein in patients. *Neurology* 1993; **43**: 403–407.

35. Steck A, Murray N, Meier C *et al*. Demyelinating neuropathy and monoclonal IgM antibody to myelin-associated glycoprotein. *Neurology* 1988; **33**: 19–23.

36. Steck AJ, Murray N, Justafre JC *et al*. Passive transfer studies in demyelinating neuropathy with IgM monoclonal antibodies to myelin-associated glycoprotein. *J Neurol Neurosurg Psychiatry* 1985; **48**: 927–929.

37. Banki K, Colombo E, Sia F *et al*. Oligodendrocyte-specific expression and autoantigenicity of transaldolase in multiple sclerosis. *J Exp Med* 1994; **180**: 1649–1663.

38. van Noort JM, van Sechel AC, Bajramovic JJ *et al*. The small heat-shock protein αB-crystallin as candidate autoantigen in multiple sclerosis. *Nature* 1995; **375**: 798–801.

39. Allegretta M, Nicklas JA, Sriram S *et al*. T Cells responsive to myelin basic protein in patients with multiple sclerosis. *Science* 1990; **247**: 718–721.

40. Allegretta M, Albertini RJ, Howell MD *et al.* Homologies between T cell receptor junctional sequences unique to multiple sclerosis and T cells mediating experimental allergic encephalomyelitis. *J Clin Invest* 1994; **94:** 105–109.

41. Zhang J, Markovic-Plese S, Lacet B *et al.* Increased frequency of interleukin 2-responsive T cells specific for myelin basic protein in peripheral blood and cerebrospinal fluid of patients with multiple sclerosis. *J Exp Med* 1994; **179:** 973–984.

42. Tsuchida T, Parker KC, Turner RV *et al.* Autoreactive CD8+ T-cell responses to human myelin protein-derived peptides. *Proc Natl Acad Sci USA* 1994; **91:** 10859–10863.

43. Selmaj K, Brosnan CF, Raine CS. Colocalization of lymphocytes bearing gamma delta T-cell receptor and heat shock protein hsp65+ oligodendrocytes in multiple sclerosis. *Proc Natl Acad Sci USA* 1991; **88:** 6452–6456.

44. Wucherpfennig KW, Newcombe J, Li H *et al.* Gamma delta T cell receptor repertoire in acute multiple sclerosis lesions. *Proc Natl Acad Sci USA* 1992; **89:** 4588–4592.

45. Rivers TM, Sprunt DH, Berry GP. Observations on attempts to produce acute disseminated encephalomyelitis in monkeys. *J Exp Med* 1933; **58:** 39–53.

46. Lassmann H. Comparative neuropathology of chronic experimental allergic encephalomyelitis and multiple sclerosis. Berlin: Heidelberg, New York: Springer 1983.

47. Wekerle H, Kojima K, Lannes-Vieira J *et al.* Animal models. *Ann Neurol* 1994; **36:** S47–S53.

48. Swanborg RH. Experimental allergic encephalomyelitis. *Meth Enzymol* 1988; **162:** 413–421.

49. Lindsey JW. Characteristics of initial and reinduced experimental autoimmune encephalomyelitis. *Immunogenetics* 1996; **44:** 292–297.

50. Mokhtarian F, McFarlin DE, Raine CS. Adoptive transfer of myelin basic protein-sensitized T cells produces chronic relapsing demyelinating disease in mice. *Nature* 1984; **309:** 356–358.

51. Jouvin-Marche E, Trede NS, Bandeira A *et al.* Different large deletions of T cell receptor Vβ genes in natural populations of mice. *Eur J Immunol* 1989; **19:** 1921–1926.

52. Padula SJ, Lingenheld EG, Stabach PR *et al.* Identification of encephalitogenic V beta-4-bearing T cells in SJL mice. Further evidence of the V region disease hypothesis? *J Immunol* 1991; **146:** 879–883.

53. Sakai K, Sinha AA, Mitchell DJ *et al.* Involvement of distinct murine T-cell receptors in the autoimmune encephalitogenic response to nested epitopes of myelin basic protein. *Proc Natl Acad Sci USA* 1988; **85:** 8608–8612.

54. Genain CP, Lee-Parritz D, Nguyen M-H *et al.* In healthy primates, circulating autoreactive T cells mediate autoimmune disease. *J Clin Invest* 1994; **94:** 1339–1345.

55. Massacesi L, Genain CP, Lee-Paritz D *et al.* Active and passively induced experimental autoimmune encephalomyelitis in common marmosets: a new model for multiple sclerosis. *Ann Neurol* 1995; **37:** 519–530.

56. Morrissey SP, Stodal H, Zettl U *et al.* In vivo MRI and its histological correlates in acute adoptive inflammation and oedema. *Brain* 1996; **119:** 239–248.

57. Bosma GC, Carroll AM. The SCID mouse mutant: Definition, characterization, and potential uses. *Annu Rev Immunol* 1991; **9:** 323–350.

58. Jones RE, Bourdette DN, Whitham RH *et al.* Induction of experimental autoimmune encephalomyelitis in severe combined immunodeficient mice reconstituted with allogeneic or xenogeneic hematopoietic cells. *J Immunol* 1993; **150:** 4620–4629.

59. Ben Nun A, Wekerle H, Cohen IR. The rapid isolation of clonable antigen-specific T lymphocyte lines capable of mediating autoimmune encephalomyelitis. *Eur J Immunol* 1981; **11:** 195–199.

60. Wekerle H, Lassmann H. Contra: Evidence against a primary lesion in the target organ in autoimmune disease. *Int Arch Allergy Immunol* 1994; **103:** 328–331.

61. Baron JL, Madri JA, Ruddle NH *et al.* Surface expression of α4 integrin by CD4 T cells is required for their entry into brain parenchyma. *J Exp Med* 1993; **177:** 57–68.

62. Yednock TA, Cannon C, Fritz LC *et al.* Prevention of experimental autoimmune

encephalomyelitis by antibodies against α4β1 integrin. *Nature* 1992; **356**: 63–66.

63. Fritz RB, McFarlin DE. Encephalitogenic epitopes of myelin basic protein. *Chem Immunol*, 1989; **46**: 101–125.

64. McRae BL, Kennedy MK, Tan LJ *et al*. Induction of active and adoptive relapsing experimental autoimmune encephalomyelitis (EAE) using an encephalitogenic epitope of proteolipid protein. *J Neuroimmunol* 1992; **38**: 229–240.

65. Bhardwaj V, Kumar V, Grewal IS *et al*. T cell determinant structure of myelin basic protein in B10.PL, SJL/J, and their F_1s. *J Immunol* 1994; **152**: 3711–3719.

66. Greer JM, Sobel RA, Sette A *et al*. Immunogenic and encephalitogenic epitope clusters of myelin proteolipid protein. *J Immunol* 1996; **156**: 371–379.

67. Sercarz EE, Lehmann PV, Ametani A *et al*. Dominance and crypticity of T cell antigenic determinants. *Annu Rev Immunol* 1993; **11**: 729–766.

68. Lehmann PV, Forsthuber T, Miller A *et al*. Spreading of T-cell autoimmunity to cryptic determinants of an autoantigen. *Nature* 1992; **358**: 155–157.

69. Lehmann PV, Sercarz EE, Forsthuber T *et al*. Determinant spreading and the dynamics of the autoimmune T-cell repertoire. *Immunol Today* 1993; **14**: 203–208.

70. Yu M, Johnson JM, Tuohy VK. A predictable sequential determinant spreading cascade invariably accompanies progression of experimental autoimmune encephalomyelitis: a basis for peptide-specific therapy after onset of clinical disease. *J Exp Med* 1996; **183**: 1777–1788.

71. Linington C, Berger T, Perry L *et al*. T cells specific for the myelin oligodendrocyte glycoprotein mediate an unusual autoimmune inflammatory response in the central nervous system. *Eur J Immunol* 1993; **23**: 1364–1372.

72. Linington C, Bradl M, Lassmann H *et al*. Augmentation of demyelination in rat acute allergic encephalomyelitis by circulating mouse monoclonal antibodies directed against a myelin/oligodendrocyte glycoprotein. *Am J Pathol* 1988; **130**: 443–454.

73. Kojima K, Berger T, Lassmann H *et al*. Experimental autoimmune panencephalitis and uveoretinitis transferred to the Lewis rat by T lymphocytes specific for the S100β molecule, a calcium binding protein of astroglia. *J Exp Med* 1994; **180**: 817–829.

74. Berger BC, Leopold IH. The incidence of uveitis in multiple sclerosis. *Am J Ophthalmol* 1968; **62**: 540–545.

75. Lucarelli MJ, Pepose JS, Arnold AC *et al*. Immunopathological features of retinal lesions in multiple sclerosis. *Ophthalmology* 1991; **98**: 1652–1656.

76. Vassalli P. The pathophysiology of tumor necrosis factors. *Annu Rev Immunol* 1992; **10**: 411–452.

77. Hofman FM, Hinton DR, Johnson K *et al*. Tumor necrosis factor identified in multiple sclerosis brain. *J Exp Med* 1989; **170**: 607–612.

78. Selmaj K, Raine CS, Cannella B *et al*. Identification of lymphotoxin and tumor necrosis factor in multiple sclerosis lesions. *J Clin Invest* 1991; **87**: 949–954.

79. Cannella B, Raine CS. The adhesion molecule and cytokine profile of multiple sclerosis lesions. *Ann Neurol* 1995; **37**: 424–435.

80. Held W, Meyermann R, Qin Y *et al*. Perforin and tumor necrosis factor α in the pathogenesis of experimental allergic encephalomyelitis: comparison of autoantigen induced and transferred disease in Lewis rats. *J Autoimmunity* 1993; **6**: 311–322.

81. Renno T, Krakowski M, Piccirillo C *et al*. TNF-α expression by resident microglia and infiltrating leukocytes in the central nervous system of mice with experimental encephalomyelitis. *J Immunol* 1995; **154**: 944–953.

82. de Kossodo S, Houba V, Grau GE *et al*. Assaying tumor necrosis factor concentrations in human serum. A WHO International Collaborative Study. *J Immunol Meth* 1995; **182**: 107–114.

83. Beck J, Rondot P, Catinot L *et al*. Increased production of interferon gamma and tumor necrosis factor precedes clinical manifestation in multiple sclerosis: Do cytokines trigger off exacerbations? *Acta Neurol Scand* 1988; **78**: 318–323.

84. Sharief MK, Hentges R. Association between tumor necrosis factor-α and disease progression in chronic progressive multiple sclerosis. *N Engl J Med* 1991; **325**: 467–472.

85. Spuler S, Yousry T, Scheller A *et al.* Multiple sclerosis: prospective analysis of TNF-α and 55 kDa TNF receptor in CSF and serum in correlation with clinical and MRI activity. *J Neuroimmunol* 1996; **66**: 57–64.

86. Rieckmann P, Albrecht M, Kitze B *et al.* Tumor necrosis factor-α messenger RNA expression in patients with relapsing-remitting multiple sclerosis is associated with disease activity. *Ann Neurol* 1995; **37**: 82–88.

87. Selmaj K, Raine CS. Tumor necrosis factor mediates myelin and oligodendrocyte damage in vitro. *Ann Neurol* 1988; **23**: 339–346.

88. Zajicek JP, Wing M, Scolding NJ *et al.* Interactions between oligodendrocytes and microglia. A major role for complement and tumor necrosis factor in oligodendrocyte adherence and killing. *Brain* 1992; **115**: 1611–1631.

89. Powell MB, Mitchell D, Lederman J *et al.* Lymphotoxin and tumor necrosis factor-alpha production by myelin basic protein-specific T cell clones correlates with encephalitogenecity. *Int Immunol* 1990; **2**: 539–544.

90. Kuchroo VK, Martin CA, Greer JM *et al.* Cytokines and adhesion molecules contribute to the ability of myelin proteolipid protein-specific T cell clones to mediate experimental allergic encephalomyelitis. *J Immunol* 1993; **151**: 4371–4382.

91. Chung IY, Norris JG, Benveniste EN. Differential tumor necrosis factor alpha expression by astrocytes from experimental allergic encephalomyelitis-susceptible and -resistant rat strains. *J Exp Med* 1991; **173**: 801–811.

92. Zipp F, Weber F, Huber S *et al.* Genetic control of multiple sclerosis: Increased production of lymphotoxin and tumor necrosis factor-α by HLA-DR2+ T cells. *Ann Neurol* 1995; **38**: 723–730.

93. Ruddle NH, Bergman CM, McGrath KM *et al.* An antibody to lymphotoxin and tumor necrosis factor prevents transfer of experimental allergic encephalomyelitis. *J Exp Med* 1990; **172**: 1193–1200.

94. Selmaj K, Raine CS, Cross AH. Anti-tumor necrosis factor therapy abrogates autoimmune demyelination. *Ann Neurol* 1991; **30**: 694–700.

95. Selmaj K, Papierz W, Glabinski A *et al.* Prevention of chronic relapsing experimental autoimmune encephalomyelitis by soluble tumor necrosis factor receptor I. *J Neuroimmunol* 1995; **56**: 135–141.

96. Rott O, Cash E, Fleischer B. Phosphodiesterase inhibitor pentoxifylline, a selective suppressor of T helper type 1- but not type 2-associated lymphokine production, prevents induction of experimental autoimmune encephalomyelitis in Lewis rats. *Eur J Immunol* 1993; **23**: 1745–1751.

97. Semmler J, Wachtel H, Endres S. The specific type IV phosphodiesterase inhibitor rolipram suppresses tumor necrosis factor-alpha production by human mononuclear cells. *Int J Immunopharmacol* 1993; **15**: 409–413.

98. Genain CP, Roberts T, Davis RL *et al.* Prevention of autoimmune demyelination in non-human primates by a cAMP-specific phosphodiesterase inhibitor. *Proc Natl Acad Sci USA* 1995; **92**: 3601–3605.

99. Sommer N, Martin R, Scott DE *et al.* A novel treatment of chronic relapsing experimental autoimmune encephalomyelitis (EAE) by the antidepressant rolipram. *J Neurol* 1995; **242**: S38.

100. Sommer N, Löschmann P-A, Northoff GH *et al.* The antidepressant rolipram suppresses cytokine production and prevents autoimmune encephalomyelitis. *Nature Med* 1995. **1**: 244–248.

101. Moreau T, Coles A, Wing M *et al.* Transient increase in symptoms associated with cytokine release in patients with multiple sclerosis. *Brain* 1996; **119**: 225–237.

102. Panitch HS, Hirsch RL, Schindler J *et al.* Treatment of multiple sclerosis with gamma interferon: Exacerbations associated with activation of the immune system. *Neurology* 1987; **37**: 1097–1102.

103. Neighbor PA, Miller AE, Bloom BR. Interferon responses of leucocytes in multiple sclerosis. *Neurology* 1981; **31**: 561–566.

104. Vervliet G, Claeys H, VanHaver H *et al.* Interferon production and natural killer cell

(NK) activity in leukocyte cultures from multiple sclerosis patients. *J Neurol Sci* 1983; **60**: 137–150.

105. Brod SA, Khan M, Bright J *et al*. Decreased CD3-mediated interferon-γ production in relapsing-remitting multiple sclerosis. *Ann Neurol* 1995; **37**: 546–549.

106. Voorthuis JAC, Uitdehaag BMJ, De Groot CJA *et al*. Suppression of experimental allergic encephalomyelitis by intraventricular administration of interferon-gamma in Lewis rats. *Clin Exp Immunol* 1990; **81**: 183–188.

107. Krakowski M, Owens T. Interferon-γ confers resistance to experimental allergic encephalomyelitis. *Eur J Immunol* 1996; **26**: 1641–1646.

108. Ferber I, Brocke S, Taylor-Edwards C *et al*. Mice with a disrupted IFN-γ gene are susceptible to the induction of experimental autoimmune encephalomyelitis (EAE). *J Immunol* 1996; **156**: 5–7.

109. Stoll G, Müller S, Schmidt B *et al*. Localization of interferon-γ and Ia-antigan in T cell line-mediated experimental autoimmune encephalomyelitis. *Am J Pathol* 1993; **142**: 1866–1875.

110. Simmons RD, Willenborg DO. Direct injection of cytokines into the spinal cord causes autoimmune encephalomyelitis-like inflammation. *J Neurol Sci* 1990; **100**: 37–42.

111. Hofman FM, von Hanwehr RI, Dinarello CA *et al*. Immunoregulatory molecules and IL 2 receptors identified in multiple sclerosis brain. *J Immunol* 1986; **136**: 3239–3245.

112. Adachi K, Kumamoto T, Araki S. Elevated soluble interleukin-2 receptor levels in patients with active multiple sclerosis. *Ann Neurol* 1990; **28**: 687–691.

113. Fesenmeier JT, Whitaker JT, Herman PK *et al*. Cerebrospinal fluid levels of myelin protein-like material and soluble interleukin-2 receptor in multiple sclerosis. *J Neuroimmunol* 1991; **34**: 77–80.

114. Gallo P, Piccino M, Pagni S *et al*. Interleukin-2 levels in serum and cerebrospinal fluid of multiple sclerosis patients. *Ann Neurol* 1988; **24**: 795–797.

115. Hartung H-P, Hughes RAC, Taylor WA *et al*. T cell activation in Guillain–Barré syndrome and in MS: elevated serum levels of soluble IL-2 receptors. *Neurology* 1990; **40**: 215–218.

116. Trotter JL, Clifford DB, Anderson CB *et al*. Elevated serum interleukin-2 levels in chronic progressive multiple sclerosis (letter). *N Engl J Med* 1988; **318**: 1206.

117. Shaw CE, Dunbar PR, Macaulay HA *et al*. Measurement of immune markers in the serum and cerebrospinal fluid of multiple sclerosis patients during clinical remission. *J Neurol* 1995; **242**: 53–58.

118. Peter JB, Boctor FN, Tourtelotte WW. Serum and CSF levels of IL-2, sIL-2R, TNF-alpha, and IL-1-beta: expected lack of clinical utility. *Neurology* 1991; **41**: 121–123.

119. Renno T, Lin JY, Piccirillo C *et al*. Cytokine production by cells in cerebrospinal fluid during experimental allergic encephalomyelitis in SJL/J mice. *J Neuroimmunol* 1994; **49**: 1–7.

120. Racke MK, Bonomo A, Scott DE *et al*. Cytokine-induced immune deviation as a therapy for inflammatory autoimmune disease. *J Exp Med* 1994; **180**: 1961–1966.

121. Racke MK, Burnett D, Pak S-H *et al*. Retinoid treatment of experimental allergic encephalomyelitis. IL-4 production correlates with improved disease course. *J Immunol* 1995; **154**: 450–458.

122. Racke MK, Dhib-Jalbut S, Cannella B *et al*. Prevention and treatment of chronic relapsing experimental allergic encephalomyelitis by transforming growth factor-β1. *J Immunol* 1991; **146**: 3012–3017.

123. Kuruvilla AP, Shah R, Hochwald GM *et al*. Protective effect of transforming growth factor β1 on experimental autoimmune diseases in mice. *Proc Natl Acad Sci USA* 1991; **88**: 2918–2921.

124. Johns LD, Flanders KC, Ranges GE *et al*. Successful treatment of experimental allergic encephalomyelitis with transforming growth factor-β1. *J Immunol* 1991; **147**: 1792–1796.

125. Racke MK, Cannella B, Albert P *et al*. Evidence of endogenous regulatory function of transforming growth factor-β1 in experimental allergic encephalomyelitis. *Int Immunol* 1992; **4**: 615–620.

126. Schluesener HJ, Lider O. Transforming growth factors B₁ and B₂: cytokines with

identical immunosuppressive effects and a potential role in the regulation of autoimmune T cell function. *J Neuroimmunol* 1989; **24**: 249–258.

127. Schluesener HJ. Transforming growth factors type B_1 and B_2 suppress rat astrocyte autoantigen presentation and antagonize hyperinduction of class II major histocompatibility complex antigen expression by interferon-γ and tumor necrosis factor-α. *J Neuroimmunol* 1990; **27**: 41–47.

128. Santos LM, al Sabbagh A, Londono A *et al*. Oral tolerance to myelin basic protein induces regulatory TGF-beta-secreting T cells in Peyer's patches in SJL mice. *Cell Immunol* 1994; **157**: 439–447.

129. Mokhtarian F, Shi A, Shirazian D *et al*. Defective production of anti-inflammatory cytokine, TGF-β by T cell lines of patients with active multiple sclerosis. *J Immunol* 1994; **152**: 6003–6010.

130. McCarron RM, Wang L, Racke MK *et al*. Cytokine-regulated adhesion between encephalitogenic T lymphocytes and cerebrovascular endothelial cells. *J Neuroimmunol* 1993; **43**: 23–30.

131. Gijbels K, Van Damme J, Proost P *et al*. Interleukin 6 production in the central nervous system during experimental autoimmune encephalomyelitis. *Eur J Immunol* 1990; **20**: 233–235.

132. Leonard JP, Waldburger KE, Goldman SJ. Prevention of experimental autoimmune encephalomyelitis by antibodies against interleukin 12. *J Exp Med* 1995; **181**: 381–386.

133. Kennedy MK, Torrance DS, Picha KS *et al*. Analysis of cytokine mRNA expression in the central nervous system of mice with experimental autoimmune encephalomyelitis reveals that IL-10 mRNA expression correlates with recovery. *J Immunol* 1992; **149**: 2496–2505.

134. Cash E, Minty A, Ferrara P *et al*. Macrophage-inactivation IL-13 suppresses experimental autoimmune encephalomyelitis in rats. *J Immunol* 1994; **153**: 4258–4267.

135. Kabat EA, Freedman DA, Murray JP *et al*. A study of the cristalline albumin, gamma globulin and total protein in the cerebrospinal fluid of one hundred cases of multiple sclerosis and in other diseases. *Am J Med Sci* 1950; **219**: 55–64.

136. Sawcer S, Jones HB, Feakes R *et al*. A genome screen in multiple sclerosis reveals susceptibility loci on chromosome 6p21 and 17q22. *Nature Genet* 1996; **13**: 464–468.

137. The Multiple Sclerosis Genetics Group. A complete genomic screen for multiple sclerosis underscores a role for the major histocompatibility complex. *Nature Genet* 1996; **13**: 469–471.

138. Ebers GC, Kukaway K, Bulman DE *et al*. A full genome search in multiple sclerosis. *Nature Genet* 1996; **13**: 472–476.

7

Does trauma make multiple sclerosis worse?
William A Sibley

Introduction

Hundreds of trials of therapy have been conducted in multiple sclerosis (MS) patients during the past several decades,[1] using a wide variety of treatments, but relatively little attention has been given to influences which might worsen the disease. One of the best examples of an agent with this capability was intrathecal tuberculin, which caused an excess of exacerbations, compared to controls, often in association with a florid pleocytosis.[2] In retrospect, it is reasonable to suspect that this was due to the elaboration of interferon gamma by the many activated and transformed T lymphocytes likely present in the cerebrospinal fluid.[3,4]

Identifying risk factors

A prospective study by Sibley and co-workers was designed to identify risk factors in the environment.[5] The only clearly identifiable risk factor, among those studied, was clinical viral infections (see Panitch, Chapter 9).[6] Since then, several other prospective studies have confirmed that viral infections are important triggers of new MS attacks, and thus new central nervous system lesions.[7–9] A possible explanation, again, is the fact that virally infected T lymphocytes elaborate interferon gamma, a cytokine known to enhance antigen recognition,[3] and reported to increase the frequency of MS exacerbations.[4]

This prospective study was done in patients with a confirmed diagnosis of MS, and was unable to find any relationship between trauma and exacerbations or progression of disability. This was true both for the entire study, and for each variety of trauma studied. The methodology and detailed results of the trauma analysis have been published elsewhere.[10–13] To recapitulate briefly, in an eight-year study from 1976 to 1984, 170 MS patients and 134 age- and sex-matched controls were questioned at monthly intervals. The patients were examined every three months, or whenever new symptoms suggesting exacerbation occurred. During the monthly contacts inquiry was made about such things as changes in medication or diet, infections, physical trauma of various kinds, stressful life events, and a variety of other things. During the eight-year period a number of patients had head injuries, sprains, major and minor surgery, fractures, burns, dental work, abrasions and bruises. The results of this study were that during either three- or six-month periods at-risk (AR) after traumatic episodes, most patients remained unchanged. Some had exacerbations during periods AR for trauma, but no more frequently than the same group of patients had at other times when trauma had not occurred, periods not-at-risk (NAR). Exacerbations occurring AR were randomly distributed in time during the AR period: i.e. they were not clustered after

Period	No. of exacerbations /years at risk	No. of exacerbations /years not at risk	Exacerbations per year at risk	Exacerbations per year not at risk	χ^2
3 Mos.	86/285	160/603	0.30	0.27	0.9 n.s.
6 Mos.	115/440	131/448	0.26	0.29	0.8 n.s.

Table 7.1
Influence of duration of period at-risk (all traumas).

the traumatic episodes. For example 15 of the 86 exacerbations occurring during a three-month period AR occurred during the first two weeks after the traumatic episode, only one more than would be expected by chance.[10] The results were similar using both a three month and six month AR period (*Table 7.1*).

There were 140 head injuries during the term of the study, occurring in 67 patients. Eleven of these were associated with loss of consciousness, or probable loss of consciousness, lasting for seconds or minutes. None had prolonged loss of consciousness. Nine exacerbations occurred during a cumulative 28.4 year period AR, and 75 exacerbations occurred in this same group of patients when NAR during 251.5 patient-years (exacerbation rate 0.32 per year AR, 0.30 per year NAR).

In contrast to the substantial number of head injuries during the study, there were only five neck sprains in a total of 93 episodes of sprain. Two of these five patients had an exacerbation during a three-month AR period following the injury. These small numbers, of course, were not statistically significant. Importantly, moreover, the form of the exacerbation in the two cases having exacerbation did not suggest that the new lesion causing the exacerbation occurred in the cervical spinal cord. In one case, a left optic neuritis occurred

20 days after injury, and in the other case weakness and numbness of the arm and trunk, exclusively on the right side, occurred 52 days later and was more likely due to a new cerebral lesion. The conclusion of this study was that trauma of the type studied was not a risk factor in MS, and that patients sustaining trauma had no more rapid progression of disability than those not having trauma.

These results were subsequently corroborated in a smaller independent study at the Mayo Clinic in a delineated cohort of 164 MS patients residing in Olmsted County, Minnesota, on December 1, 1991 (prevalence cohort).[14] This group included 122 residents of the county at the time of diagnosis (between 1905 and 1991), and an additional 42 patients whose MS had had its onset elsewhere, but who had been resident in the county for at least a year. From careful review of clinical records of these patients, it was found that 54 fractures had occurred in 39, including small and long bone, pelvic, hip and spinal fractures. Exacerbations occurred no more commonly in six-month periods after trauma than in similar periods prior to trauma. Also, progression of disability was no greater in patients who had trauma than in those who had not.

One conclusion of these two studies is that peripheral trauma, including trauma to the

Type trauma	Pts.	Epis.	Exac/AR	Time AR (yrs)	Exac/NAR	Time/NAR (yrs)	Rate/yr/AR	Rate/yr/NAR
Major and Minor Surg. Fractures	56	160	7	33.9	97	216.8	0.21	0.45
Dental Sprains Burns Head inj. Ab/con.	93	716	79	143.5	157	324.5	0.55	0.48

Chi square on the occurrences in the first row = 4.04 ($p < 0.05$); chi square for the second row = 0.91, N.S.

Ab/con = abrasions, contusions.

This table is adapted from *Table 4* of the primary publication[10] and includes only the 95 patients having one or more exacerbations during the study, AR period = 3 months.

Table 7.2
Exacerbation rates when at risk for surgical procedures and fractures, compared to other types of trauma.

extremities, face, and dental trauma, is not a risk factor in MS. The prospective study of Sibley *et al.* examined numerous instances of such injuries, and both studies included many fractures of bone. As a matter of fact, in this investigation there was a significant inverse relationship between fractures and surgical procedures and exacerbation rates (*Table 7.2*). Even the leading proponent of the hypothesis that trauma may worsen MS, Charles Poser, now concedes that peripheral trauma is an unlikely cause.[13] This was not always so. In the 1960s Henry Miller of Newcastle noted instances of peripheral trauma, followed by MS symptoms in the same part of the body. He cited, for example, the case of a soccer player who was hit in the face by a soccer ball, and a few days later developed numbness of the same side of the face due to MS.[15] This idea that peripheral trauma might somehow trigger MS attacks involving the traumatically affected part, was first espoused during the era of poliomyelitis epidemics. In that disease, it was alleged that when a patient with poliomyelitis developed limb paralysis, it was more likely to involve a limb that had recently been injected with vaccines, or vigorously exercised. Localized changes in the circulation of the spinal cord in response to these external factors were thought to be responsible for this phenomenon.[16] Our own experience suggests that such trauma site and lesion level correlations are fortuitous.[10–11]

A second conclusion, from the Sibley *et al.* study, is that minor head injuries are not risk factors for exacerbation or worsening of MS. Some have criticized this study because not enough serious head and neck injuries were studied.[17] There is some validity to the latter criticism: there were no serious head injuries in the study, and no episodes of prolonged unconsciousness, although there were 11 episodes of concussion manifest by brief loss of consciousness for seconds or a few minutes. Nonetheless, it is these minor head and neck injuries, the latter often called 'whiplash' in court proceedings, which form the subject of most litigation. We believe, moreover, that the number of mild head injuries (140) was sufficient to test the hypothesis that they result in an excess of exacerbations due to blood–brain barrier (BBB) breakdown. As noted, the results were negative: there was no tendency to increased exacerbation rates whatsoever.

Despite these studies, the idea that trauma might be responsible for worsening of MS, in some instances, persists. The idea is an old one, fueled by anecdotal case reports of worsening of established cases of MS shortly after trauma, or, in a few instances, the onset of the first symptoms of MS after trauma. In our experience with several such cases, it is not the MS that is new, but rather the diagnosis that is new. Many patients, upon review of old medical records, have had suggestive symptoms of MS in the past which were not recognized or properly investigated. The traumatic event served the purpose of bringing the patient to the attention of a neurologist and a magnetic resonance imaging (MRI) scanner. Most such cases have multiple lesions characteristic of MS on the first cranial MRI scan taken after the trauma, suggesting that the MS had pre-existed the trauma by several years. In a few cases, no credible symptom of MS can be discovered on review of pre-trauma records, and the MRI scan reveals only a few lesions, consistent with recent onset.

Modern understanding of the frequency of clinical and MRI activity of MS,[18–20] suggests that coincidence is a likely explanation for many of these post-traumatic worsenings in MS patients. US Public Health Service statistics indicate that one-third of the population has a memorable trauma each year.[21] Cases of alleged traumatic exacerbation are usually those with a short interval between the trauma and new MS symptoms, and they are selected, by the legal process, from a large population pool which contains many examples of trauma without subsequent exacerbation. For example, if only one-third of the approximately 300,000 patients with MS in the US[22] had a single annual exacerbation, 8333 MS exacerbations would occur monthly. During this same year one-third would experience a memorable trauma, or 2777 traumas per month. In fact, this estimate of trauma rate is probably low, because the frequency of trauma in MS patients is 2–3 times higher than in age-matched controls (*Table 7.3*).[10] To avoid any coincidental occurrence of exacerbation after trauma, including a few closely related in time, would require that trauma prevents exacerbation.

Even when new cases of MS follow trauma, coincidence must be considered a likely explanation for the same reasons: the frequency of trauma, and the fact that about 10,000 new cases of MS occur in the US each year. If the crude incidence rate of about 6 per 100,000 population, found in Rochester, Minnesota, is applicable to the entire country, 15,000 new MS cases a year would be predicted.[23]

	Patient annual rate (mean)	Control annual rate (mean)	Ratio patient/control
Dental	0.18	0.11	1.6
Minor surgery	0.17	0.06	2.8
Major surgery	0.06	0.06	1.3
Burns	0.18	0.005	36.0
Sprains	0.11	0.06	1.8
Fracture	0.06	0.03	2.0
Head injury	0.16	0.06	2.6
AB/LAC/CON	0.66	0.20	3.3

Table 7.3
Frequency of various types of trauma in MS patients and controls.[10]

Does trauma accelerate the appearance of symptomatic MS?

The idea that trauma might actually cause a disease as complex as MS is probably no longer an issue. Both empiric and scientific evidence is available refuting this point of view. Included in the empiric evidence is the fact that patients with traumatic paraplegia, the worst form of spinal injury, rarely develop MS.[24] The same is true of head injuries. Large cohorts of patients with moderate to serious head injuries from both World Wars have been observed for many years. The experienced senior neurologist, Bryan Mathews, has said that ... 'personal experience of a large series of veterans who have survived penetrating head wounds has not revealed any instance of multiple sclerosis.'[25] If the frequency of MS was increased in such subjects, it would be well known.

This empiric evidence is bolstered by scientific studies from the Department of Health Sciences Research at the Mayo Clinic. This large clinic has a unique ability to 'prospectively' follow retrospectively identified cohorts of patients who have experienced significant trauma, because it has provided both primary and tertiary care to the population of Olmsted County since the turn of the century. These records have been indexed in detail and are readily available for retrieval.[26] A recent study from this institution identified a cohort of 819 patients sustaining moderate to severe head injuries during the past 30 years, all at a time when the patients were in the proper age group to be susceptible to MS. A follow-up of this cohort in clinic records showed that none of these patients developed MS within six months, although two developed MS at lengthy intervals following the head injury – 3 and 21 years – a number consistent with the expected incidence of MS in this number of patients, even if trauma had not occurred.[14] Likewise, only one of 973 patients having lumbar or cervical disc surgery, followed a mean of 10 years, developed MS.[26] In another cohort of 561 patients suffering from cervical radiculopathy, none had a later diagnosis of MS.[27] Thus, in the total of 2353 patients represented in these trauma cohorts, it is clear that there were no more new MS cases than would be expected by chance following these known specified types of physical stress to the nervous system, by individual group, or for all combined.

The possibility that trauma causes the onset of symptomatic MS has become less controversial in recent years as a result of prospective follow-up of these large historically identified cohorts of trauma patients. In addition four negative case control studies lend no support to this hypothesis.[28–31] Since prospective and historical cohort studies are the most valid ways of examining the hypothesis that trauma makes MS worse,[26] the essentially negative findings of such studies has convinced most neurologists that trauma is not a significant factor causing worsening of MS.[10,14,32]

The blood–brain barrier hypothesis

Poser suggests that trauma may adversely affect the course of MS only in cases in which head or spinal cord trauma leads to a localized breakdown in the BBB.[33,34] He argues that, since a breakdown in the BBB is a constant feature prior to new lesions of MS, new

lesions of any kind causing BBB breakdown may cause the formation of new MS lesions at the sites of such damage. He even states that, once the BBB is broken by trauma, patients may progress in their disability more rapidly in the ensuing months and years, and be permanently worse than they would have been without the trauma. Poser cites case reports in which traumatic events have been followed in a short time interval by new symptoms of MS. While some of these patients have had known MS in the past, others have apparently had 'silent' MS, since, at the time of their first post-trauma cranial MRI scan, they have multiple cerebral lesions typical of MS. The argument is made that such patients might have remained clinically silent had they not had the trauma.

Surely it is common experience, however, that the majority of all patients in whom a new diagnosis of MS is made come from this same population pool of patients with silent MS, since they have multiple old MS lesions on the first cranial MRI scan. The exact size of the silent pool of patients remains speculative, but Engell estimates it to be approximately one-fourth the number of diagnosed cases.[35] The idea that *any* lesion which causes a breakdown in the BBB can result in a new MS lesion in the brain or spinal cord has not been confirmed. Pathologists do not see rims of demyelination surrounding incidental brain disease in MS patients, such as infarcts or tumors, as would be predicted by this hypothesis.[11]

Brain and Wilkinson described a number of cases of coexisting cervical spondylosis and MS, and suggested that compression of the spinal cord by spondylitic ridges determined the appearance of adjacent MS lesions in the spinal cord.[36] Oppenheimer, a neuropathologist, determined that MS lesions were about twice as common in the cervical cord as in the rest of the spinal cord.[37] He pointed out, however, that MS lesions in the cervical cord were just as common in patients without spondylosis as in patients who had it. He studied in great detail the spinal cords of 20 patients with chronic MS, three of whom had severe spondylosis. Oppenheimer speculated that the common appearance of fan-shaped lesions in the lateral columns of the cervical cord might be due to traction on the cord at the attachment site of denticulate ligaments, during neck flexion, perhaps by alteration of the blood–brain barrier in this area. His publication includes detailed drawings of the distribution and pattern of plaques in the lower four cervical segments in 18 of the 20 patients. In 12 of the 18 patients the lesion pattern included roughly symmetrical bilateral lateral column lesions, and in another six there were predominantly unilateral lateral column plaques. Eleven of the patients also had prominent bilateral dorsal column plaques, however, and two cases were excluded from the analysis because of severe edema of the entire cervical cord in one, and total demyelination in another: such cases are not readily explained by the denticulate ligament hypothesis. Since 1978, when Oppenheimer proposed his idea that MS patients should avoid full neck flexion, we are not aware of any confirmatory data. In our experience MS patients who engage in athletic activities and physical conditioning programs do no worse than others. While the cervical spine is more mobile than the thoracic spine, it is not clear whether this is the reason for the increased frequency of MS lesions in the cervical cord. There are undoubtedly more important unknown factors determining the distribution of MS lesions, probably similar to those responsible for the increased frequency of lesions in the optic nerves and periventricular areas.

In order to prove that trauma worsens MS it would first be necessary to prove that exacerbations occur more commonly after trauma than at other times, i.e. that it is a risk factor. Those who purport to believe in a relationship between trauma and worsening of MS have never conducted studies to prove that trauma, even head and neck trauma, is a risk factor. Only anecdotal cases are reported. No counts are made of patients having similar trauma without experiencing exacerbations of the illness. We are asked to believe in the reality of traumatic exacerbations simply using *post hoc, ergo propter hoc* reasoning, and because a possible, but unproven, mechanism exists whereby this might occur.

The effect of moderate or severe head or spine trauma on the course of MS remains largely unknown. We are not aware of any case series or even individual case reports dealing with the effect of moderate or severe non-surgical head injuries in MS patients. Proponents of the idea that *any* breakdown of the BBB may cause new lesions point to the report of Gonsette and colleagues, describing fresh demyelination surrounding the path of trocars introduced into the brain to produce lesions in the thalamus to control tremor, in some, but not all patients at *post mortem* examination.[38] As noted in a previously published examination of this subject,[11] the Gonsette report was made in the pre-MRI era, and it is possible that the trocars could not be introduced without encountering lesions already present. Another possible example of the same phenomenon was reported in a single case by Reichert *et al.*, although these authors conceded that is was possible that the lesion near the trocar was coincidental, because of the multiplicity of MS lesions in the brain of their patient, although they favoured a causative hypothesis.[39]

In contrast, in recent years there have been numerous instances in which brain surgery has been performed on MS patients, usually to biopsy a solitary large demyelinating lesion.[40–44] John Kepes, a neuropathologist reporting a series of 31 such cases,[40] is not aware of any instance in which the surgery was associated with new MS lesions at the surgical site (personal communication). None of the other reports mention any adverse effect of the surgery in terms of causing new lesions, or worsening of the patients' clinical condition. In most such instances, once the biopsy diagnosis of demyelinating lesion was made, patients have been given corticosteroids, and have made a relatively good improvement. In one case a large MS lesion in a cerebellar hemisphere prompted resection of the hemisphere because of a pre-operative diagnosis of neoplasm. The patient is said to have tolerated this procedure well, and to be still doing well at seven months post-operatively, although two small additional lesions were then seen by MRI in one cerebral hemisphere.[42] No new lesions were described adjacent to the resection.

The idea that a traumatic breach of the BBB could have some special long-term adverse effect on the course of MS seems insupportable in the light of the many natural history studies in recent years, employing serial MRI studies of MS patients using gadolinium enhancement. These studies indicate that BBB breakdown occurs very frequently as part of the natural history of the disease. Some studies report as many as 20 new enhancements per patient per year in the cranial MRI scan.[20] Bastianello *et al.* reported an even higher frequency of some 40 enhancements per patient-year on the basis of a three-month serial study.[45] Some believe that all such gadolinium enhancements represent the precursor of a new demyelinating lesion, although this concept has not been confirmed. Miller *et al.* reviewed enhancing lesions, and then reviewed the unenhanced scans on the same patients, in

a serial study, and found that in about half the instances, no new T_2 weighted lesions could be identified at the site of areas of gadolinium enhancement.[46]

Rather, it is now apparent that inflammation of veins and venules in the central nervous system (CNS) of MS patients is frequent, and that in many such instances, but probably not all, these periods of inflammation are followed by new demyelinating lesions. Indeed, periodic venular inflammation and increased permeability of veins also occurs in the retina in about 25 per cent of MS patients, and even here appears to be a fundamental part of MS pathology.[47–50] A number of studies have shown periodic breakdown in the blood–retinal barrier, usually around veins at the site of perivenous sheathing, although in three cases sheathing has been described also about arterioles in the retina, often at the site where arterioles and veins cross.[48] This was the case in one of our patients (RG), who had periodic fluorescein angiography prior to the MRI era: *Fig. 7.1* shows perivascular leakage of fluorescein into the vitreous in this case.[49] This

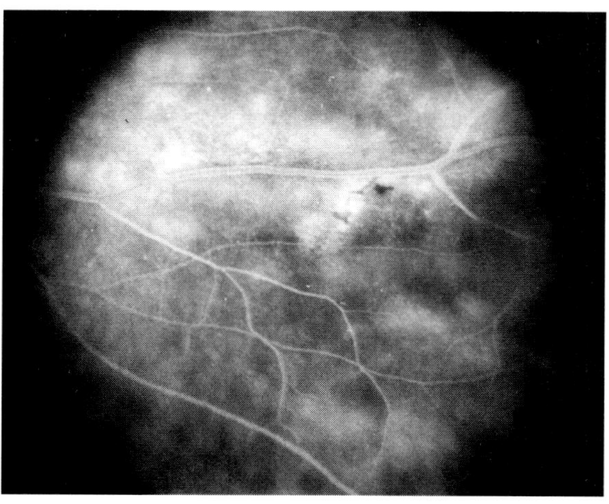

Fig. 7.1
Perivascular leakage of fluoroscein into the vitreous humour.

patient, who also had pars planitis and perivenous sheathing in the retina, had clinically inactive MS at the time of this retinal angiogram, but had a clinical exacerbation of MS several months prior to this and about a year later as well.

A careful six-month prospective study was recently reported, in which 23 MS patients had both monthly fluorescein retinal angiograms and cranial MRI scans with gadolinium enhancement. Six instances of perivenous sheathing were seen in these patients, and retinal angiography showed leakage in three cases, all of whom had perivenous sheathing; during the same time period 204 new areas of gadolinium enhancement in cranial MRI scans occurred in 22 of the 23 patients.[50]

Conclusion

The preponderance of scientific evidence suggests that peripheral trauma and mild head injuries do not worsen existing MS. This conclusion is based on the results of a prospective study in patients with established MS, and was corroborated by a careful record review in a delineated prevalence cohort of MS patients at the Mayo Clinic. Likewise, similar 'prospective' follow-up, in medical records, of several retrospectively identified trauma cohorts at the same institution, has shown no greater frequency of development of symptomatic MS than would be expected by chance. Anecdotal case reports describing instances of a brief interval between traumatic episodes and MS symptoms are selected from a large population pool in which such a relationship is not noted, and are probably best explained by coincidence. The effect of moderate and severe central nervous system trauma on MS remains unknown, but the concept that *any* breakdown in the BBB results in new MS lesions is not proven, nor is it supported by the recent neurosurgical literature.

References

1. Sibley WA. Therapeutic Claims Committee of the International Federation of Multiple Sclerosis Societies, 4th edn., New York: Demos Vermande 1996.
2. Kelly RE, Jellinek EH. Intrathecal tuberculin in disseminated sclerosis. *Br Med J* 1961; **ii**: 421–424.
3. Mannering GJ, Deloria LB. The pharmacology and toxicology of the interferons. *Ann Rev Pharmocol Toxicol* 1986; **26**: 455–515.
4. Panitch HS, Hirsch RL, Haley AS *et al*. Exacerbation of multiple sclerosis in patients treated with gamma interferon. *Lancet* 1987; **1**: 893–895.
5. Sibley WA. Risk factors in multiple sclerosis. In: Raine CS, McFarland HF, Tourtellotte WW, eds. *Multiple Sclerosis: Clinical and Pathogenetic Basis*, London: Chapman and Hall 1997, 141–148.
6. Sibley WA, Bamford CR, Clark K. Clinical viral infections and multiple sclerosis. *Lancet* 1985; **1**: 1313–1315.
7. Narod S, Johnson-Lussenburg CM, Zheng Q *et al*. Viral infections and MS (letter). *Lancet* 1985; **2**: 165.
8. Panitch HS. Influence of infection on exacerbations of multiple sclerosis. *Ann Neurol* 1994; **36**: S25–S28.
9. Andersen O, Lygner P, Bergstrom T *et al*. Viral infections trigger multiple sclerosis relapses: a prospective seroepidemiological study. *J Neurol* 1993; **240**: 417–422.
10. Sibley WA, Bamford CR, Clark K *et al*. A prospective study of physical trauma and multiple sclerosis. *J Neurol Neurosurg Psychiatry* 1991; **54**: 584–589.
11. Sibley WA. Physical trauma and multiple sclerosis (editorial). *Neurology* 1993; **43**: 1871–1874.
12. Kurland LT, Rodriguez M, O'Brien PC *et al*. Physical trauma and multiple sclerosis (letter). *Neurology* 1994; **44**: 1362–1364.
13. Sibley WA, Bamford CR, Clark K *et al*. A prospective study of physical trauma and multiple sclerosis [letter]. *J Neurol Neurosurg Psychiatry* 1992; **55**: 524–525.
14. Siva A, Radhakrishnan K, Kurland LT *et al*. Trauma and multiple sclerosis: a population-based cohort study from Olmsted County, Minnesota. *Neurology* 1993; **43**: 1878–1882.
15. Miller H. Trauma and multiple sclerosis. *Lancet* 1964; **1**: 848–850.
16. Trueta J, Hodes R. Provoking and localising factors in poliomyelitis; an experimental study. *Lancet* 1954; **1**: 998.
17. Jellinek EH. Trauma and multiple sclerosis [editorial]. *Lancet* 1994; **343**: 1053.
18. Willoughby EW, Grochowski E, Li DBK *et al*. Serial magnetic resonance scanning in multiple sclerosis: a second prospective study in relapsing patients. *Ann Neurol* 1989; **25**: 43–49.
19. Koopmans RA, Li DKB, Oger J *et al*. Chronic progressive multiple sclerosis: serial magnetic resonance brain imaging over 6 months. *Ann Neurol* 1989; **26**: 248–256.
20. McFarland HF, Frank JA, Albert PS *et al*. Using gadolinium-enhanced magnetic resonance imaging lesions to monitor disease activity in multiple sclerosis. *Ann Neurol* 1992; **32**: 758–766.
21. Collins JG. National Center for Health Statistics. Types of injuries and impairments due to injuries. United States Vital Statistics, Series 10, No. 159, DHHS No. (PHS) 871587. Washington, DC: Public Health Service, US Government Printing Office 1986; 24.
22. Anderson DW, Ellenberg JH, Leventhal CM *et al*. Revised estimate of the prevalence of multiple sclerosis in the United States. *Ann Neurol* 1992; **31**: 333–336.
23. Wynn DR, Rodriguez M, O'Fallon WM *et al*. A reappraisal of the epidemiology of multiple sclerosis in Olmsted County, Minnesota. *Neurology* 1990; **40**: 780–786.
24. Burke DC, Cheshire DJE. Neuromyelitis optica: A review of the literature and a report of a case which followed traumatic paraplegia. *Paraplegia* 1968; **6**: 79–89.

25. Matthews WB. *McAlpine's Multiple Sclerosis*, 2nd edn., Edinburgh: Churchill Livingstone 1990; 113.

26. Kurland LT. Trauma and multiple sclerosis. *Ann Neurol* 1994; **36**: S33–S37.

27. Sunku J, Kurland LT. Multiple sclerosis and trauma [letter]. *Neurology* 1994; **44**: 2416.

28. Kurland LT, Westlund KB. Epidemiologic factors in the etiology and prognosis of multiple sclerosis. *Ann NY Acad Sci* 1954; **58**: 682–701.

29. Bobowick R, Kurtzke JF, Brody J *et al*. Twin study of multiple sclerosis: an epidemiologic inquiry. *Neurology* 1978; **28**: 978–987.

30. Von Wilhelm E. Beziehungen Zwischen Erkrankungen ins Kindesalter und Multiple Scklerose Erkrankung. *Schweiz Arch Neurol Neurochi Psychiat* 1970; **106**: 311–317.

31. Alter M, Speer J. Clinical evaluation of possible etiologic factors in multiple sclerosis. *Neurology* 1968; **18**: 109–116.

32. Statement of the Medical Advisory Board of the National MS Society New York, re: trauma and MS, 1994.

33. Poser CM. Trauma and multiple sclerosis: an hypothesis. *J Neurol* 1987; **234**: 155–159.

34. Poser CM. Multiple sclerosis. Observations and reflections—a personal memoir. *J Neurol Sci* 1992; **107**: 127–140.

35. Engell T. A clinical patho-anatomical study of clinically silent multiple sclerosis. *Acta Neurol Scand* 1989; **79**: 428–430.

36. Brain R, Wilkinson M. The association of cervical spondylosis and disseminated sclerosis. *Brain* 1957; **80**: 456–478.

37. Oppenheimer DR. The cervical cord in multiple sclerosis. *Neuropathol Appl Neurobiol* 1978; **4**: 151–162.

38. Gonsette R, Andre-Balisaux G, Delmotte P. La permeabilite des vaisseaux cerebraux VI: demyelinisation experimentale provoquee par des substances agissant sur la barriere hemato-encephalique. *Acta Neurol Belg* 1966; **66**: 247–262.

39. Reichert T, Hassler R, Mundinger F *et al*. Pathologic-anatomic findings and cerebral localisation in stereotactic treatment of extrapyramidal motor disturbance in MS. *Confinia Neurologica* 1975; **37**: 24–40.

40. Kepes JJ. Large focal tumor-like demyelinating lesions of the brain; intermediate entity between multiple sclerosis and acute disseminated encephalomyelitis? A study of 31 patients. *Ann Neurol* 1993; **33**: 18–27.

41. Nesbit GM, Forbes GS, Scheithauer BW *et al*. Multiple sclerosis: histopathologic and MR and/or CT correlation in 37 cases at biopsy and three cases at autopsy. *Radiology* 1991; **180**: 467–474.

42. Rusin JA, Vezina LG, Chadduck WM *et al*. Tumoral multiple sclerosis of the cerebellum in a child. *Am J Neuroradiol* 1995; **16**: 1164–1166.

43. Chakrabortty S, Nagashima T, Saitoh M *et al*. Intracerebral ring-enhancing lesions in a patient with multiple sclerosis: a case report. *Surg Neurol* 1995; **43**: 591–594.

44. Estes ML, Rudick RA, Barness GH *et al*. Stereotactic biopsy of an active multiple sclerosis lesion. *Arch Neurol* 1990; **47**: 1299–1303.

45. Bastianello S, Pozzilli C, Bernardi S *et al*. Serial study of gadolinium-DTPA MRI enhancement in multiple sclerosis. *Neurology* 1990; **40**: 591–595.

46. Miller DH, Barkhof F, Nauta JJP. Gadolinium enhancement increases the sensitivity of MRI in detecting disease activity. *Brain* 1993; **116**: 1077–1094.

47. Younge BR. Fluorescein angiography and retinal venous sheathing in multiple sclerosis. *Can J Ophthalmol* 1976; **11**: 31–36.

48. Kerrison JB, Flynn T, Green WR. Retinal pathologic changes in multiple sclerosis. *Retina* 1994; **14**: 445–451.

49. Bamford CR, Ganley JP, Sibley WA *et al*. Uveitis, perivenous sheathing and multiple sclerosis. *Neurology* 1978; **28**: 119–124.

50. Birch MK, Barbosa S, Blumhardt LD, *et al*. Retinal venous sheathing and the blood-retinal barrier in multiple sclerosis. *Arch Ophthalmol* 1996; **114**: 34–39.

8

Does pregnancy make multiple sclerosis better or worse?

Michael Hutchinson

The short response to the question posed in the title is that probably pregnancy does improve the course of multiple sclerosis (MS) but there is a counterbalancing deterioration in the puerperium. When both pregnancy and the post-partum period are considered, then the overall effect on the course of MS is probably neutral. The aim of this chapter is to validate this conclusion.

The ideal study of the effect of pregnancy in MS has not been, and could not be, performed. The problem with all studies, including recent cohort studies, is the difficulty in obtaining valid control patients. It is probable that women with MS who decide to have children have a milder form of MS than women who do not do so. It is clear from several studies that MS influences marriage rate (reduced), divorce rate (increased), and fertility (reduced).[1,2] It could be argued that MS does not affect biological fertility but favours the decision not to have children.[1] In a Swedish study of onset bouts the fecundity of the MS population before onset was lower than the Swedish population.[2] There appears to be a greater frequency of induced abortions in pregnant MS women than might be expected.[1,3] The reasons for medical termination may include a desire not to have children on a mistaken belief, stemming from the older literature, that pregnancy has an adverse effect on the course of MS. The frequency of spontaneous abortions and malformations does not differ between before- or after-onset of MS in a given population.[1]

The ideal study of the effect of pregnancy in MS would be to prospectively recruit women who may be contemplating pregnancy and to randomly assign them to a pregnancy and non-pregnancy group. The former group would be asked to become pregnant, the latter group not to do so, and one would follow both groups prospectively for the year prior to pregnancy, the pregnancy period, and for at least one year after pregnancy. Such a study would require to be multicentred and clearly would be impossible to perform. Given these difficulties, various authors of both cohort and retrospective studies have used control groups consisting of either the pregnant women under study during the non-pregnancy periods, or a group of matched non-pregnant women followed for the same time period. To support the hypothesis that it is not valid to attempt to match the pregnant MS with non-pregnant MS patients it should be noted that in two recent studies the relapse rates of the pregnant MS women during non-pregnancy periods were lower at 0.51 and 0.63 relapses per year compared to the relapse rates of the non-pregnant women of 0.86 and 0.82 relapses per year respectively.[3,4]

Relapse rates in pregnancy and the puerperium

Until the study of Tillman, reports of the effect of gestation on MS had been anecdotal and usually adverse in conclusions. Tillman and others found no evidence for any negative effect of pregnancy in MS.[5,6] It is with the study of Millar and his colleagues that the first systematic studies of the effects of pregnancy and MS began.[7] All studies to date from 1959 are summarized in *Tables 8.1* and *8.2*. The studies can be grouped into retrospective,[7–12] cohort,[3,4,13,14] and prospective reports.[15] The main criterion of disease activity measured was the relapse rate which, although relatively easy to measure, is confounded by the fact that retrospective assessment of relapse rates misses many relapses.[16] The relapse rate for women at the age at which pregnancy is being contemplated, and for their controls, should be approximately 0.5 relapses per year.[17] In the group of retrospective studies deemed 'unacceptable' the relapse rates during non-pregnancy years varied from 0.075 to 0.32 relapses per year and in the non-pregnant control years between 0.104 and 0.29 relapses per year (*Table 8.1*). For this reason the five studies listed in *Table 8.1* are deemed unacceptable because of the low rate of ascertained relapses.[7–11] All these studies did show, however, that the relapse rate in the three months post-partum was significantly higher than the relapse rate during pregnancy. In four of these studies the relapse rate in the post-partum three months was higher than the relapse rate in the same patients during non-pregnant periods (self-controls).[7–10] In the Israeli study it was noted that the relapse rate fell steadily during all three trimesters of pregnancy; these authors also found an increased relapse rate in the fourth to sixth month post-partum.[10] Only the study of Schapira and colleagues suggested

that pregnancy in MS might have a non-significant adverse effect on disability;[8] in two other retrospective studies no effect on disability was found.[7,9] The overall effect on the relapse rate in the pregnancy year (nine months of pregnancy and three months post-partum) was unfavourable in three studies[7–9] when compared to non-pregnancy periods and not significantly different in one study.[10]

Acceptable pregnancy studies

Since 1988 there has been one retrospective study with acceptable control relapse rates,[12] and four cohort studies in which a group of MS patients who became pregnant were followed as a cohort in a clinic setting.[3,4,13,14] Although called prospective by the authors in two papers, it has been argued cogently and persuasively that these are cohort rather than truly prospective studies.[18] There is a small prospective study of eight patients in one centre which demonstrated unconvincingly no relapses during pregnancy, with six of the eight patients having relapses in the three months post-partum.[15]

The five acceptable retrospective and cohort studies are detailed in *Table 8.2*. The conclusions from individual studies vary considerably one from another. Sadovnik *et al.* and Bernardi *et al.* found a fall in the relapse rate during pregnancy, but in the former study the only period in which the relapse rate was significantly different from controls was the third trimester of pregnancy.[4,13] In two of these recent studies the relapse rate was actually reported to rise in the third trimester compared to other trimesters of pregnancy.[3,12] Overall relapse rates during the nine months of pregnancy were not noted to be reduced in three studies[3,4,14] but, in two, were significantly reduced in comparison to control rates.[12,13] In

Study (ref)	Number of pregnancies (women)	Relapses observed				Annualized relapse rates		
		Pregnancy	3 month post-partum	Pregnancy	Post-partum	Pregnancy year	Self control	Non-pregnant control
Millar et al.[7]	170 (70)	6	39	0.047	0.92	0.27	0.075	0.104
Schapira et al.[8]	124 (220)	12	19	0.13	0.61	0.25	0.17	NA
Ghezzi and Caputo[9]	206 (119)	34	91	0.22	1.76	0.61	0.32	0.29
Korn-Lubetski et al.[10]	199 (66)	20	41	0.13	0.82	0.31	0.29	0.28
Nelson et al.[11]	191 (111)	19	44	0.13	0.9	0.33	NA	NA
ALL STUDIES	890	91	234	0.14	1.05	0.37	–	–

Table 8.1

A summary of data on relapses and annualized relapse rates with control rates in five early studies in which control rates are unacceptably low or absent. Annualized relapse rate is the number of relapses observed for the period divided by the number of patients and corrected for the time period (for example, for the three month post-partum the rate is multiplied by four). NA = not available. Control rates are given for the same patients during non-pregnancy periods (self controls) and for other non-pregnant patients.

| | | Relapses observed | | | | Annualized relapse rates | | |
Study (ref)	Number of pregnancies (women)	Pregnancy	3 month post-partum	Pregnancy	Post-partum	Pregnancy year	Self control	Non-pregnant control
Frith and McLeod[12]	85 (50)	19	14	0.29	0.66	0.39	0.53	NA
Bernardi et al.[13]	66 (52)	5	16	0.10	0.97	0.32	0.65	NA
Roullet et al.[3]	32 (33)	19	13	0.61	1.62	1.0	0.51	0.86
Sadovnik et al.[4]	58 (47)	20	14	0.46	0.96	0.59	0.63	0.82
Worthington et al.[14]	14 (14)	5	6	0.48	1.7	0.78	0.57	0.5
ALL STUDIES	255	68	63	0.36	0.98	0.51	–	–

Table 8.2
A summary of data on relapses and annualized relapse rates
with control rates in the five most recent studies in which
control rates are at acceptable values. For explanation of
headings and abbreviations see Table 8.1.

the three month post-partum period a rise in the relapse rate was noted in all studies but this was not significant in comparison to control relapse rates in two,[4,12] whereas in three studies a significant post-partum rise in relapse rate was noted.[3,13,14]

The effect of the 'pregnancy year' (nine months pregnancy + three months post-partum) on relapse rates in comparison to controls was significantly favourable in one study,[13] but in the four others the rates were non-significantly favourable in one,[12] similar to controls in two[3,4] and non-significantly greater than controls in one.[14]

A unique contribution to the study of disease activity during pregnancy came from a fortuitous examination, by magnetic resonance imaging (MRI), of two women who became pregnant in the course of a study of serial MRI findings in MS.[19] Disease activity was measured by the occurrence of new lesions or the enlargement of pre-existing lesions on MRI. During pregnancy this measure of disease activity decreased and returned during the post-partum period to pre-pregnancy levels. The study demonstrated also the marked discrepancy between the frequent new lesions seen by MRI and the relative paucity of clinically evident relapses.

The difficulty with the above analysis of individual studies is that the number of patients in each study is small and there is a risk that important differences in relapse rates might be missed due to a type II error. A summary of all the data from these five studies (*Table 8.2*) does, however, indicate an overall trend (which had also been noted in the previous earlier reports – (*Table 8.1*):

- a fall in relapse rate in the nine months of pregnancy
- a marked rise in the relapse rate in the three months post-partum

- overall, no significant difference between relapse rates for the 'pregnancy year' in comparison to reported rates for the same patients during non-pregnancy periods.

Disability and pregnancy in MS

Given the above overall neutral effect of pregnancy and the post-partum period on the relapse rate in MS, it is not surprising that the overwhelming majority of studies have not demonstrated any negative or positive effect of pregnancy on disability.[3,5–7,9] In an early study from the UK a non-significantly unfavourable effect of pregnancy on disability was suggested[8] but more rigorous studies, including a community-based population study,[20] and others, have not shown any effect.[21–22] As argued above, it is unlikely that such a study of disability in pregnancy is possible; MS patients who become pregnant probably are self-selected from patients with less severe forms of the disease and adequate control studies are impossible or at least of suspect validity. The lack of relationship between relapse frequency and disability in natural history studies, suggests that increased disability is unlikely to be caused by the increased post-partum relapse rate.[23] The commonly used tool to measure disability, the Kurtzke Expanded Disability Status Scale (EDSS)[24] is relatively insensitive to change over a short period of time in the range of impairments seen in women contemplating pregnancy.[25,26]

Only one study has suggested that pregnancy may have a favourable effect on disability.[2] In an incidence cohort study of 100 women aged 15–50 years in Goteborg the authors found that non-pregnant patients had a 3.2 times higher risk (95 per cent CI; 1.01–10.3) of entering the progressive phase than MS patients who had been pregnant.

The PRIMS study

Given the problems inherent in previous small studies, and the contradictory findings, a sub-committee of the European Committee for Research in MS (ECTRIMS) planned a prospective study of pregnancy in MS (PRIMS).[27] This was funded by the European Union Biomed Programme under the direction of Professor Christian Confavreux in Lyon, France. A set of data-collection forms using the EDMUS system[28] covering the pre-pregnancy period, the pregnancy and two years post-partum, was prepared and circulated to interested neurologists in 12 European countries. Two local coordinators in each country were responsible for ensuring recruitment, and at the end of recruitment in July 1995 260 pregnancies in 251 women with MS were entered in the study. The local secretariat in Lyon were responsible for ensuring that data were collected in time and that reporting was internally consistent. No external auditing of individual data collection forms was performed.

The aim of the study was to examine the natural history of MS before, during and after pregnancy by measurement of relapse rate and residual disability. The latter was measured using the EDSS[24] and the EDMUS Impairment Scale.[28] Relapse severity was not assessed because no valid method is presently available. There was no control group for the reasons described above; the argument is that there is no valid control group for these patients. The hypothesis was that the relapse rate would fall during pregnancy in comparison to the retrospectively assessed pre-pregnancy year and would rise in the post-partum period of three months in comparison to all other periods. The control periods for assessment of the non-pregnancy relapse rate were the pre-pregnancy year (retrospective) and the year following the post-partum year (prospective).

Initial analysis of 250 pregnancies revealed a steady relapse rate in the pre-pregnancy year of 0.69 relapses per year per person which was maintained in the first two trimesters of pregnancy and fell significantly in the third trimester. A marked rise in the relapse rate occurred in the first three months post-partum and thereafter the relapse rate appeared to return to the same rate as noted in the pre-pregnancy year. Overall, the relapse rate in the pregnancy year was the same as in the year prior to pregnancy.[29]

Breast feeding and the MS post-partum period

Only a few studies have addressed the question of the effects of breast feeding on the post-partum period and no definite answers emerge.[11,21] In an American study the relapse rates in the 36 breast feeding and the 29 non-breast feeding mothers were 38 per cent and 31 per cent, respectively.[11] The authors found that the mean time to exacerbation in the post-partum period was the same for breast feeding and non-breast feeding mothers.[11] One German study found that MS mothers breast fed their infants less often during the disease than before onset.[21] The PRIMS study is examining, in a prospective manner, the issue of the effect of breast feeding on the occurrence of post-partum relapses.[29]

Mechanisms of the protective effect of pregnancy in MS

The state of immunosuppression which accompanies pregnancy, and the loss of this state in the post-partum period, is generally assumed to explain the changes observed in the relapse rate in MS.[30] Experimental allergic encephalomyelitis is suppressed by pregnancy.[31]

Other auto-immune diseases such as rheumatoid arthritis demonstrate improvement or remission during gestation and, after delivery, arthritis activity predictably returns.[32]

The mechanism of pregnancy immunosuppression, by which the semi-allogenic foetus escapes rejection and amelioration of auto-immune diseases occurs, is one of the major unsolved problems in immunology. Most of the important studies have concerned the mechanisms of remission of rheumatoid arthritis. Immunosuppressive substances in pregnancy include alpha-2-fetoprotein, pregnancy-associated plasma protein, pregnancy-associated alpha-glycoprotein and chorionic gonadotrophic hormone.[30] It has been hypothesized that peptides from HLA class II molecules of the foetus temporarily interrupt auto-immunity which has occurred because of a defect in the presentation or recognition of HLA self-peptides in the patient.[33] The roles of oestrogen as an immunosuppressive agent and even testosterone have been proposed.[34] Increasing understanding of the role of various cytokines in pregnancy suggests that the feto-placental unit redirects maternal immunity away from cell-mediated towards enhanced humoral responsiveness. There is evidence that T_H1 cytokines (interleukin(IL)-2, interferon-γ(IFN-γ) and tumour necrosis factor (TNF)) have deleterious effects on pregnancy leading to fetal loss. This may be inhibited by T_H2 cytokines produced from the placenta down-regulating the harmful cytokines.[35] For a fuller discussion the reader is directed to various reviews.[30,33,35,36]

Advice to a woman with MS contemplating pregnancy

The evidence from the studies quoted in this review is reassuring. Women can be advised that there will be an amelioration of their disease activity with a reduction in the risk for relapse during pregnancy and that, although there is an increased relapse rate in the three post-partum months, the overall effect of the pregnancy year is no different from the non-pregnancy period.

The increased risk of relapse in the puerperium might be controlled by the (re-)introduction of treatment of interferon-β (IFN-β) as soon as possible after delivery.[37] Although there is no direct evidence that IFN-β will prevent or reduce the risk of relapse in this period this does seem a logical method of attempting to alter the post-partum flare-up of activity. IFN-β cannot be used if breast feeding is contemplated and, of course, its use must be stopped well before conception, probably at least three months before initiating a pregnancy.

For a woman with MS the decision to have a child or further pregnancies should not be influenced by ill-judged negative advice from the neurologist or physician. There is no evidence that pregnancy and the puerperium overall will have any deleterious effect on the course of MS and, with the use of IFN-β following delivery, a reduction in the post-partum relapse risk may be possible.

References

1. Poser S, Raun NE, Wikstrom J *et al.* Pregnancy, oral contraceptives and multiple sclerosis. *Acta Neurol Scand* 1979; **59**: 108–118.
2. Runmarker B, Andersen O. Pregnancy is associated with a lower risk of onset and a better prognosis in multiple sclerosis. *Brain* 1995; **118**: 253–261.
3. Roullet E, Verdier-Taillefer M-H, Amarenco P *et al.* Pregnancy and multiple sclerosis: a longitudinal study of 125 remittent patients. *J Neurol Neurosurg Psychiatry* 1993; **56**: 1062–1065.
4. Sadovnik AD, Eisen K, Hashimoto SA *et al.* Pregnancy and multiple sclerosis: a prospective study. *Arch Neurol* 1994; **51**: 1120–1124.
5. Tillman AJB. The effect of pregnancy on multiple sclerosis and its management. *Res Publ Assoc Nerv Ment Dis* 1950; **28**: 548–582.
6. McAlpine D, Compston N. Some aspects of the natural history of disseminated sclerosis. *Q J Med* 1952; **21**: 135–167.
7. Millar JHD, Allison RS, Cheesman EA *et al.* Pregnancy as a factor influencing relapse in disseminated sclerosis. *Brain* 1959; **82**: 417–426.
8. Schapira K, Poskanzer DC, Newell DJ *et al.* Marriage, pregnancy and multiple sclerosis. *Brain* 1966; **89**: 419–428.
9. Ghezzi A, Caputo D. Pregnancy: a factor influencing the course of multiple sclerosis? *Eur Neurol* 1981; **20**: 517–519.
10. Korn-Lubetski I, Kahona E, Cooper G *et al.* Activity of multiple sclerosis during pregnancy and the puerperium. *Ann Neurol* 1984; **16**: 229–231.
11. Nelson LM, Franklin GM, Jones MC. Risk of multiple sclerosis exacerbation during pregnancy and breast feeding. *J Am Med Ass* 1988; **259**: 3441–3443.
12. Frith JA, McLeod JG. Pregnancy and multiple sclerosis. *J Neurol Neurosurg Psychiatry* 1988; **51**: 495–498.
13. Bernardi S, Grasso MG, Bertollini R *et al.* The influence of pregnancy on relapses in multiple sclerosis: a cohort study. *Acta Neurol Scand* 1991; **84**: 403–406.
14. Worthington J, Jones R, Crawford M *et al.* Pregnancy and multiple sclerosis – a three year prospective study. *J Neurol* 1994; **241**: 228–233.
15. Birk K, Ford C, Smeltzer S *et al.* The clinical course of multiple sclerosis during pregnancy and the puerperium. *Arch Neurol* 1990; **47**: 738–742.
16. Matthews WB. *McAlpine's Multiple Sclerosis*, Edinburgh: Churchill Livingstone 1991, 144–145.
17. Lhermitte F, Marteau R, Gazengel J *et al.* The frequency of relapse in multiple sclerosis: a study based on 245 cases. *J Neurol* 1973; **205**: 47–59.
18. Ruddick RA. Pregnancy and multiple sclerosis. *Arch Neurol* 1995; **52**: 849–850.
19. Waldererveen van MAA, Tas MW, Barkhof, F *et al.* Magnetic resonance evaluation of disease activity during pregnancy in multiple sclerosis. *Neurology* 1994; **44**: 327–329.
20. Weinshenker BG, Hader W, Carriere W *et al.* The influence of pregnancy on disability from multiple sclerosis; a population-based study in Middlesex County, Ontario. *Neurology* 1989; **39**: 1438–1440.
21. Poser S, Poser W. Multiple sclerosis and gestation. *Neurology* 1987; **33**: 1422–1427.
22. Thompson DS, Nelson LM, Burns A *et al.* The effects of pregnancy in multiple sclerosis; a retrospective study. *Neurology* 1986; **36**: 1097–1099.
23. Runmarker B, Anderson O. Prognostic factors in a multiple sclerosis incidence cohort with twenty five years of follow-up. *Brain* 1993; **116**: 117–134.
24. Kurtzke JF. Rating neurological impairment in multiple sclerosis: an expanded disability status scale (EDSS). *Neurology* 1983; **33**: 1444–1452.
25. Weinshenker BG, Bass B, Rice GPA *et al.* The natural history of multiple sclerosis; a geographically based study. 2. Predictive value of the early clinical course. *Brain* 1989; **112**: 1419–1428.

26. Weinshenker BG, Ebers GC. The natural history of multiple sclerosis. *Can J Neurol Sci* 1987; **14**: 255–264.

27. Hutchinson M. Pregnancy and multiple sclerosis [editorial]. *J Neurol Neurosurg Psychiatry* 1993; **56**: 1043–1045.

28. Confavreux C, Compston DAS, Hommes OR *et al*. EDMUS, a European database for multiple sclerosis. *J Neurol Neurosurg Psychiatry* 1992; **55**: 671–676.

29. Hours M, Cortinovis-Tourniaire P, Moreau T *et al*. The influence of pregnancy on multiple sclerosis, a European multicentric prospective study. First results. *J Neurol* 1996; **243**: S2 (abstract).

30. Duquette P, Girard M. Hormonal factors in susceptibility to multiple sclerosis. *Curr Opinion Neurol Neurosurg* 1993; **6**: 195–201.

31. Evron S, Brenner T, Abramsky O. Suppressive effect of pregnancy on the development of experimental allergic encephalomyelitis in rabbits. *Am J Reprod Immunol* 1984; **5**: 109–113.

32. Persellin RH. The effect of pregnancy on rheumatoid arthritis. *Bull Rheum Dis* 1977; **27**: 922–927.

33. Ostensen M, Nelson JL. Bits and pieces in a puzzle – rheumatoid arthritis and pregnancy. *Br J Rheumatol* 1995; **34**: 1–3.

34. James WH. Rheumatoid arthritis, the contraceptive pill and androgens. *Ann Rheum Dis* 1993; **52**: 470–474.

35. Wegmann TG, Lin H, Guilbert L *et al*. Bidirectional cytokine interactions in the maternal-fetal relationship: is successful pregnancy a T_H2 phenomenon?. *Immunol Today* 1993; **14**: 353–356.

36. Hedge UC. Immunomodulation of the mother during pregnancy. *Med Hypotheses* 1991; **35**: 159–164.

37. The IFNB Multiple Sclerosis Study Group. Interferon β-1b is effective in relapsing-remitting multiple sclerosis 1. Clinical results of a multicenter, randomised, double-blind, placebo-controlled trial. *Neurology* 1993; **43**: 655–661.

9

The importance of viral infections and vaccinations in multiple sclerosis

Hillel Panitch

Introduction

The idea that multiple sclerosis (MS) may be caused by a virus or other infectious agent is far from new. Shortly after the original clinical and pathologic descriptions of the disease by Charcot, his student and protégé, Pierre Marie, proposed an infectious etiology for MS, and suggested that it might be prevented by vaccination.[1,2] Over 100 years later, the causative agent of MS has not yet been identified; however, it is still thought likely that infection plays a prominent role in the pathogenesis of the disease. On the basis of multiple lines of genetic, epidemiologic, pathologic, and immunologic evidence, MS is generally considered to be an immune-mediated disease in which an autoimmune response to myelin proteins is triggered by one or more exogenous agents in a genetically susceptible host.[3,4] Although bacterial infection is not a likely possibility, recent identification of the bacteria which cause conditions such as peptic ulcer and Lyme arthritis,[5] as well as the association of preceding bacterial infection with some cases of Guillain–Barré syndrome,[6] leaves open the possibility of a role for such an agent in MS. Novel agents such as the prions responsible for Creutzfeldt–Jakob disease should also not be overlooked. Nevertheless, the evidence for viral involvement is more compelling from several points of view: viruses can cause inflammatory demyelinating diseases both in animals and in humans,[7] can remain latent in the central nervous system (CNS),[8] and can also trigger exacerbations of MS.[9–11]

The recent success of interferon-beta (IFN-β) therapy in the treatment of MS[12–14] also raises the possibility that virus infection is involved in the disease. In fact, the earliest IFN treatment studies[15,16] were undertaken, at least in part, to take advantage of the antiviral activity of the interferons. It now appears, however, that the interferons act principally via their immunomodulatory rather than their antiviral properties to modify relapse rate, disease progression, and magnetic resonance imaging (MRI) activity in MS.[17,18]

This review will concentrate on the evidence for virus infection, and immune responses to virus infection, as potentially important factors in the etiology and pathogenesis of MS. If a viral cause were identified, vaccination to prevent the disease would, of course, be feasible. However, it might not be advisable if the immune response to the virus were to cross-react with myelin proteins, a mechanism for which evidence has recently appeared.[19,20] We will also address the more practical question of whether or not vaccinations such as the 'flu vaccine', commonly given to reduce the severity of influenza, are hazardous to MS patients.

Is MS caused by a virus?

Arguments for and against a viral etiology of MS are summarized in *Table 9.1*. Numerous viruses have been implicated in MS, either by serologic techniques, by isolation from brain tissue, or more recently by the polymerase chain reaction (PCR) technique to identify viral genetic material. To date, these observations have remained unconfirmed and inconclusive. However, there are other ways in which a virus can initiate disease, the most probable in this case being to activate auto-reactive T cells which enter the CNS, recognize myelin components, and begin the inflammatory process which results in demyelination. Evidence for viral involvement, though circumstantial, comes from pathologic, serologic, and epidemiologic studies.

The pathology of MS, with perivascular lymphocytic infiltrates of mononuclear cells and demyelinated gliotic plaques, is consistent with an infectious process. Similar changes can be seen in chronic viral infections in animals, such as canine distemper, caused by a paramyxovirus similar to measles; visna in

Pro:
  Pathology of MS consistent with a viral and/or autoimmune disease
  Elevated levels of IgG and oligoclonal bands in CSF
  Effect of migration between high and low risk areas
  Mini-epidemics of MS, e.g. in the Faroe Islands
  Seasonal variation of MS attack rate
  Ability of viral infections to trigger exacerbations of MS
  Isolation of viruses from brain tissue of MS patients
  Animal and human models of virus-induced inflammatory demyelination
  Similarities between MS and post-infectious or post-vaccinal encephalomyelitis
  Localization of viral antigens by immunostaining or *in situ* hybridization
  Detection of viral genomic or mRNA sequences in MS by PCR
  Molecular mimicry with activation of myelin-specific T cells by viral peptides

Con:
  Numerous unconfirmed isolations of different viruses over past 50 years
  Failure of CSF IgG or oligoclonal bands to react with specific viruses
  High frequency of antibodies to candidate agents in control populations
  Beneficial effect of corticosteroids and immunosuppressive drugs
  Effect of environmental factors minimal in some population studies
  Failure to transmit disease to animals with CNS tissue
  Induction of relapsing EAE by immunological means alone
  Molecular mimicry implicates viruses of questionable relevance to MS

Table 9.1
Arguments for and against a viral etiology of MS.

sheep, caused by a retrovirus; and Theiler's murine encephalomyelitis virus infection, caused by a picornavirus. Many of these conditions have been studied extensively as animal models of MS.[7] There are also similarities between MS and chronic human encephalitides including subacute sclerosing panencephalitis (SSPE), a late complication of measles; progressive multifocal leukoencephalopathy (PML), caused by an opportunistic papovavirus in immunosuppressed patients; the CNS complications of human immuno-deficiency virus (HIV) infection; and tropical spastic paraparesis caused by the HTLV-1 virus.[5,7] However, the pathology of MS is distinct from each of these, and is much more reminiscent of acute disseminated encephalomyelitis (ADEM) or post-infectious encephalomyelitis, a T cell-mediated autoimmune disease which can follow various viral infections and immunizations.[2]

ADEM was not uncommon as a complication of measles, occurring in one of every thousand cases prior to the advent of measles vaccination in the 1960s. It has also been described following other exanthematous diseases of childhood, and after a variety of immunizations. Several days after the primary viral infection or vaccination, patients typically develop acute symptoms of alteration of consciousness, seizures, and multifocal neurological signs. Sometimes the disease can present as acute transverse myelitis with the abrupt onset of paraplegia. Pathologically, there are perivenous mononuclear cell infiltrates with demyelination of the white matter, similar to that seen in MS. However, the virus does not persist in nervous tissue, and in the case of measles there is good evidence that it may never invade the CNS, but instead may activate autoreactive T lymphocytes which then cross the blood–brain barrier (BBB) and initiate the disease.[21] The disease is monophasic, and does not recur in those patients who

recover, although approximately 5 per cent of patients with acute transverse myelitis go on to develop MS, and an unusual variant called 'relapsing transverse myelitis' has been described.[22] In some cases ADEM may be indistinguishable from the initial attack of MS, especially in patients with typical white matter lesions on MRI scans, who have a greatly increased risk of progressing to clinically definite MS.[23]

Striking parallels exist between ADEM and experimental allergic encephalomyelitis (EAE), the classic immunologic animal model of MS, which suggest that similar autoimmune processes may be involved in both conditions. Furthermore, several animal models of virus-induced demyelination appear to include an EAE-like component, i.e. the virus infection induces an autoreactive T cell response, directed against myelin basic protein (and possibly other myelin antigens), which may be responsible for immune-mediated demyelination and other features of the disease. Examples of this phenomenon have been described in experimental coronavirus infection[24] and measles virus infection[25] of rats, as well as in Theiler's virus infection of mice.[7] However, their relevance to MS remains controversial.

Evidence for and against virus infection

Serologic studies of serum and cerebrospinal fluid (CSF) have helped to fuel the viral hypothesis of MS, although they have not resulted in its clarification. In the 1940s Kabat and co-workers[26] showed that MS patients had elevated levels of immunoglobulin G (IgG) in their CSF, and in 1962 Adams and Imagawa[27] reported elevated measles antibody titers in MS serum. In the ensuing decades, numerous investigators examined serum and CSF for viral antibodies, and found them, usually in higher titers than in control subjects.[2] Increased antibody levels were also reported for vaccinia, Epstein–Barr virus (EBV), rubella, *herpes simplex* virus (HSV), and other viruses, in some cases more than one viral titer being elevated in the same patient. The discovery of oligoclonal IgG bands in the CSF, which were not present in the serum, aroused a great deal of interest because similar bands had been described in SSPE, neurosyphilis, and other neurological diseases of known cause in which there was intrathecal synthesis of antibodies.[28] In those cases, the bands almost always reacted with the specific viral or bacterial antigen, and could be removed by absorption. Unfortunately, extensive attempts to characterize the oligoclonal bands in MS by several different techniques have failed,[29] and their identity remains a mystery.

Epidemiologic studies of MS have also contributed to the perception that it may be etiologically associated with an infectious agent. The well known north–south gradient in MS prevalence in North America and Western Europe, and a mirror-image gradient in Australia and New Zealand, suggest that exposure to an environmental factor associated with latitude may play a role in the disease. A consistent effect of migration from areas of higher to lower prevalence and vice-versa has also been described,[30] with migrants tending to maintain the risk of their country of origin, or to assume the risk of their new environment, depending on whether they move before or after the age of 12–15 years. It has been suggested that this indicates an abnormal immune response to exposure to an infectious agent at that age, with subsequent development of MS years later.[31] Clusters of MS and miniepidemics have also been reported, the most famous being the Faroe Islands 'epidemic'

which occurred from 1943 to the mid-1970s. This unique phenomenon was extensively investigated and documented by Kurtzke,[30] who described four separate outbreaks of the disease over the course of 30 years, all attributed to an agent termed the primary MS affection (PMSA), introduced by British troops during their occupation of the Faroes in World War II. Despite Kurtzke's careful documentation of clinical cases, no viral, genetic, or immunologic studies have been done, and the putative PMSA, as well as other susceptibility factors in the population, remains unknown.

Genetic factors are also thought to play a part in MS susceptibility, although it is not clear if 'susceptibility' refers to acquisition of a particular infectious agent, or to the likelihood of mounting an aberrant immunologic response to that agent. The most careful prospective studies of twins show a concordance rate of only 31 per cent in identical twins, versus 5 per cent in dizygotic twins, even with long-term follow-up and MRI studies to evaluate subclinical disease,[32] indicating that genetic factors alone are insufficient to account for the majority of cases of MS. Recent genomic screening studies, in which the entire complement of genomic DNA was searched for MS-associated sequences, were notably disappointing in that no strong linkages were identified by any of four research teams, the most consistent association being with the major histocompatibility locus on chromosome 6.[33] On the other hand, in a study of MS patients who had been adopted in infancy,[34] the risk of MS in the adoptive family was no greater than in the general Canadian population, indicating that heredity, rather than common exposure to a transmissible agent, was the principal factor in the development of MS in these patients. At present, we are left with conflicting findings about the relative contributions of genetics and environment in MS, and with a large volume of undigested data on many viruses suggesting their possible viability as candidate etiologic agents which may activate the disease.

Candidate viruses in MS

There is no assurance that MS is initiated by a known virus, or that the virus persists in the nervous system in recognizable form. In view of the difficulty of isolating such an agent thus far, it seems more probable that the primary infective agent does not persist, even in a latent state.[5] Nevertheless, over a dozen viruses have been identified in MS, either by serologic techniques, direct isolation in tissue culture, or by PCR.[2] Others are considered possible candidates for epidemiologic reasons, or because of their ability to induce MS-like inflammatory demyelination in both animals and humans. *Table 9.2* summarizes a short list of agents currently thought to be leading contenders for the title of 'MS-associated virus.'

Measles virus has probably received more scrutiny than any other agent because it fulfills so many of the requirements for an MS virus: its association with elevated antibody levels in the serum and CSF of MS patients, its ability to persist in the CNS as in SSPE, its association with a post-infectious demyelinating disease, and its effects on the immune system. In addition, some investigators have identified measles virus genetic material in brain tissue of MS patients. However, the epidemiology of measles does not correlate with that of MS, and widespread measles vaccination in developed countries has not led to a decrease in the incidence of MS, as it has in SSPE.[35]

Canine distemper virus (CDV), a neurotropic paramyxovirus similar to measles, also has its adherents as a possible causative agent of MS.[5,8,36] In its natural host, the virus can persist in the brain, causing a relapsing or progressive demyelinating disease which is pathologically similar to MS. Furthermore, there have been reports of increased exposure to dogs with CDV or similar illnesses among MS patients, and 'epidemics' of MS in the Faroe Islands and in Iceland have been linked to

Family	Examples
Paramyxovirus	Measles, canine distemper
Herpes virus	HSV-1 and 2, Epstein–Barr, HHV-6
Coronavirus	229E
Retrovirus	HTLV-1
Adenovirus	Type 2

Table 9.2
Viruses currently considered good candidates as etiologic or relapse-inducing agents in MS.

outbreaks of CDV. Because of strong antigenic similarities between measles and CDV, it has not been possible to detect CDV-specific antibodies in humans. Recently, however, Cook and co-workers[37] synthesized CDV peptides which do not cross-react with measles, and were able to show a moderately increased frequency of serum antibodies to these peptides in MS patients when compared to controls. Although these findings tend to support an association of CDV and MS, the virus has not been recovered from MS patients, it has not been detected by immunohistochemical or *in situ* hybridization techniques in MS tissue, and it has not been shown to induce a cellular immune response to myelin antigens in any species.[7] Thus its role in MS remains uncertain.

Several other viruses which have recently appeared in the literature and aroused the interest of MS investigators as possibly being implicated in MS include the HTLV-1 retrovirus, human coronavirus 229E, EBV, HSV, and human herpes virus type 6 (HHV-6). These will be discussed briefly, since they all have their pros and cons as potential candidates.

With the discovery of human retroviruses, and occurrence of the AIDS epidemic, it was natural to inquire whether MS might be associated with a retrovirus. HIV, HTLV-1 and visna, a retrovirus of Icelandic sheep, can all cause CNS demyelinating lesions. Early serologic and PCR studies[38,39] suggested that HTLV-1, the causative agent of tropical spastic paraparesis, was present in MS brain tissue. Subsequent attempts to confirm this finding were inconclusive until a large carefully controlled study[40] showed that HTLV-1 was not associated with MS, and that previous false positive results arose from the extreme sensitivity and ease of contamination of the PCR method. An association between MS and an unknown retrovirus, perhaps similar to visna, remains a possibility, but seems unlikely at the present time.

The murine JHM coronavirus causes demyelination, and has been shown to activate myelin basic protein-reactive lymphocytes which can transfer an EAE-like disease to normal recipient animals.[24] Two human coronaviruses have been identified, which are responsible for perhaps a third of common upper respiratory infections, and one of these (229E) has been implicated in MS both serologically and by detection of viral genomic sequences in patients by PCR.[41] Furthermore, T cell lines from MS patients were recently shown[42] to cross-react with myelin basic protein and coronavirus 229E antigens, providing strong evidence for molecular mimicry between this common viral pathogen and a major component of myelin.

The herpes viruses EBV and HSV have long been considered as potential culprits in MS. Several studies have shown higher titers of antibodies to EBV antigens in MS patients than in controls, and in one small study several patients with neurological complications of EBV infection subsequently developed an MS-like disease.[43] However, a clear-cut association with MS will be extremely difficult to prove, as antibody positivity is nearly universal in the normal adult population, and thus far EBV DNA has not been detected in MS brain tissue.[5] HSV is a reasonable candidate for an MS-associated virus because of its strong neurotropism, ability to establish latency in the nervous system, and association with demyelination in animal models.[7,44,45] Recently, Tourtellotte and co-workers[46] studied MS and control brain tissue for HSV-1 and HSV-2 gene sequences, and found them at a somewhat higher frequency in MS brain. However, the results were not statistically significant, and must be considered inconclusive.

HHV-6 is a recently described, nearly ubiquitous agent that causes roseola in children. It remains latent in the brain and other tissues,

Direct infection and apoptosis of oligodendroglia
Cell-mediated cytotoxicity with lysis of infected oligodendroglia
Immune response to virus with bystander demyelination
Molecular mimicry with cross-reactive immune response to myelin proteins
Activation of myelin-specific T cells with release of proinflammatory cytokines
Stimulation of auto-reactive T cells by a viral 'superantigen'

Table 9.3
Possible mechanisms of viral-induced demyelination.

usually with no untoward consequences. Most individuals are seropositive for the virus. In 1995, a flurry of interest in HHV-6 was aroused by the report[47] that it could be identified by PCR in brains of MS patients, was localized to plaques, and appeared prominently by immunohistochemical staining in the nuclei of oligodendrocytes. The principal difficulty with this study was the choice of controls, which included very few brains of patients with inflammatory diseases of the CNS. As Cook *et al.* have pointed out,[5] HHV-6 could be activated non-specifically by an inflammatory response, or possibly by immunosuppressive agents commonly used to treat MS. Further confirmation is needed before this virus can be seriously considered as a pathogenetic agent in MS.

Possible mechanisms of viral induction of autoimmunity in MS

How might these viruses activate the auto-immune processes responsible for the clinical features and inflammatory demyelination in MS? Several possibilities are listed in *Table* 9.3. Persistent or latent infection of oligodendroglia with apoptosis is a possibility, as is cell-mediated anti-viral cytotoxicity causing inflammatory demyelination. These have been extensively sought with negative results. It is more probable that viral infection of glial cells is transient, if it occurs at all, and probably takes place years before the onset of clinical disease as part of a systemic viral infection. During that initial phase, T cells are activated, including cells which recognize myelin antigens such as myelin basic protein (MBP), proteolipid protein (PLP), or myelin oligodendrocyte glycoprotein (MOG). These memory T cells then persist in the peripheral immune system (and possibly within the CNS as well), until activated by an appropriate stimulus, possibly another viral infection, acting through release of proinflammatory cytokines such as IFN-γ,[48] interleukin 12, tumor necrosis factor-alpha (TNF-α), or other soluble mediators. Virus-associated proteins can also act as 'superantigens' which may non-specifically activate autoreactive T cells.[49] The hypothetical scenario is similar in many respects to post-infectious ADEM, but on a much longer time scale, and with the additional feature of genetically based immunoregulatory dysfunction, so that the disease continues to relapse and progress.

The most probable mechanism of T-cell activation, both at the initiation of disease and subsequently, is currently thought to be the phenomenon of molecular mimicry. Mimicry has been proposed in the past by investigators who identified viral peptide sequences homologous to those of myelin antigens.[19,50] However, the observations were not pursued further until recently, when Wucherpfennig and Strominger,[20] using a more sophisticated approach, screened a large number of viral and bacterial peptides to select a panel of peptides with the appropriate amino acid side chains required for binding to the major histocompatibility complex (MHC) class II molecule, and for activating T-cell receptors specific for the immunodominant region of MBP. Of 129 peptides which fit the criteria, seven viral and one bacterial sequence were able to activate MBP-specific T-cell clones derived from MS patients. The viral peptides which give the greatest activation were specific for HSV, EBV, adenovirus type 12, influenza A, and human papillomavirus, not all of which have previously been recognized as possible MS-associated agents. Three of the T-cell clones were activated by more than one peptide. This study provides convincing evidence for molecular mimicry as a mechanism of T-cell activation, and also suggests that a single virus is probably not responsible for initiating the autoimmune response in MS.

Influence of virus infection on MS exacerbations

Numerous exogenous factors have been proposed as triggers for exacerbations of MS, including physical trauma, psychological stress, infection, immunization, and exposure to toxins. Anecdotal reports implicating minor trauma have enjoyed a degree of popularity in the legal community. However, the only relapse-associated factors documented with any degree of rigor are infection, trauma from electrical shock or penetrating injury to the CNS, and delivery after pregnancy; and even some of these remain controversial (see Sibley, Chapter 7 and Hutchinson, Chapter 8). The few prospective studies of viral infections as triggering events which have appeared[9–11,51,52] are summarized in *Table 9.4*. Perhaps the most important of these was reported by Sibley and co-workers,[9] who studied 170 MS patients and 134 healthy controls over an eight-year period to assess the influence of selected environmental events, including infection, on MS attacks. The subjects were followed by monthly questionnaires and frequent clinic visits for up to eight years, and attack rates were calculated for periods at risk (AR, from two weeks before to five weeks after the onset of upper respiratory or gastrointestinal symptoms consistent with virus infection), and for the remaining time designated not at risk (NAR). Although the AR periods accounted for only 12 per cent of the study time, 27 per cent of attacks occurred during those periods. The AR attack rate (0.64 per year) was nearly three times the NAR attack rate (0.23 per year). The median time from onset of infection to attack was eight days, and all types of viral infection (respiratory, gastrointestinal, and herpetic) gave similar results, whereas bacterial urinary tract infections were not associated with an increased risk of exacerbation. Unfortunately, no serological studies were done as part of this trial.

A similar study performed in 60 MS patients in Sweden[10] yielded similar results, although the relative risk in the AR period was not as great. Relapses tended to occur one to two weeks after the onset of upper respiratory

Reference	No. of patients	Attacks associated with URIs	URIs followed by attacks
Sibley and Foley[51]	69	48%	NA
Sibley *et al.*[9]	170	27%	8.6%
Narod *et al.*[52]	39	32%	15%
Andersen *et al.*[10]	60	NA (RR = 1.3)	NA
Panitch[11]	30	68%	32%

NA = not available; RR = relative risk.

Table 9.4
Studies of clinical viral infection and exacerbations of MS.

infections, with marked seasonal variation, the peak frequency of infections and AR relapses occurring in the spring and fall. An additional feature of this study was the inclusion of serological testing for several common respiratory viruses, resulting in a significant increase in adenovirus type 2 antibody titers in patients having relapses during AR periods. Moreover, the authors found several homologous amino acid sequences between adenovirus and both MBP and PLP, suggesting that molecular mimicry might be involved.

The most recent study on the role of infection as a trigger of MS attacks[11] was performed in conjunction with the multicenter trial of IFN-β-1b which resulted in approval of the drug for treatment of relapsing–remitting MS.[12] Thirty patients at a single clinical center kept daily logs, noting upper respiratory infection (URI) symptoms in themselves, family members, and co-workers for two years. They were examined every three months and at each relapse, and were tested periodically for antibodies to several common upper respiratory pathogens. MS attacks were classified as major or minor, and relapse rates were calculated for AR and NAR periods as in the Sibley and Andersen studies. The principal difference between this and the previous trials, was that the patients were treated either with IFN-β-1b (one-third with 8 million units, and one-third with 1.6 million units) or with placebo, given every other day by subcutaneous injection. The results were consistent with the trials described above, and also provided some insights about the effect of interferon therapy on MS activity. There was marked seasonal variation in URIs, but this was not reflected in the occurrence of MS attacks, probably because of the effect of treatment. As in the other studies, the peak attack frequency occurred one to two weeks

	Placebo	Low dose	High dose
MS attacks	41	30	24
URIs	55	50	62
Ratio	0.75	0.60	0.39

Thirty MS patients were followed for two years in the interferon beta-1b treatment trial.[11] The reduced ratios of attacks to URIs indicate that treatment with subcutaneous interferon, especially at 8 million units every other day, reduced attack frequency, although it did not prevent URIs[12].

Table 9.5
*MS attacks and upper respiratory infections
(URIs) in patients treated with interferon beta-1b.*

after the onset of URIs. A strong correlation was found between MS attacks and URIs, with approximately one-third of URIs resulting in attacks, and nearly two-thirds of attacks occurring in temporal association with URIs. Attack rates were 2.92 per year in AR periods compared to 1.16 in NAR periods ($p < 0.001$). High dose interferon treatment reduced the frequency of MS attacks, and increased the proportion of attack-free patients in the high dose group, but had no effect on the number of URIs, which remained approximately the same in all three treatment groups. Disappointingly, no serologic association with adenovirus or any other specific virus was found, except for EBV antibodies, which were thought to be elevated non-specifically during acute attacks. Perhaps if acute and convalescent titers had been obtained with each MS relapse, or if antibodies to rhinoviruses and coronaviruses had been measured, the results

would have been more compelling. Although a specific virus could not be incriminated, the importance of respiratory infections as an important trigger of MS attacks was confirmed. Finally, this study provided evidence that reduction of the relapse rate by IFN-β-1b is not simply the secondary effect of a reduction in viral infections. Rather, it is more likely that it modulates immune responses to viral infection, such as activation of myelin-reactive T cells and release of proinflammatory cytokines, which would otherwise lead to renewed clinical disease activity.

Vaccination in MS

The occurrence of ADEM after vaccinations, and the fact that MS exacerbations can be precipitated by activation of the immune system,[48] have raised questions about the safety of immunization against viral infections in

MS. Some reports have suggested that occasional patients may develop their initial symptoms of MS, or relapses of pre-existing MS, shortly after vaccination.[53] In the first prospective study, Sibley and colleagues[54] followed a group of patients receiving influenza vaccine, and found no significant increase in relapses. Similarly, patients vaccinated with the swine influenza vaccine, which caused an outbreak of Guillain–Barré syndrome in 1976, appeared to have no increase in MS symptoms.[55,56]

Miller *et al.*[57] recently attempted to address this question in a prospective study of 104 patients who were evaluated for neurologic status and development of influenza-like symptoms over a six-month period after receiving either influenza vaccine or placebo. Although the vaccinated patients had twice as many relapses as those in the placebo group (11 versus 5), the differences were not statistically significant, either in terms of MS attacks or influenza-like illness. Furthermore, seven patients in the vaccinated group developed symptoms consistent with influenza. One wonders what the results would have been had the study been conducted in a larger group of patients, and if MRI scans and viral serology had been performed in addition to the clinical observations.

The question of whether or not MS patients should receive 'flu vaccine' recurs every year, and the answer is still unclear. Most authorities feel that vaccination poses no undue risk, and is far less likely to induce a relapse than is influenza itself, which can be a severe febrile illness. We routinely recommend that patients at risk for influenza, such as health care personnel and individuals with compromised pulmonary function, receive the vaccine. The risks of other vaccines, especially those developed recently for conditions such as varicella-zoster chickenpox, hepatitis A and B, and pneumococcal pneumonia, have not been studied at all in MS. One must bear in mind the principle of molecular mimicry described above, by means of which even a killed vaccine could theoretically activate myelin reactive T cells. However, the risk to benefit ratio of these immunizations is probably low, if used in the appropriate clinical setting.

References

1. Marie P. Sclérose en plaques et maladies infectueuses. *Prog Med* 1884; **12**: 287–289.
2. Johnson RT. The virology of demyelinating disease. *Ann Neurol* 1994; **36**: S54–S60.
3. McFarlin DE, McFarland HF. Multiple sclerosis. *N Engl J Med* 1982; **307**: 1183–1188, 1246–1251.
4. Cook SD, Rohowsky-Kochan C, Bansil S *et al*. Evidence for multiple sclerosis as an infectious disease. *Acta Neurol Scand* 1995; **161**: 34–42.
5. Cook SD, Rohowsky-Kochan C, Bansil S *et al*. Evidence for a viral etiology of multiple sclerosis. In: Cook SD, ed. *Handbook of Multiple Sclerosis*, 2nd edn., New York: Marcel Dekker, Inc 1996; 97–119.
6. Enders U, Karch H, Toyka KV *et al*. The spectrum of immune responses to *Campylobacter jejuni* and glycoconjugates in Guillain–Barré syndrome and in other neuroimmunological disorders. *Ann Neurol* 1993; **34**: 136–144.
7. Dal Canto MC. Experimental models of virus-induced demyelination. In: Cook SD, ed. *Handbook of Multiple Sclerosis*, 2nd edn., New York: Marcel Dekker, Inc 1996; 53–96.
8. Cook SD, Dowling PC. Multiple sclerosis and viruses: an overview. *Neurology* 1980; **30**(2): 80–91.
9. Sibley WA, Bamford CR, Clark K. Clinical viral infections and multiple sclerosis. *Lancet* 1985; **1**: 1313–1315.
10. Andersen O, Lygner P-E, Bergström T *et al*. Viral infections trigger multiple sclerosis relapses: a prospective seroepidemiological study. *J Neurol* 1993; **240**: 417–422.
11. Panitch HS. Influence of infection on exacerbations of multiple sclerosis. *Ann Neurol* 1994; **36**: S25–S28.
12. IFNB Multiple Sclerosis Study Group. Interferon beta-1b is effective in relapsing-remitting multiple sclerosis. I. Clinical results of a multicenter, randomized, double-blind, placebo-controlled trial. *Neurology* 1993; **43**: 655–661.
13. IFNB Multiple Sclerosis Study Group and University of British Columbia MS/MRI Analysis Group. Interferon beta-1b in the treatment of multiple sclerosis: Final outcome of the randomized controlled trial. *Neurology* 1995; **45**: 1277–1285.
14. Jacobs L, Cookfair D, Rudick R *et al*. Intramuscular interferon beta-1a for disease progression in relapsing multiple sclerosis. *Ann Neurol* 1996; **39**: 285–294.
15. Jacobs L, O'Malley J, Freeman A *et al*. Intrathecal interferon reduces exacerbations of multiple sclerosis. *Science* 1981; **214**: 1026–1028.
16. Knobler RL, Panitch HS, Braheny SL. Controlled clinical trial of systemic alpha interferon in multiple sclerosis. *Neurology* 1984; **34**: 1273–1279.
17. Panitch H, Milo R. Interferon therapy for multiple sclerosis. *Int MS J* 1995; **2**: 13–25.
18. Weinstock-Guttman B, Ransohoff RM, Kinkel RP *et al*. The interferons: Biological effects, mechanisms of action, and use in multiple sclerosis. *Ann Neurol* 1995; **37**: 7–15.
19. Fujinami RS, Oldstone MBA. Amino acid homology between the encephalitogenic site of myelin basic protein and virus: mechanism for autoimmunity. *Science* 1985; **230**: 1043–1045.
20. Wucherpfennig KW, Strominger JL. Molecular mimicry in T cell mediated autoimmunity: viral peptides activate human T cell clones specific for myelin basic protein. *Cell* 1995; **80**: 695–705.
21. Johnson RT, Griffin DE, Hirsch RL *et al*. Measles encephalomyelitis – clinical and immunologic studies. *N Engl J Med* 1984; **310**: 137–141.
22. Tippett DS, Fishman PS, Panitch HS. Relapsing transverse myelitis. *Neurology* 1991; **41**: 703–706.
23. Morrissey SP, Miller DH, Kendall BE *et al*. The significance of brain magnetic resonance imaging abnormalities at presentation with clinically isolated syndromes suggestive of multiple sclerosis. *Brain* 1993; **116**: 135–146.

24. Watanabe R, Wege H, ter Meulen V. Adoptive transfer of EAE-like lesions from rats with coronavirus induced demyelinating encephalomyelitis. *Nature* 1983; **305**: 150–153.

25. Liebert UG, Linington C, ter Meulen V. Induction of autoimmune reactions to myelin basic protein in measles virus encephalitis in Lewis rats. *J Neuroimmunol* 1988; **17**: 103–118.

26. Kabat EA, Freedman DA, Murray JP *et al*. A study of the crystalline albumin, gamma globulin and total protein in the cerebrospinal fluid of one hundred cases of multiple sclerosis and other diseases. *Am J Med Sci* 1950; **219**: 55–64.

27. Adams JM, Imagawa DT. Measles antibodies in multiple sclerosis. *Proc Soc Exp Biol Med* 1962; **3**: 562–566.

28. Norrby E. Viral antibodies in multiple sclerosis. *Prog Med Virol* 1978; **24**: 1–39.

29. Vartdal F, Vandvik B, Norrby E. Viral and bacterial antibody responses in multiple sclerosis. *Ann Neurol* 1979; **8**: 248–255.

30. Kurtzke JF. Epidemiologic evidence for multiple sclerosis as an infection. *Clin Microbiol Rev* 1993; **6**: 382–427.

31. Dean G. Epidemiology of multiple sclerosis. *Neuroepidemiology* 1984; **3**: 58–73.

32. Sadovnick AD, Armstrong H, Rice GPA *et al*. A population-based study of multiple sclerosis in twins: update. *Ann Neurol* 1993; **33**: 281–285.

33. Bell JI, Lathrop GM. Multiple loci for multiple sclerosis. *Nature Genet* 1996; **13**: 377–378.

34. Ebers GC, Sadovnick AD, Risch NJ *et al*. A genetic basis for aggregation in multiple sclerosis. *Nature* 1995; **377**: 150–151.

35. Bansil S, Troiano R, Dowling PC *et al*. Measles vaccination does not prevent multiple sclerosis. *Neuroepidemiology* 1990; **9**: 248–254.

36. Cook SD, Dowling PC. A possible association between house pets and multiple sclerosis. *Lancet* 1977; **1**: 980–982.

37. Rohowsky-Kochan C, Dowling PC, Cook SD. Canine distemper virus-specific antibodies in multiple sclerosis. *Neurology* 1995; **45**: 1554–1560.

38. Koprowski H, De Freitas EC, Harper ME *et al*. Multiple sclerosis and human T-cell lymphotropic retroviruses. *Nature* 1985; **318**: 154–160.

39. Reddy EP, Sandberg-Wollheim M, Mettus RV *et al*. Amplification and molecular cloning of HTLV-1 sequences from DNA of multiple sclerosis patients. *Science* 1989; **243**: 529–533.

40. Ehrlich GD, Glaser JB, Bryz-Gornia V *et al*. Multiple sclerosis, retroviruses, and PCR. *Neurology* 1991; **41**: 335–343.

41. Stewart JN, Mounir S, Talbot PJ. Human coronavirus gene expression in the brains of multiple sclerosis patients. *Virology* 1992; **191**: 502–505.

42. Talbot PJ, Paquette J-S, Ciurli C *et al*. Myelin basic protein and human coronavirus 229E cross-reactive T cells in multiple sclerosis. *Ann Neurol* 1996; **39**: 233–240.

43. Bray PF, Culp KW, McFarlin DE *et al*. Demyelinating disease after neurologically complicated primary Epstein–Barr virus infection. *Neurology* 1992; **42**: 278–282.

44. Townsend JJ. The demyelinating effect of corneal HSV infections in normal and nude (athymic) mice. *J Neurol Sci* 1981; **50**: 435–441.

45. Kastrukoff LF, Lau AS, Kim SU. Multifocal CNS demyelination following peripheral inoculation with herpes simplex virus type 1. *Ann Neurol* 1987; **22**: 52–59.

46. Sanders VJ, Waddell AE, Felisan SL *et al*. Herpes simplex virus in postmortem multiple sclerosis brain tissue. *Arch Neurol* 1996; **53**: 125–133.

47. Challoner PB, Smith KT, Parker JD *et al*. Plaque-associated expression of human herpes virus 6 in multiple sclerosis. *Proc Natl Acad Sci USA* 1995; **92**: 7440–7444.

48. Panitch HS, Hirsch RL, Haley AS *et al*. Exacerbations of multiple sclerosis in patients treated with gamma interferon. *Lancet* 1987; **1**: 893–895.

49. Rudge P. Does a retrovirally encoded superantigen cause multiple sclerosis? *J Neurol Neurosurg Psychiatry* 1991; **54**: 853–855.

50. Jahnke U, Fischer EH, Alvord EC. Sequence homology between certain viral proteins and proteins related to encephalomyelitis and neuritis. *Science* 1985; **229**: 282–284.

51. Sibley WA, Foley J. Infection and immunization in multiple sclerosis. *Ann NY Acad Sci* 1965; **122**: 457–466.

52. Narod S, Johnson-Lussenburg CM, Zheng Q et al. Clinical viral infections and multiple sclerosis (letter). *Lancet* 1985; **2**: 165–166.

53. Miller H, Cendrowski W, Schapira K. Multiple sclerosis and vaccination. *Br Med J* 1967; **2**: 210–213.

54. Sibley WA, Bamford CR, Laguna JF. Influenza vaccination in patients with multiple sclerosis. *J Am Med Ass* **236**: 1965–1966.

55. Bamford CR, Sibley WA, Laguna JF. Swine influenza vaccination in patients with multiple sclerosis. *Arch Neurol* 1978; **35**: 242–243.

56. Myers LW, Ellison GW. Swine-influenza vaccination in multiple sclerosis. *N Engl J Med* 1976; **295**: 1204.

57. Miller AE, Morgante LA, Buchwald LY et al. A multi-center, randomized, double-blind, placebo-controlled trial of influenza immunization in multiple sclerosis. *Neurology* 1997; **48**: 312–314.

10

Immunotherapy of multiple sclerosis: what are the implications of disease heterogeneity?

Reinhard Hohlfeld

Introduction

This chapter does not intend to provide a detailed review but rather to discuss briefly general aspects of the immunotherapy of multiple sclerosis (MS). The major theme is that the more refined and differentiated therapies available in the future will require more detailed knowledge of the pathogenesis, course and prognosis of MS in order to establish categories for the (re-)classification of MS and MS variants. Recent general overviews of the immunotherapy of MS may be found in the references.[1–7]

Disease heterogeneity: Implications for therapy

In MS, as in other diseases, rational treatment depends on a thorough understanding of the aetiology and pathogenesis of the disease. The history of medicine provides numerous examples of diseases which were initially defined as clinical syndromes but had to be reclassified and often subdivided into distinct entities as more and more details of their pathogenetic processes were unravelled. Research into the pathogenesis of MS, and especially the rapidly growing number of different animal models, are beginning to reveal a remarkable heterogeneity and complexity of the pathogenetic mechanisms of inflammatory demyelinating central nervous system (CNS) disease.[8,9] In view of these developments, it seems likely that much more refined classifications can be developed in the future for the disease we today call MS. Clearly, this will dramatically improve the chances for a more differentiated therapeutic approach.

For the time being, however, our knowledge is still limited. As attempted in *Table 10.1*, subtypes of MS can be defined only by very crude, preliminary criteria which may prove totally false. Despite such limitations, *Table 10.1* can serve as a guide for the subsequent discussion.

Viral versus autoimmune aetiology

The evidence for an immunopathogenesis of MS is strong but mostly indirect, because much of it has been derived from autoimmune animal models.[9] It is still unclear whether virus(es) or other infectious agents play a role. In principle, there are three possibilities

- viruses are not involved in MS
- a primary early viral infection triggers a secondary autoimmune reaction, e.g. by 'molecular mimicry'
- or MS is caused by a persistent viral infection of the CNS.

Although numerous viruses have been incriminated over the years, most of these claims have not been substantiated. This is not

I. Aetiology		II. Pathophysiology		III. Course		IV. Stage		V. Activity		VI. Severity		VII. Other factors	
A.	Virus infection (persistent? trigger?)	A.	T-cell mediated effector mechanism	A.	Relapsing–remitting	A.	Early	A.	Active (clinical? MRI? immunological?)	A.	Mild	A.	Male
B.	Autoimmune reaction (primary? secondary?)	B.	Antibody-mediated effector mechanism	B.	Primary progressive	B.	Intermediate	B.	Inactive	B.	Moderate	B.	Female
C.	Different (unknown?) mechanism	C.	Combination of A and B	C.	Secondary progressive	C.	Late		etc.	C.	Severe	a.	HLA-DR2+
etc.		etc.		D.	Progressive–relapsing		etc.		etc.		etc.	b.	HLA-DR2−
				etc.								α.	Mitochondrial mutation+
		a.	Target autoantigen: MBP									β.	Mitochondrial mutation−
		b.	MOG										etc.
		c.	PLP										
		d.	S-100β										
		etc.											

Table 10.1
Provisional classification of MS types according to different criteria.

surprising as it is extremely unlikely that a single virus would be involved in all forms of MS. It is not so unlikely, however, that subtypes or 'variants' of MS are related to viral infection. For example, subacute leukoencephalomyelitis caused by CNS infection with human herpes virus 6 can manifest as acute MS.[10] Clearly, for appropriate treatment it is essential to identify such cases.

Although acute or persistent viral infection is probably not causative of most cases of MS, viral infection could trigger a secondary autoimmune response. It is now accepted that potentially autoaggressive T lymphocytes specific for myelin basic protein (MBP) or other autoantigens of the central nervous system pre-exist in the normal immune system of rodents[11] and primates.[12,13] One of the first hypothetical events in the pathogenesis of MS is the activation of these autoreactive, potentially autoaggressive T cells in the 'periphery' outside the CNS. This activation could occur via 'molecular mimicry' during viral (or bacterial) infection. Many bacterial and viral proteins share short sequence homologies with autoantigens.

Apart from molecular mimicry, there are several other mechanisms by which *autoreactive* T cells might be activated and thus be converted into frankly *autoaggressive* cells. For example, the T cells could be activated by stimulation with a viral or bacterial 'superantigen'. Superantigens stimulate T cells by crosslinking their T-cell receptor (TCR) β-chain with an HLA class II molecule expressed on another cell.[14–17] Because the superantigen-binding site of the TCR β-chain is shared between many different T-cell clones, superantigens can activate large numbers of T-cell clones specific for many different antigens, including autoantigens.

Autoreactive T cells could also be stimulated by completely non-specific mechanisms, such as exposure to high local concentrations of cytokines secreted in the course of unrelated inflammatory reactions. Furthermore, the loss of self-tolerance could result from a change in autoantigen expression or by crossing an anatomical barrier. Experimental support has been provided for most of these mechanisms, and it is likely that different human autoimmune diseases (and different forms of MS?) are triggered by different mechanisms. In addition, different mechanisms may operate at different stages of the same disease. It is obvious that identification of the aetiology in individual cases is not an academic problem but of the utmost practical relevance for therapy.

Cell-mediated versus antibody-mediated effector mechanisms

Although transfer experiments demonstrate that autoreactive T cells are critically important in the immunopathogenesis of experimental autoimmune encephalomyelitis (EAE) (and, by analogy, probably also MS), it is becoming increasingly clear that B cells and their products – antibodies – are equally important, especially for demyelination (see *Fig. 10.1* for a current scheme of MS pathogenesis). The lesions of classic myelin basic protein-(MBP) induced EAE in Lewis rats, which are produced by the transfer of purified MBP-specific T cells alone, are mainly inflammatory, not demyelinating. If, however, a monoclonal antibody specific for myelin oligodendrocyte glycoprotein (MOG) is co-injected with the T cells, large demyelinating lesions develop.[18,19] The fact that the transfer of T cells is necessary, but by no means sufficient for demyelination, has been observed not only with MBP-specific T cells, but also with T cells specific for other CNS autoantigens, such as MOG and S-100β. Demyelinating lesions develop also in these models after co-injection

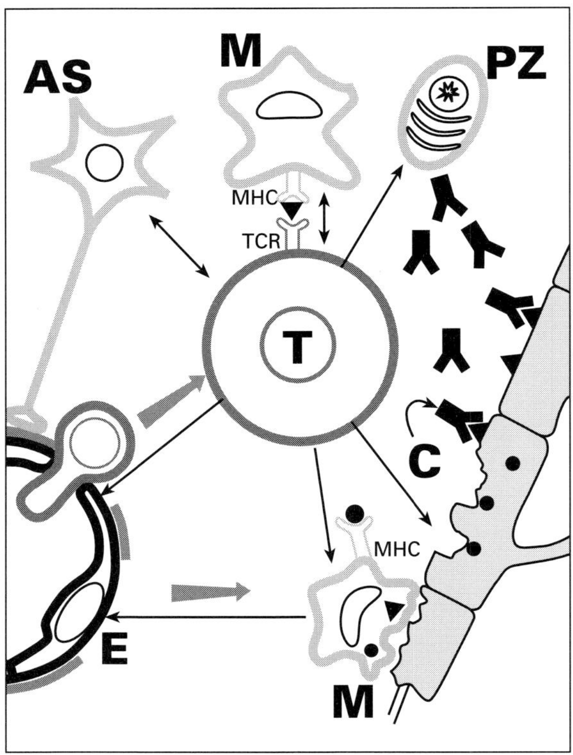

Fig. 10.1
Crucial steps in MS pathogenesis. *Pre-existing autoreactive T cells (T) are activated outside the central nervous system. The activated T cells traverse the blood–brain barrier (left; E = endothelial cell) and are locally reactivated when they recognize 'their' antigen on the surface of local antigen-presenting cells (centre). The activated T cells secrete cytokines which stimulate microglia cells (M) and astrocytes (AS), recruit additional inflammatory cells, and induce antibody production by plasma cells (PZ). Antimyelin antibodies and activated macrophages/microglia (M) are thought to cooperate in myelin destruction (right). Further abbreviations: C = complement; MHC = major histocompatibility complex; TCR = T-cell receptor for antigen.*

of anti-MOG antibody.[20,21] These observations support the concept that T cells specific for various CNS autoantigens initiate inflammation and disturb the blood–brain barrier (BBB), whereas autoantibodies against surface antigens of myelin or oligodendrocytes are required to produce demyelination.[9,22]

Very little information is available on the exact mechanisms of antibody-mediated demyelination. There is evidence that after binding to the myelin surface, demyelinating autoantibodies activate complement and attract macrophages and microglia.[23–25] The macrophages contribute to demyelination not only by physically 'stripping' the myelin, but also by directed release of inflammatory mediators, including reactive oxygen species and eicosanoids. Furthermore, macrophages secrete tumour necrosis factor (TNF-α), also thought to participate in myelin injury.[26–28] In addition, some mediators and cytotoxic factors are presumably provided by activated glial cells, thus contributing to myelin injury.[29,30]

Obviously, the relative role of the different effector mechanisms (T cells, B cells and antibodies, and others) and autoantigens (MBP, MOG, PLP, S-100β, and others) is a critical factor for immunotherapy. Extensive efforts have recently been made to tilt pathogenic T-cell responses from TH1-type to TH2-type. The rationale behind this strategy is that TH1 T cells, which produce proinflammatory cytokines such as interferon(IFN)-γ and TNF-α, often act as disease-mediating inflammatory cells, whereas TH2 T cells, which produce interleukin(IL)-4 and IL-10 and provide help for antibody-producing B cells, are often beneficial and can ameliorate autoimmune disease. As discussed above, both TH1 and TH2 cells seem to play a pathogenic role in MS. This role may vary in different forms and cases. Thus, tilting the T-cell response may have unforeseen deleterious, rather than the expected beneficial, consequences.[31]

An important, still unresolved, problem is how the relative importance of the different autoantigens and effector mechanisms can be established in an individual patient. Histological studies provide evidence for pathogenic heterogeneity. For example, Lucchinetti *et al.* presented a new classification scheme of lesional activity based on the composition of myelin degradation products in macrophages.[8] These criteria allow one to distinguish between different patterns of demyelination, including demyelination with relative preservation of oligodendrocytes, myelin destruction with concomitant, complete destruction of oligodendrocytes, and primary destruction of oligodendrocytes with secondary demyelination.[8] It would not be surprising if the lesional morphologies reflect different pathogenic mechanisms, requiring differentiated immunotherapy.

Relapsing versus progressive course

It is presently unclear whether the clinical course really provides helpful criteria to define subtypes of MS for differentiated therapy. Most ongoing clinical studies empirically differentiate (more or less rigorously) between relapsing–remitting and progressive MS, excluding primary progressive MS. More results are needed to decide whether such distinction is meaningful. A comprehensive review of primary chronic progressive MS may be found in Thompson *et al.*[32]

Early versus late stages of disease

Common sense and clinical judgement would suggest that the earlier immunotherapy is initiated, the better the chances are for preventing deficit. Arguments against very early treatment include the high cost of long-term therapy and adverse reactions, which could diminish or abolish therapeutic effectiveness at a later stage when therapy is urgently needed (e.g. development of neutralizing antibodies to IFN-β). In particular, the 'tolerance-inducing' therapies (see below) appear suitable for early therapy.

At the other end of the clinical spectrum, patients with severe impairment have an increased risk for various adverse reactions to immunotherapy. Furthermore, immunotherapy cannot be expected to reverse a pre-existing chronic deficit. Therefore, patients with advanced disease are bad candidates for immunotherapy, and aggressive immunosuppressive treatments are usually contraindicated.

Active versus inactive phases

Ideally, the intensity of immunosuppressive or immunomodulatory treatment should be adjusted to disease activity. How can disease activity be measured? One of the first lessons learned from MRI studies was that clinical activity is a very poor indicator of disease activity. It is probably unrealistic to assume that the currently available MRI techniques alone can provide reliable and feasible indicators of disease activity for therapeutic monitoring. However, the various imaging techniques have an enormous potential, and it is conceivable that they can in the future be developed into practicable and reliable tools for assessing disease activity.[33,34]

As far as laboratory markers of disease activity are concerned, the consensus is that, as yet, none of the proposed 'activity markers' (e.g. T-cell subsets, myelin degradation products, cytokine levels and expression, etc.) has proved suitable for routine monitoring of disease activity. There are many reasons for this, mostly related to limitations of the feasibility, reliability, sensitivity and specificity of the various assays. Despite the unsolved problems, it is likely that more dependable and feasible laboratory tests of disease activity will soon be developed.

Mild versus severe MS

There are presently no perfect criteria for assessing, let alone predicting, the individual course and severity of MS. Clearly, such criteria are crucial for a decision on whether and when to initiate immunomodulatory treatment. There is no need to treat benign MS, but MS cases with poor prognosis should be treated early. There is some evidence that imaging studies may help assess the severity and prognosis in individual cases,[35–37] but a precise prediction is not possible.

Immunotherapeutic strategies

The need for differentiating between distinct types of MS is underscored by the growing number of immunotherapies either already approved and available or in an advanced or early stage of clinical development. At present, there is little information on how the different therapies can be optimally applied in different types of MS.

In this section, some general aspects of immunotherapy will be addressed. Detailed reviews may be found in the references at the end of this chapter.[1–7]

Immunosuppression versus immunomodulation

It has become fashionable to speak of 'immunomodulation' rather than 'immunosuppression'. Immunomodulation suggests a gentle and sophisticated technique in contrast to a brutal and crude immunosuppression. This is certainly an oversimplification. However, because the term 'immunomodulation' is more comprehensive than 'immunosuppres-

sion', it seems more accurate. It should be remembered, however, that for most immunomodulatory therapies the mechanism of action is far from clear, and the long-term effects on the immune system are unknown. Furthermore, most immunomodulatory therapies have an immunosuppressive component, and *vice versa*. Thus, in the last analysis, the distinction is perhaps more semantic than real.

Chemical versus biological agents

Advances in biotechnology have promoted the development of a new class of biotechnological products for immunotherapy. These biotechnological agents are used to manipulate the immune system by selectively mimicking, inhibiting, or otherwise interacting with naturally occurring polypeptides or oligonucleotides (*Table 10.2*[7]). In comparison, 'chemical immunomodulators' are small (not necessarily synthetic) molecules distinct from proteins and oligonucleotides. Some of the new biotechnological agents hold the promise of an unprecedented selectivity of action. On the other hand, these agents present a number of specific problems, ranging from inconvenient application (by subcutaneous, intramuscular or intravenous injection) to immunogenicity (stimulation of neutralizing antibodies). Thus, it is obvious that biotechnological agents are not necessarily superior to chemical immunomodulators.

Monotherapy versus combination therapy

It is only logical to consider combining different immunotherapies which work via different mechanisms. A striking example for the effectiveness of combined therapy has recently been provided by anti-viral therapy in HIV infection. Obviously, the difficulty is to select the right agents to combine, as well as the right

- Therapy with cytokines and anti-cytokines
    - Interferons
    - TNF antagonists
    - Cytokine-induced 'immune deviation'
    - TGF-β
    - Interleukin-10
    - Interleukins-4 and 13
    - Interleukin-1 inhibitors
    - Chemokines
    - Other cytokines
- Anti-inflammatory agents
    - Inhibitors of matrix metalloproteinases
- Therapies directed at cell interaction and differentiation molecules, such as
    - Adhesion molecules
    - Costimulatory molecules
    - Leukocyte differentiation molecules
- Immunotherapies targeting the 'Trimolecular complex'
    - MHC inhibitors
    - Altered peptide ligands
    - Oral tolerance
    - Other strategies of tolerance induction by modification of antigen presentation
    - Copolymer-1
    - Vaccination with T cells or TCR peptides

Table 10.2
Biotechnological agents for the immunotherapy of MS.[7]

type of MS. An important potential problem is that the different immune mechanisms targeted by different agents may be interdependent, so that one agent depends on the intactness of mechanisms inhibited by another agent. Clinical trials need to look carefully for such adverse interactions, which are difficult to predict. Examples of plausible combinations (which, incidentally, present a major challenge for trial design) include IFN-β plus copolymer-1, or IFN-β plus azathioprine.

Tolerance-inducing versus permanent immunotherapy

Ideally, immunotherapy would not have to be applied indefinitely, but only for a limited, short time to achieve a permanent result. Such tolerance-inducing therapy has indeed been achieved in experimental situations, especially transplantation models. For example, permanent xenograft tolerance has been induced by a somewhat drastic approach: mice were thymectomized, purged *in vivo* with monoclonal antibodies specific for T cells and natural killer cells, given whole body irradiation, and then grafted with fetal pig thymus and liver tissues. The immune system of these mice appeared functional but permanently tolerated skin transplants from the porcine father of the fetal donors.[38] While these experiments have only indirect relevance for MS, they demonstrate that it is possible to achieve a state of permanent and selective immune tolerance by combining different immunological manipulations. By analogy, it may be possible to 'silence' an ongoing immune reaction permanently by combining different immunotherapies. Possible approaches include combinations of anti-leukocyte differentiation antigens, combinations of anti-costimulatory agents, and various strategies for 'immune deviation'.[7]

Selective versus non-selective therapies

Selective, antigen-specific immunotherapies target the trimolecular complex (TMC) of T-cell stimulation.[39,40] In principle, each component of the TMC can be targeted. The major histocompatibility (MHC) molecule could be blocked by anti-MHC antibodies or 'blocking peptides'; the antigen (or antigenic peptide) could be applied in such a way that the autoreactive T cells are inhibited rather than stimulated; and the TCR could be targeted with anti-TCR antibodies or by T cell or TCR peptide vaccination.[7]

The concept of antigen-selective immunotherapy is very attractive, but it poses special practical problems. For example, it has been shown that the T-cell response against various candidate CNS autoantigens is much more

complex in humans than it is in certain inbred rodent strains. This implies that selective immunotherapy needs to be 'individualized' (tailored for individual patients). Furthermore, there is growing evidence that the autoimmune response is not static but dynamic. For example, new autoantigens may be recruited over time. Conceivably, this 'antigen spreading' might not be slowed but accelerated by certain immunotherapies.

The first approved agent with alleged selectivity for myelin autoantigens (MBP, PLP, MOG) is copolymer-1.[41] However, as long as the exact mechanisms of action are unknown, it is difficult to judge how antigen-specific copolymer-1 therapy really is.

Conclusion: Prospects for a differentiated immunotherapy of MS

In order to make optimal use of the increasing number of immunotherapies, it is essential to improve our understanding of the pathogenic and clinical heterogeneity of MS. Eventually, it must be possible to classify and stage the disease in order to design the therapy for each individual patient. We are presently at a relatively early stage of this development. While our current therapies are clearly better than those of only a few years ago, they may appear almost primitive in the near future.

Acknowledgement

I am grateful to Mrs Judy Benson for valuable comments and for a critical reading of the manuscript.

References

1. Ebers GC. Treatment of multiple sclerosis. *Lancet* 1994; **343**: 275–280.
2. Noseworhty JH. Immunosuppressive therapy in multiple sclerosis: Pros and cons. *Int MS J* 1994; **1**: 79–89.
3. Weiner HL, Hohol MJ, Khoury SJ *et al*. Therapy for multiple sclerosis. *Neurol Clinics* 1995; **13**: 173–196.
4. Polman CH, Hartung H-P. The treatment of multiple sclerosis: Current and future. *Curr Opin Neurol* 1995; **8**: 200–209.
5. Hommes OR, Sandberg M, Silberberg D. Emerging treatments in multiple sclerosis. *Multiple Sclerosis* 1996; **1**: 306–403.
6. Thompson AJ, Noseworthy JH. New treatments for multiple sclerosis: A clinical perspective. *Curr Opin Neurol* 1996; **9**: 187–198.
7. Hohlfeld R. Biotechnological agents for the immunotherapy of multiple sclerosis: Principles, problems, and perspectives. *Brain* 1997; **120**: 865–916.
8. Lucchinetti CF, Brück W, Rodriguez M *et al*. Distinct patterns of multiple sclerosis pathology indicates heterogeneity in pathogenesis. *Brain Pathol* 1996; **6**: 259–274.
9. Wekerle H, Kojima K, Lannes-Vieira J *et al*. Animal models. *Ann Neurol* 1994; **36**: S47–S53.
10. Carrigan DR, Harrington D, Knox KK. Subacute leukoencephalitis caused by CNS infection with human herpesvirus-6 manifesting as acute multiple sclerosis. *Neurology* 1996; **47**: 145–148.
11. Schluesener HJ, Wekerle H. Autoaggressive T lymphocyte lines recognizing the encephalitogenic region of myelin basic protein: In vitro selection from unprimed rat T lymphocyte populations. *J Immunol* 1985; **135**: 3128–3133.
12. Burns J, Rosenzweig A, Zweiman B *et al*. Isolation of myelin basic protein-reactive T cell lines from normal human blood. *Cell Immunol* 1983; **81**: 435–440.
13. Genain CP, Lee-Parritz D, Nguyen M-H *et al*. In healthy primates, circulating autoreactive T cells mediate autoimmune disease. *J Clin Invest* 1994; **94**: 1339–1345.
14. Marrack P, Kappler JW. The staphylococcal enterotoxins and their relatives. *Science* 1990; **248**: 705–710.
15. Scherer MT, Ignatowicz L, Winslow GM *et al*. Superantigens: Bacterial and viral proteins that manipulate the immune system. *Annu Rev Cell Biol* 1993; **9**: 101–128.
16. Fleischer B. Superantigens. *Acta Pathol Microbiol Immunol Scand [C]* 1995; **102**: 3–12.
17. Kotzin BL, Leung DYM, Kappler J *et al*. Superantigens and their potential role in human disease. *Adv Immunol* 1995; **54**: 99–166.
18. Linington C, Bradl M, Lassmann H *et al*. Augmentation of demyelination in rat acute allergic encephalomyelitis by circulating mouse monoclonal antibodies directed against a myelin/oligodendrocyte glycoprotein. *Am J Pathol* 1988; **130**: 443–454.
19. Genain CP, Nguyen M-H, Letvin NL *et al*. Antibody facilitation of multiple sclerosis-like lesions in a nonhuman primate. *J Clin Invest* 1995; **96**: 2966–2974.
20. Linington C, Berger T, Perry L *et al*. T cells specific for the myelin oligodendrocyte glycoprotein (MOG) mediate an unusual autoimmune inflammatory response in the central nervous system. *Eur J Immunol* 1993; **23**: 1364–1372.
21. Kojima K, Berger T, Lassmann H, *et al*. Experimental autoimmune panencephalitis and uveoretinitis in the Lewis rat transferred by T lymphocytes specific for the S100β molecule, a calcium binding protein of astroglia. *J Exp Med* 1994; **180**: 817–829.
22. Lassmann H, Vass K. Are current immunological concepts of multiple sclerosis reflected by the immunopathology of its lesions? *Springer Semin Immunopathol* 1995; **17**: 77–87.
23. Compston A, Scolding N, Wren D *et al*. The pathogenesis of demyelinating disease: Insights

from cell biology. *Trends Neurosci* 1991; **14:** 175–182.

24. Hartung H-P, Archelos JJ, Zielasek J *et al.* Circulating adhesion molecules and inflammatory mediators in demyelination: A review. *Neurology* 1995; **45** (suppl 6): S22–S32.

25. Brosnan CF, Raine CS. Mechanisms of immune injury in multiple sclerosis. *Brain Pathol* 1996; **6:** 243–257.

26. Brosnan CF, Selmaj K, Raine CS. Hypothesis: A role for tumor necrosis factor in immune-mediated demyelination and its relevance to multiple sclerosis. *J Neuroimmunol* 1988; **18:** 87–94.

27. Selmaj KW, Raine CS. Tumor necrosis factor mediates myelin and oligodendrocyte damage in vitro. *Ann Neurol* 1988; **23:** 339–346.

28. Selmaj K, Raine CS, Farooq M *et al.* Cytokine cytotoxicity against oligodendrocytes. Apoptosis induced by lymphotoxin. *J Immunol* 1991; **147:** 1522–1529.

29. Selmaj K, Raine CS, Cannella B *et al.* Identification of lymphotoxin and tumor necrosis factor in multiple sclerosis lesions. *J Clin Invest* 1991; **87:** 949–954.

30. Cannella B, Raine CS. The adhesion molecule and cytokine profile of multiple sclerosis lesions. *Ann Neurol* 1995; **37:** 424–435.

31. Genain CP, Abel K, Belmar N *et al.* Late complications of immune deviation therapy in a nonhuman primate. *Science* 1996; **274:** 2054–2057.

32. Thompson AJ, Polman CH, Miller DH *et al.* Primary progressive multiple sclerosis: A review. *Brain* 1997; **120:** 1085–1096.

33. Miller, DH. Magnetic resonance imaging and spectroscopy in multiple sclerosis. *Curr Opin Neurol* 1995; **8:** 210–215.

34. Miller DH, Albert PS, Barkhof F *et al.* Guidelines for the use of magnetic resonance techniques in monitoring the treatment of multiple sclerosis. *Ann Neurol* 1996; **39:** 6–16.

35. Filippi M, Horsfeld MA, Morrissey SP *et al.* Quantitative brain MRI lesion load predicts the course of clinically isolated syndromes suggestive of multiple sclerosis. *Neurology* 1994; **44:** 635–641.

36. Truyen L, van Waesberghe JHTM, van Walderveen MAA *et al.* Accumulation of hypointense lesions ("black holes") on T1 spin-echo MRI correlates with disease progression in multiple sclerosis. *Neurology* 1996; **47:** 1469–1476.

37. Losseff NA, Webb SL, O'Riordan JI *et al.* Spinal cord atrophy and disability in multiple sclerosis. A new reproducible and sensitive MRI method with potential to monitor disease progression. *Brain* 1996; **119:** 701–708.

38. Zhao Y, Swenson K, Sergio JJ *et al.* Skin graft tolerance across a discordant xenogeneic barrier. *Nat Med* 1996; **2:** 1211–1216.

39. Hohlfeld R. Neurological autoimmune disease and the trimolecular complex of T-lymphocytes. *Ann Neurol* 1989; **25:** 531–538.

40. Wraith DC, McDevitt HO, Steinman L *et al.* T cell recognition as the target for immune intervention in autoimmune disease. *Cell* 1989; **57:** 709–715.

41. Arnon R. The development of Cop-1 (Copaxone®), an innovative drug for the treatment of multiple sclerosis. *Immunol Lett* 1996; **50:** 1–15.

11

Do steroids have a long-term benefit?

Xavier Montalban

Adrenocorticotrophic hormone (ACTH) and glucocorticosteroids (GCs) were introduced as therapeutic agents in the late 1940s and remain the mainstay of treatment for many autoimmune disorders including multiple sclerosis (MS). Since then, many uncontrolled and controlled trials have been conducted to determine optimal therapy. These trials have been extensively reviewed, and for more detailed discussion the interested reader is referred elsewhere.[1–6] The primary effect of ACTH results from the secretion of adrenocorticosteroids. A direct effect of ACTH on the immune system is not clear. Furthermore, some patients with MS exhibit a variable response to ACTH.[7] For all these reasons I am not going to review this agent in this chapter, and only the randomized controlled trials will be mentioned.

What are steroids?

Steroids are adrenocorticohormones, which are divided into GCs and mineralocorticoids based on their biological activity. GCs are produced by the adrenal cortex under the regulatory influence of ACTH. The latter is produced by corticotrophs of the anterior pituitary, in turn, under the regulatory influence of hypothalamic corticotrophin-releasing hormone (CRH) and arginine vasopressin (AVP). In the resting state, basal levels of CRH, AVP, ACTH, and cortisol, are released in a pulsatile and circadian fashion. At these baseline levels, the main function of cortisol is to sustain normal blood glucose levels and to prevent arterial hypotension. Whether and to what extent the immunosuppressive effects of cortisol are relevant at resting state levels in humans is still unknown. GCs modulate a large number of metabolic, cardiovascular, immune, and behavioural functions and they prevent or suppress inflammation and other immunologically mediated processes at pharmacologic doses. They are among the most potent anti-inflammatory agents and exert most of their effects through specific, ubiquitously distributed intracellular receptors. The anti-inflammatory potency, quantitated in a bioassay which measures the suppression of swelling of rat paw or rabbit ear induced by an irritant, parallels the glucocorticoid potency (*Table 11.1*).

GCs circulate in blood, either in the free form or in association with cortisol-binding globulin. The former, as lipophilic substances, can readily cross the cell membrane to interact with high affinity with the glucocorticoid receptors. This unliganded receptor is part of a multiprotein complex which consists of the receptor, two molecules of hsp90, and one molecule each of hsp70, and hsp56, an immunophilin of the FK506 binding class. In addition, and depending on the stringency of the extraction conditions, other, less well characterized proteins have occasionally been

	Glucocorticoid activity	Mineralocorticoid activity	Biological half-life (hours)
Cortisol	1	1	8–12
Prednisone	4	0.8	24–36
Methylprednisolone	5	0.5	24–36
Dexamethasone	25	0	56–96

Table 11.1
Biological activity of commonly used GCs.

found to participate in this complex. Experimental evidence supports a model of constant bidirectional shuttling of the complex between the cytosol and the nucleus. The exact composition of the complex may determine the predominant direction of this movement. When the ligand binds, the receptor dissociates from the rest of the hetero-oligomer and is no longer able to reassociate with it. Inside the nucleus, the hormone-receptor complexes bind to specific glucocorticoid responsive elements within DNA. These elements can act both positively and negatively on transcription, depending on the gene on which the complex acts. In addition to modulating transcription, GCs also have effects on later cellular events, including RNA translation, protein synthesis, and secretion (*Fig. 11.1*).

What are the effects of GCs?

Anti-inflammatory and immunosuppressive effects

GCs inhibit the access of leukocytes to inflammatory sites, interfere with their function and suppress the production and the effects of humoral factors. Although GCs affect many, if not all, the cells and tissues of the body, in general, leukocyte traffic is more susceptible to alteration by GCs than is cellular function; in turn, cellular immunity is more susceptible than humoral immunity. Several factors influence the magnitude of these effects, including

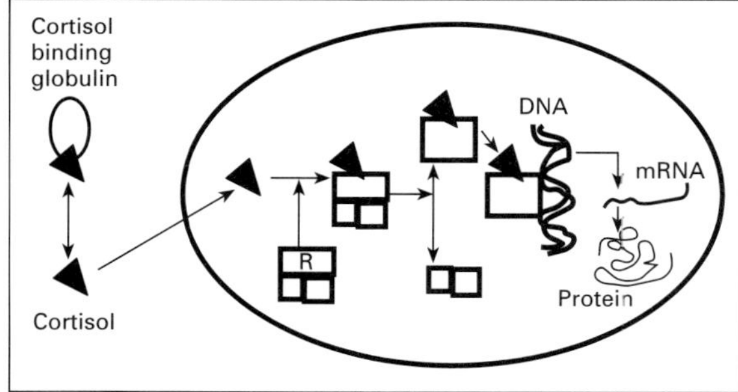

Fig. 11.1
Schematic mechanism of action of GCs.

the dose and route of administration, as well as the type and differentiation state of the target cell population. There are also several important host variables which modify the anti-inflammatory response to GCs. Some patients with systemic lupus erythematosus (SLE) appear to have an increase in glucocorticoid catabolism. Target tissue resistance may also exist in SLE and rheumatoid arthritis. These factors may explain the variable therapeutic responses observed in different patients and diseases.

Non-lymphoid inflammatory cells

Macrophages   GCs inhibit expression of class II major histocompatibility complex (MHC) antigens induced by interferon (IFN)-γ, block the release of cytokines, such as interleukin (IL)-1 IL-6 and tumour necrosis factor (TNF)-α, depress production and release of pro-inflammatory prostaglandins and leukotrienes and depress macrophages activity.

Neutrophils   The major effect is inhibition of neutrophil adhesion to endothelial cells; this is probably the explanation for the characteristic neutrophilia.

Endothelial cells   GCs have profound effects on the activation and subsequent function of endothelial cells. They inhibit up-regulation of the expression of class II major histocompatibility complex (MHC) antigens as well as endotoxin-induced up-regulated expression of the adhesion molecules endothelial leukocyte adhesion molecule-1 (ELAM-1 or CD62-E) and intercellular cell adhesion molecule-1 (ICAM-I or CD54), which are critical to leukocyte localization.

Lymphocytes

A single dose of GC produces a marked but transient lymphocytopenia. The mechanism involves the redistribution of circulating lymphocytes to other lymphoid compartments, particularly the bone marrow and, in some cases, apoptosis of immature human T cells and activated T cells.

GCs also inhibit T-cell activation, IL-2 and IFN-γ production, among others. Thus GCs inhibit cytotoxic, helper and suppressor T cells. Ramirez *et al.* showed an increase in IL-4 production and IL-4, IL-10, and IL-13 mRNA levels and a decrease in IFN-γ and TNF synthesis on reactivated rat CD4+ T cells which had previously been cultured for one week in the presence of dexamethasone.[8] On the other hand, B cells are relatively resistant to the immunosuppressive effects of GCs. A brief course of daily high-dose prednisone decreases serum immunoglobulin levels. T cells are therefore affected more than B cells and helper cells more than suppressor cells.

For more detailed discussion of the pharmacology of GCs the interested reader is referred elsewhere.[9,10]

What immunological parameters do GCs modify in MS?

High dose intravenous methylprednisolone (IVMP) decreases central nervous system (CNS) immunoglobulin G (IgG) synthesis within 3–6 days after treatment and for up to 60 days following treatment in patients with MS.[11] Treatment with IVMP significantly reduces CSF myelin basic protein (MBP) and anti-MBP antibody levels in patients with MS.[12] In some studies oligoclonal bands have been noted to disappear in some patients with MS.[11] Rosenberg and colleagues suggested that steroids may improve capillary function by reducing activity of gelatinase B and urokinase type plasminogen activator and increasing levels of tissue inhibitor to metalloproteinases.[13] The improvement of all of these pathologic parameters could be a non-specific effect of steroid treatment, since a cause-and-effect relationship between normalized laboratory values and clinical remission has never been established.

Hypothalamic–pituitary–adrenal axis function in MS

Inflammatory cytokines acutely and chronically stimulate the hypothalamus to activate pituitary–adrenal function, with resultant glucocorticoid-mediated restraint of the immune system. After administration of MBP, Lewis rats, which do not have the ability to increase adequately the secretion of CRH after exposure to an inflammatory agent, developed experimental autoimmune encephalomyelitis (EAE) which can be prevented by the administration of GCs, whereas EAE-resistant strains of rats can be made susceptible by adrenalectomy.[14] Patients with MS have significantly higher plasma cortisol levels at baseline, but more normal plasma ACTH responses to CRH and blunted ACTH responses to AVP.[15] Purba *et al.* showed a significant increase in the number of CRH-expressing neurons in the paraventricular nucleus of the hypothalamus of MS patients.[16] Grasser and co-workers showed an heterogeneity of the hypothalmic–pituary–adrenal (HPA) system function, most likely at the corticosteroid receptor level, which may have clinical implications for all those treatments which affect HPA system and the course of MS.[17] Whether HPA axis activity may have contributed to the initial susceptibility to MS or to the continuation of the ongoing process is still unknown.

Are GCs useful in acute exacerbation of MS?

CSF concentrations of MP are high six hours after high-dose IVMP treatment.[18] Several studies and clinical experience clearly indicate that GCs hasten the rate of recovery from acute exacerbations of MS. It has not been shown definitively, however, that these drugs enhance the degree of recovery.

Clinical trials

Durelli *et al.* conducted a double-blind placebo-controlled trial of high-dose IVMP (15 mg/kg/day on days 1–3, 10 mg/kg/day on days 4–6, 5 mg/kg/day on days 7–9, 2.5 mg/kg/day on days 10–12, and 1 mg/kg/day on days 13–15) on 23 patients with MS in acute relapse. Bout duration was significantly lower in the IVMP group patients at the 15th day. They also concluded, through an uncontrolled one year follow-up, that this therapy was ineffective in modifying the long-term natural history.[11]

Milligan and colleagues carried out a randomized double-blind, placebo-controlled trial of high dose IVMP (500 mg daily for five days) in 22 patients with MS in acute relapse. The IVMP treated patients showed significant decreased disability scores at one and four weeks after treatment compared to controls.[19]

Since gastrointestinal absorption of corticosteroids is excellent, the same effect might be obtained from the more feasible and comparable dose of oral corticosteroids. Alam *et al.* performed a randomized double-blind placebo-controlled trial of IVMP versus oral MP at an equivalent high dose (500 mg/day for five days) on 35 MS patients with an acute relapse. Although a type II error (false negative) due to small sample size cannot be ruled out, oral treatment was as effective as intravenous treatment in acute relapse of MS, and no major adverse events were seen in either group, including no increase in gastrointestinal symptoms in the oral group.[20] However, a comparison of intravenous and oral absorption efficacy using 1000 mg doses suggests individual variability with the oral absorption ranging from 70 to 80 per cent of the levels from intravenous administration.[21]

How do GCs modify magnetic resonance imaging (MRI)?

A breakdown of the blood–brain barrier (BBB) in association with inflammation is the earliest detectable event in the development of the new lesion in MS.[22] BBB impairment in MS lesions can now be readily detected and monitored by gadolinium-diethylene triamine pentaacetic acid (Gd-DTPA) enhanced MRI (*Fig. 11.2*). Consistent and rapid suppression of MRI enhancement during GC treatment has been widely demonstrated. Route of administration can be less important than dose. Troiano *et al.* performed 50 computed tomography scans on 36 patients within four months of a clinical relapse to determine the effect on lesion enhancement of high dose GC therapy (prednisone 60–120 mg/day), low-dose GC therapy (prednisone 10–50 mg/day or up to 100 mg every other day), or no GC therapy. Multiple enhancing lesions were seen in 75 per cent of positive scans in the untreated group and in 70 per cent of positive scans in the low-dose group. In the high-dose group, however, multiple enhancing lesions were not found.[23]

Burnham *et al.* reported on the effects of IVMP (1000 mg/day) for four to eight days on Gd-enhancing lesions in seven patients with acute demyelinating diseases and compared pretreatment brain MRIs with studies obtained one to four days after treatment. Five patients had complete suppression and two had significant suppression of Gd enhancement.[24]

Barkoff *et al.* also showed a significant reduction in the number of Gd-enhancing lesions after high dose IVMP (1000 mg/day for ten days).[25,26] Interestingly, it was uncommon for a lesion which stopped enhancing to show enhancement on a subsequent examina-

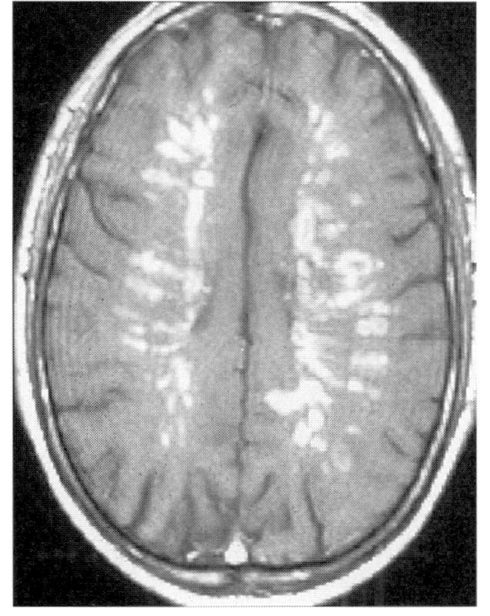

(a)

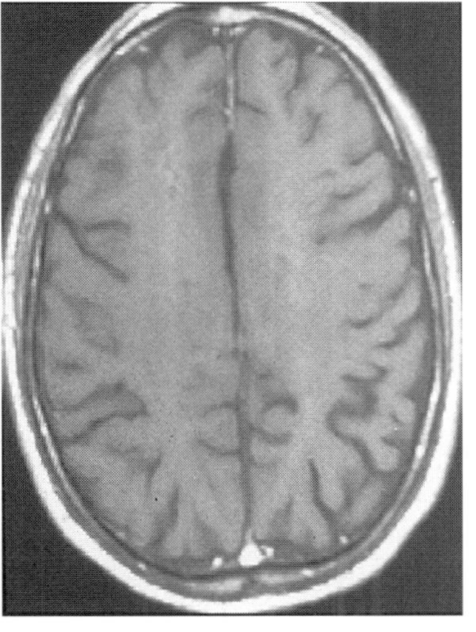

(b)

Fig. 11.2
Dramatic reduction in the number of Gd-enhancing lesions after high dose IVMP therapy. (a) Diffuse-enhanced and (b) no enhancement.

tion. The authors concluded that the effect of MP is temporary (on average 9.7 weeks).[26]

Miller and colleagues also showed a rapid reduction of BBB abnormalities in 96 per cent of enhancing lesions after a three-day course of high dose IVMP (1000 mg/day for three days). Nevertheless these authors showed that many lesions re-enhanced within a few days of stopping IVMP and new lesions appeared within one month.[27]

What are the side effects of a single bolus of high dose IVMP?

Adverse effects during short-term, high-dose IVMP are usually minor. A facial flush may suddenly appear and a facial erythema may persist throughout the period of treatment. A metallic taste during the infusion and acne in the days or weeks following are also common.

Other less common adverse effects are euphoria, insomnia, restlessness, hallucination, paranoid ideation, psychoses or seizures. They are probably secondary to the binding of GCs to receptors in the brain. Sleep disturbance, mild mood change, stomach upset and facial flushing were significantly more frequent in the Optic Neuritis Treatment Trial (ONTT) treated patients. Serious side effects were rare, one patient developed severe depression on the third day of the IV treatment and another developed acute pancreatitis.[28] Some studies showed normal hypothalamic–pituitary–adrenal axis function after IVMP bolus therapy, suggesting that GC coverage is not required.[29] A single high dose pulse of IVMP does not reduce bone density in fully ambulatory patients and multiple pulses seem not to have a cumulative effect on bone density.[30] Anaphylaxis reactions and sudden death have anecdotally been reported following IVMP.[31,32]

Does a single dose of GC have long-lasting effects on the natural history of MS?

Optic Neuritis Treatment Trial

In December 1993, Beck *et al.* reported the latest and most important finding from the ONTT.[33] Intravenous methylprednisolone (1 g/day for three days), followed by oral prednisone (1 mg/kg/day for 11 days), prescribed for patients with acute, isolated optic neuritis, reduced the two-year incidence of definite MS by more than 50 per cent. Visual acuity recovered faster in the patients who received IVMP than in controls. No differences were observed after six months. Visual field, colour sense and contrast sensitivity also recovered somewhat faster in the methylprednisolone group than in controls, though slight advantage in these aspects persisted at six months but no long-term visual benefit was observed.

Among the 389 patients in the ONTT who did not have MS at study entry, 10 (7.5 per cent) of 134 intravenously treated patients developed at least one neurological event, thus being diagnosed MS within two years, compared with 21 (16.7 per cent) of 126 placebo-treated patients. This was a significant reduction ($p = 0.063$) in the MS conversion rate at the two-year stage. No differences were observed between patients treated with oral prednisone (14.7 per cent) and placebo. Did the incidence of MS in placebo-treated patients conform to that of other studies? The two-year rate of development of clinically defined multiple sclerosis in the placebo group approximated that of other reported series. Therefore the ONTT intravenous group fared better than expected. On the other hand, a higher recurrence rate of optic neuritis in the prednisone group compared with the placebo group was found in a previous ONTT report.[34] This protective effect began to lessen after two years. It was among patients who had multiple MRI signal abnormalities (two or more 3 mm diameter) that IVMP treatment had its greatest protective effect (36 versus 16 per cent). Those patients whose scans were normal did not appear to benefit from treat-

	Acute relapse of MS			Natural history of MS		
	Clinical evidence	*Lab. evidence*	*MRI evidence*	*Clinical evidence*	*Lab. evidence*	*MRI evidence*
High dose IVMP	Strong[11,19]	Strong[11,12]	Strong[24–27]	Mild[33,37]	Mild[11]	Mild[26,36]
Regular pulses of high dose IVMP				Mild[44]	None	None
Low oral dose of GC	None	None	None	None	None	None

Table 11.2
Clinical, laboratory and MRI evidence that GC can improve or modify the natural course of MS.

ment. In fact, the rate of development of clinical definite MS in patients with a normal scan was so very low that therapeutic efficacy for these patients could not be judged. By the end of the third year of follow-up, the cumulative incidence of definite MS in each group was similar: 17.3 per cent in the intravenous group, 21.3 per cent in the placebo group and 24.7 per cent in the prednisone group.[35]

Criticisms of ONTT

The principal criticism is that the ONTT was designed by ophthalmologists primarily to determine the effects of corticosteroid treatment on visual outcome, not on other neurological events. The long-term development of MS was a planned secondary outcome variable.

Another controversial point is that there was no matched placebo-treated, hospitalized, treatment arm to control for the methylprednisolone arm. Thus the trial was only partly blind.

Abnormal cerebro-spinal fluid (CSF) at the time of ON and certain HLA types also appear to predict clinical dissemination. No data were presented by Beck *et al.* on the proportion of patients in the three treatment arms with abnormal CSF, or with particular HLA types.

Although the statistical analyses are thorough, the actual number of patients in whom MS developed was small: 18 in the placebo group, 19 in the oral prednisone group and 10 in the intravenous methylprednisolone group.

In the original study cohort, patients with probable and definite MS were included. These patients were eliminated from the ONTT. However, the eliminated patients were equally distributed in all three treatment arms and thus did not create a bias.

Follow-up MRI data were not collected; it is not known whether IVMP had an effect in reducing the number of new lesions, including those which were asymptomatic.

Recommendations from the ONTT results

The message of the ONTT report is as follows: oral prednisone is not useful, and may even be contraindicated in the first episode of ON; MRI scans are necessary at the onset of ON, if the scans are pathological (two or more 3 mm diameter signal abnormalities), then IVMP is advised. This can be true in patients who meet ONTT criteria (18–46 years, onset within the previous eight days, no previous corticosteroid treatment or MS diagnosis). There is some evidence that clinical expression of ON between adults and children is different, bilateral ON being relatively common in the latter, so ONTT treatment recommendations may not be applicable to children.

Speculation from the ONTT results

The extrapolation of the ONTT results might lead to the use of a pulse of IVMP for the first episode of any neurologic event suggestive of a clinical demyelinating episode when the MRI is abnormal. Mild sensory attacks in MS typically are not treated. Should patients with subjective sensory complaints, but with an abnormal MRI, be treated? Whether the results of the ONTT therefore have implications for the treatment of acute episodes of MS is unknown.

There are no guidelines as to whether retreatment would be beneficial. Studies are needed to determine whether patients with MS should receive pulse corticosteroid therapy at regular intervals.

Other studies

Smith *et al.* reported a decrease in the rate of new enhancing lesion formation, but not in the total number of enhancing lesions after six months of high dose IVMP treatment. The authors suggest that initiation of enhancing lesions was affected more than the persistence of enhancing lesions.[36]

Cazzato *et al.* performed a double blind, placebo-controlled, randomized crossover trial of high-dose IVMP (1 g/day for five days followed by oral prednisone therapy for four days) in 35 patients with a primary progressive form of MS. A statistically significant improvement of Extended Disability Status Score (EDSS) in IVMP treated patients was recorded at 90 days and disappeared at 120 days.[37]

Is there any rationale for the beneficial effect of intravenous corticosteroids on the development of MS?

There is no known mechanism to explain the two-year effect of a brief treatment with cortiocosteroids. Long-term benefit of the ONTT is more than questionable because of the extremely variable interval, from months to years, between the first and second manifestations in those in whom MS develops. Nevertheless, Weishenker reported that patients with a high attack rate (more than five clinical attacks in the first two years), a short first interattack interval (less than two years), among other factors, are more likely to achieve a DSS rating of 6.0 than those without these clinical characteristics.[38] Therefore, preventing the relapses in the first two years of disease could have a protective long-term effect. Frequin *et al.* reported the results of an unblinded, uncontrolled, prospective study on 56 MS patients who were treated with high-dose IVMP, on ten consecutive days with 1000 mg IVMP daily. This study did not show a significant clinical benefit. Interestingly, the authors found persistent and prolonged decreased levels of the CSF variables (decreased intrathecal IgG synthesis and MBP levels) two years after IVMP treatment.[39] Brinkmann and Kristofic suggested that GC may be more efficient in blocking recruitment and clonal expansion of T cells in response to a primary antigenic stimulus, rather than in suppressing proliferation of recall of already primed memory T cells. These authors also suggested that prolonged T-cell receptor (TCR)/CD3 stimulation of human CD4 T cells reduces the sensitivity to the antiproliferative effects of GC.[40] These results may reflect the situation in many chronic inflammatory diseases, including MS, where excessive stimulation of antigen-specific T cells may occur as a result of a persistence of antigens in the body over prolonged time periods, and can also explain the loss of effectiveness of GC treatment in chronic forms of MS. As we mentioned earlier, Ramirez *et al.* showed an increase in IL-4 production and IL-4, IL-10 and IL-13 mRNA levels, and a decrease in IFN-γ and TNF synthesis on reactivated rat CD4+ T cells which had been previously cultured for one week in the presence of dexamethasone. These results suggest that steroid-induced cytokine Th2 phenotype is long lasting and it does not return to a Th1 baseline.[8] Another theoretical mechanism is the hypothetical primary neuroprotective mechanism of action of IVMP. A 24-hour IVMP treatment was shown to be effective in enhancing neurological recovery in spinal cord injured patients. An inhibition oxygen-free radical-induced lipid peroxidation mechanism has been hypothesized.[41] Whether this mode of action plays a role in MS is unknown.

Is chronic GC treatment useful in MS?

Anecdotal experience and limited clinical studies indicate that 'pulse' GC also provides improvement in a substantial percentage of patients in the chronic–progressive phase of the disease. Clearly, chronic use of GC is not effective in preventing acute exacerbations or chronic progression.

Miller and colleagues performed a double blind randomized trial on 86 patients with MS using prednisolone, 15 mg/day p.o. for the first eight months and 10 mg/day p.o. for another ten months. No benefit was observed in either the number of acute exacerbations, or progression of chronic disability.[42]

Tourtellotte *et al.* performed a double blind randomized trial on 76 MS patients using methylprednisolone 8–12 mg/day p.o. for 18 months. The authors concluded that pyramidal, cerebellar and bladder functions worsened more in the placebo group. Nevertheless, only a few statistically significant differences were found to support these findings.[43]

Whithan and Bourdette reported on 23 MS patients treated with IVMP pulse therapy receiving four-weekly infusions for one year. In chronic progressive MS patients, no beneficial clinical effect was found, but in relapsing MS patients a reduction in the relapse rate was noted.[44]

What are the side effects of chronic treatment with GC?

The mineralocorticoid effects may cause sodium and water retention which may result in oedema, hypertension and even congestive heart failure.

The androgenic effects may cause acne from rashes, hirsutism, loss of scalp hair and menstrual irregularities.

The glucocorticoid effects may cause hyperglycaemia and redistribution of body fat. The catabolism of proteins observed in prolonged GC administration can produce thinning of the skin, myopathy, neuropathy, cataracts and osteoporosis. Aseptic necrosis of bone has been reported in 1 per cent of patients. Ulceration of the gastrointestinal tract is a relatively rare complication.

The frequency of adverse effects is correlated with the dose, frequency and route of administration, duration of therapy, and underlying disease state.[45] In general, split-dose GC regimens are more toxic than alternate-day treatment protocols. Interestingly, Polman *et al.* performed an unblinded study in ten patients with chronic progressive MS. No signs of cushingoid appearance, behavioural changes, hypertension, changes in bone mass or bone metabolism, or adrenal suppression, were observed after nine monthly IVMP pulses.[46]

Do steroids and IFN-β interact?

IFN-β reduces the number of exacerbations in MS. The therapeutic mechanism of action responsible for the beneficial effects of IFNs in MS is not known. Despite large doses of intravenous or intramuscular IFN, increased serum cortisol levels, 9 or 45 MUI every other day do not seem to elevate serum or urine cortisol in MS patients.[47] On the other hand, Crockard and colleagues have recently shown that monocytes from normal subjects and MS patients pre-treated *in vitro* with methylprednisolone, expressed significantly less HLA-DR after stimulation with IFN-β. In contrast, IFN-β induced HLA-DR expression was not down-regulated following subsequent *in vitro* treatment with methylprednisolone. These authors suggest that the immunomodulatory effects of IVMP could be attenuated in MS patients receiving regular IFN-β therapy.[48] This effect has not been described in clinical practice. In fact, Gasperini *et al.* showed, in a small number of patients treated with IFN-β,

that the mean number and volume of enhancing lesions found during a clinical attack were similar to those found in the same patients before IFN-β treatment. Moreover, reduction of the active plaques after IVMP was higher during IFN-β therapy.[49]

Conclusions

High dose IVMP hastens the rate, but not the degree, of recovery from acute exacerbations of MS. Side effects are uncommon. Clearly the optimum regimen is unknown. We commonly administer 1 g/day for 3–5 days of IVMP in our patient facility where a nurse, physician and medical supplies for treating anaphylaxis or cardiovascular collapse, are immediately available. Consensus is lacking regarding prednisone tapering after high-dose IVMP; although prednisone taper is not necessary to avoid HPA axis insufficiency, it could help prevent immediate relapses after discontinuing IVMP. IVMP is advised in first episodes of optic neuritis if the MRI is abnormal, although other confirmatory studies are needed. Another issue to be addressed is whether all patients with a first attack of MS should receive initial treatment with high-dose GC. Clearly, the chronic use of low doses of oral GC is not effective in preventing acute exacerbations or chronic progression. Because of the adverse effects caused by the chronic use of these agents and their lack of efficacy such regimens should not be used. Regular pulses of high-dose IVMP could have a positive effect in MS. Placebo-controlled, double-blind, randomized clinical trials are needed to demonstrate such an effect.

References

1. Troiano R, Cook SD, Dowling PC. Corticosteroid therapy in acute multiple sclerosis. In: Cook SD, ed. *Handbook of Multiple Sclerosis*. New York, Dekker 1990; 351–369.
2. Ellison GW. Chronic progressive multiple sclerosis steroids and immunosuppressive drugs. In: Cook SD, ed. *Handbook of Multiple Sclerosis*. New York, Dekker 1990; 371–402.
3. Myers LW. Treatment of multiple sclerosis with ACTH and corticosteroids. In: Rudick RA and Goodkin DE, eds. *Treatment of Multiple Sclerosis. Trial Designs, Results and Future Perspectives*. London, Chapman and Hall 1992; 135–156.
4. Thompson AJ, Kennard C, Swash M *et al*. Relative efficacy of intravenous methylprednisolone and ACTH in the treatment of acute relapse in MS. *Neurology* 1989; **39**: 969–971.
5. Troiano R, Cook SD, Dowling PC. Steroid therapy in multiple sclerosis. *Arch Neurol* 1987; **44**: 803–807.
6. Poser CM. Corticotropin is superior to corticosteroids in the treatment of MS. *Arch Neruol* 1989; **46**: 946.
7. Snyder BD, Lakatua DJ, Poe RP. ACTH-induced cortisol production in multiple sclerosis. *Ann Neurol* 1981; **10**: 388–389.
8. Ramirez F, Fowell DJ, Puklavec M *et al*. Glucocorticoids promote a Th2 cytokine response by CD4+ T cells in vitro. *J Immunol* 1996; **156**: 2406–2412.
9. NIH Conference. Glucocorticoid therapy for immune-mediated disease. Basic and clinical correlates. *Ann Intern Med* 1993; **119**: 1198–1208.
10. Bamberger CM, Schulte HM, Chrousos GP. Molecular determinants of glucocorticoid receptor function and tissue sensitivity of glucocorticoids. *Endocr Rev* 1996; **17**: 245–261.
11. Durelli L, Cocito D, Riccio A *et al*. High-dose intravenous methylprednisolone in the treatment of multiple sclerosis: clinical-immunologic correlations. *Neurology* 1986; **36**: 238–243.
12. Warren KG, Catz I, Verona MJ *et al*. Effect of methylprednisolone on CSF IgG parameters, myelin basic protein and anti-myelin basic protein in multiple sclerosis exacerbations. *Can J Neurol Sci* 1986; **13**: 25–30.
13. Rosenberg GA, Dencoff JE, Correa N *et al*. Effect of steroids on CSF matrix metalloproteinases in multiple sclerosis – relation to blood-brain barrier injury. *Neurology* 1996; **46**: 1626–1632.
14. Mason D, MacPhee I, Antoni F. The role of the neuroendocrine system in determining genetic susceptibility to experimental allergic encephalomyelitis in the rat. *Immunology* 1990; **70**: 1–5.
15. Michelson D, Stone L, Galliven E *et al*. Multiple sclerosis is associated with alterations in Hypothalamic–Pituitary–Adrenal axis function. *J Clin Endocrinol Metab* 1994; **79**: 848–853.
16. Purba JS, Raadsheer FC, Hofman MA *et al*. Increased number of corticotropin-releasing hormone expressing neurons in the hypothalamic paraventricular nucleus of patients with multiple sclerosis. *Neuroendocrinology* 1995; **62**: 62–70.
17. Grasser A, Moller A, Backmund H *et al*. Heterogeneity of hypothalamic–pituitary–adrenal system response to a combined dexamethasone-CRH test in multiple sclerosis. *Exp Clin Endocrinol Diabetes* 1996; **104**: 31–37.
18. Defer GL, Barre J, Ledudal P *et al*. Methylprenisolone infusion during acute exacerbation of MS: plasma and CSF concentrations. *Eur Neurol* 1995; **35**: 143–148.
19. Milligan NM, Newcombe R, Compston DAS. A double-blind controlled trial of high dose methylprednisolone in patients with multiple sclerosis. 1. Clinical effects. *J Neurol Neurosurg Psychiatry* 1987; **50**: 511–516.
20. Alam SM, Kyriakides T, Lawden M *et al*. Methylprednisolone in multiple sclerosis: a comparison of oral with intravenous therapy at equivalent high dose. *J Neurol Neurosurg Psychiatry* 1993; **56**: 1219–1220.

21. Narang PK, Wilder R, Chatterji DC *et al.* Systemic bioavailability and pharmacokinetics of methylprednisolone in patients with rheumatoid arthritis following high-dose pulse administration. *Biopharm Drug Dispos* 1983; **4:** 233–248.

22. Kermode AG, Thompson AJ, Tofts PS *et al.* Breakdown of the blood-brain-barrier precedes symptoms and other MRI signs of new lesions in multiple sclerosis. *Brain* 1990; **113:** 1477–1489.

23. Troiano RA, Hafstein MP, Zito G *et al.* The effects of oral corticosteroid dosage on CT enhancing multiple sclerosis plaques. *J Neurol Sci* 1985; **70:** 67–72.

24. Burnham JA, Wright RR, Dreisbach J, Murray RS. The effect of high-dose steroids on MRI gadolinium enhancement in acute demyelinating lesions. *Neurology* 1991; **41:** 1349–1354.

25. Barkhof F, Hommes OR, Scheltens P *et al.* Quantitative MRI changes in gadolinium-DTPA enhancement after high-dose intravenous methylprednisolone in multiple sclerosis. *Neurology* 1991; **41:** 1219–1222.

26. Barkhof F, Was MW, Frequin STFM *et al.* Limited duration of the effect of methylprednisolone on changes on MRI in multiple sclerosis. *Neuroradiology* 1994; **36:** 382–387.

27. Miller DH, Thompson AJ, Morrisey SP *et al.* High dose steroids in acute relapses of multiple sclerosis: MRI evidence for a possible mechanism of therapeutic effect. *J Neurol Neurosurg Psychiatry* 1992; **55:** 450–453.

28. Chrousos GA, Kattah JC, Beck RW *et al. J Am Med Ass* 1993; **269:** 2110–2112.

29. Miro J, Amado JA, Pesquera C *et al.* Assessment of the hypothalamic–pituitary–adrenal axis function after corticosteroid therapy for MS relapses. *Acta Neurol Scand* 1990; **81:** 524–528.

30. Schwid SR, Goodman AD, Puzas JE *et al.* Sporadic corticosteroid pulses and osteoporosis in multiple sclerosis. *Arch Neurol* 1996; **53:** 753–758.

31. Prysee-Phillips WEM, Chandra RK, Robse B. Anaphylactoide reaction to methylprednisolone pulsed therapy. *Neurology* 1984; **34:** 1119–1121.

32. Bocanegra TS, Castaneda MO, Espinoza LR *et al.* Sudden death after methylprednisolone pulse therapy. *Ann Intern Med* 1981; **95:** 122.

33. Beck RW, Cleary PA, Trobe JD *et al.* The effect of corticosteroids for acute optic neuritis on the subsequent development of multiple sclerosis. *N Engl J Med* 1993; **329:** 1764–1769.

34. Beck RW, Cleary PA, Anderson MM *et al.* A randomized, controlled trial of corticosteroids in the treatment of acute optic neuritis. *N Engl J Med* 1992; **326:** 581–588.

35. Beck RW. The Optic Neuritis Treatment Trial: Three year follow-up results. *Arch Opthalmol* 1995; **113:** 136–137.

36. Smith ME, Stone LA, Albert SP *et al.* Clinical worsening in multiple sclerosis is associated with increased frequency and area of gadopentetate dimeglumine-enhancing magnetic resonance imaging lesions. *Ann Neurol* 1993; **33:** 480–489.

37. Cazzato G, Mesiano T, Antonello R *et al.* Double-blind, placebo-controlled, randomized, crossover trial of high-dose methylprednisolone in patients with chronic progressive form of multiple sclerosis. *Eur Neurol* 1995; **35:** 193–198.

38. Weinshenker BG. Natural history of multiple sclerosis. *Ann Neurol* 1994; **36:** S6–S11.

39. Frequin STFM, Lamers KJB, Barkhof F *et al.* Follow-up study of MS patients treated with high-dose intravenous methylprednisolone. *Acta Neurol Scand* 1994; **90:** 105–110.

40. Brinkmann V, Kristofic C. Regulation by corticosteroids of Th1 and Th2 cytokine production in human CD4+ effector cells generated from CD45RO− and CD45RO+ subsets. *J Immunol* 1995; **155:** 3322–3328.

41. Hall ED. The neuroprotective pharmacology of methylprednisolone. *J Neurosurg* 1992; **76:** 13–22.

42. Miller H, Newell DJ, Ridley A. Multiple sclerosis. Trials of maintenance treatment with prednisolone and soluble aspirin. *Lancet* 1961; **21:** 127–129.

43. Tourtellotte WW, Haerer AF, Arbor A. Use of an oral corticosteroid in the treatment of multiple sclerosis. A double-blind study. *Arch Neurol* 1965; **12:** 536–545.

44. Whithan RH, Bourdette DN. Treatment of multiple sclerosis with high dose methylpred-

nisolone pulse therapy. *Neurology* 1989; (suppl 1): 357.

45. Bennett DR, Dickinson BD, Rodgers BJ *et al.* AMA drug evaluations 1994. Chicago, American Medical Association 1993; 1877–1913.

46. Polman CH, Van Der Wiel HE, Teule GJ *et al.* A commentary on steroid treatment in multiple sclerosis. *Arch Neurol* 1991; **48**: 1011–1013.

47. Reder AT, Lowy MT. Interferon-beta treatment does not elevate cortisol in multiple sclerosis. *J Interferon Res* 1992; **12**: 195–198.

48. Crockard AD, Treacy MT, Droogan AG *et al.* Methylprednisolone attenuates interferon-beta induced expression of HLA-DR on monocytes. *J Neuroimmunol* 1996; **70**: 29–35.

49. Gasperini C, Koudriatseva T, Pozzilli C *et al.* Association of high dose of steroid with recombinant beta interferon therapy: prolonged effect on Gd-enhancing lesions in relapsing remitting MS. *Eur J Neurol*, 1996; **3** (suppl 1): 35.

12

How effective is interferon-beta in multiple sclerosis?

Fred D Lublin

Introduction

July 1993 was a seminal moment in the history of treatment for multiple sclerosis (MS). At that time interferon (IFN)-β-1b (Betaseron) was approved for use by the US Food and Drug Administration for the treatment of MS patients with the relapsing–remitting form of the disease. This was the first agent licensed for use in treating MS patients and thus signalled the beginning of the treatment era for MS. Since that time a second form of IFN-β, IFN-β-1a (Avonex IFN-β) and another agent, copolymer 1, have been approved for use. IFN-β subsequently was approved for use in Europe and in other areas of the world. Worldwide use of IFN-β is estimated at about 60,000 patients.

There are a number of properties of IFN-β which recommend its usage in MS. As with all interferons, it has anti-proliferative activity and thus inhibits lymphocyte replication.[1,2] It has antiviral activity, although this is not a likely mechanism in MS, as there is as yet no known 'MS virus' and the number of banal viral infections which could potentially trigger exacerbations of MS was no different in the placebo or interferon patients during clinical testing.[3] IFN-β inhibits the immune activating properties of interferon-γ,[1] most notably the up-regulation of the class II locus of the major histocompatibility complex (MHC) by IFN-γ. The mechanism for this action, in tissue cul-

ture experiments, appears to involve induction of an interferon stimulated gene factor.[4] As treatment with IFN-γ appeared to exacerbate MS,[5] this down-regulation could explain the beneficial effects of IFN-β. IFN-β also inhibits production of tumor necrosis factor (TNF)-α which is toxic to both myelin and oligodendrocytes *in vitro* and participates in the cell-mediated immune activation cascade.[6] Conversely, IFN-β enhances production of the immunosuppressive cytokine transforming growth factor (TGF)-β and interleukin (IL)-10.[7] IFN-β also augments the defective suppressor cell function which occurs in patients with MS.[8] It is not known which of these, or whether any of these, properties of IFN-β is responsible for its effects in MS, but the net effect of IFN-β appears to be down-regulation of the cell-mediated immune response which, in untreated patients with MS, tends to be activated.

Unlike many of the other agents recently tested in MS, little animal model data is available for IFN-β. IFN-β was tested in rats for its effect on experimental allergic encephalomyelitis (EAE), a cell-mediated autoimmune disorder which has clinical and pathologic similarities to MS. Abreu found that interferon inhibited EAE when administered systemically or when used *in vitro* on encephalitogenic cells prior to transfer into naive animals.[9,10] These data are supportive of the use of IFN-β in treating MS. The species specificity of IFNs limits the ability to test recombinant products in animal models. Further confusing the issue is the rather paradoxical affect of IFN-γ and antibodies to IFN-γ on EAE. Several studies have demonstrated that systemic administration of antibodies to IFN-γ markedly enhanced EAE, even in resistant strains of mice.[11–14] Conversely, systemic administration of IFN-γ tends to ameliorate EAE, even when administered directly into the central nervous system.[15,16] This would suggest that IFN-γ, and probably most cytokines, work in the immunologic micro-environment of the autoimmune process, making it difficult to assess therapies which employ systemic administration.

Clinical trials

Initial clinical trials with interferon utilized IFN-α preparations, both natural and recombinant. These studies produced modest to insignificant clinical effects on the course of MS.[17–19] Natural IFN-β administered intrathecally produced a reduction in relapse rate in a small, double-blind study.[20] A similarly designed study failed to confirm this, and in fact showed a worsening of the relapse rate in the intrathecal IFN-β treated group.[21] There are both theoretical issues and animal data which would suggest that intrathecal administration of IFN would not be of benefit. Administration of IFN-β intraventricularly into rats failed to ameliorate EAE, while systemic administration was effective.[10,22] Further, the inconvenience and discomfort of this administration would make it rather impractical.

The first systemic use of IFN-β in MS patients was a pilot safety and dosing study of 30 patients, using doses of IFN-β from 0.8 to 16 million Units (mU) three times weekly with a placebo control group.[23] This study demonstrated the safety of IFN-β and gave a hint of therapeutic efficacy in the higher doses. Also found was a relative intolerance of doses of 16 mU given three times weekly.

In 1988, a large, multicenter trial of IFN-β in patients with MS was initiated in North America. This study utilized a double-blind, placebo-controlled design. The inclusion criteria were patients with relapsing–remitting disease, Kurtzke Expanded Disability Status Scale (EDSS) scores of 0–5.5 and two or more exacerbations in the prior two years. Data were obtained from 372 patients randomized to receive either placebo, 1.6 mU IFN-β, or 8 mU IFN-β, subcutaneously, every other day. The primary outcome measures were reduction in annual exacerbation rate and proportion of exacerbation-free patients. At the end of the planned two year study, patients were offered re-enrollment for an additional year to assess the progression of the disease, as assessed by change in Expanded Disability Status Scale (EDSS).[3]

The results of this study, after two years, were that patients who received 8 mU of IFN-β had a significant reduction, by one-third, in the annual exacerbation rate, as compared to placebo-treated patients (0.84 versus 1.27; $p = 0.0001$). More importantly, the degree of reduction in exacerbation rate was most impressive, almost 50 per cent, in those exacerbations rated as moderate or severe. The other primary end-point, proportion of patients remaining exacerbation-free, also showed a significant difference, favoring IFN-β (8 mU IFN-β = 36, placebo = 18, $p = 0.007$). The median time to first exacerbation was significantly prolonged, nearly twice as long in the 8 mU group as compared to placebo ($p = 0.015$). Further, there were significant reductions in the number and days of hospitalization in the IFN-β treated group. The IFN-β 1.6 mU group demonstrated a dose response effect, with clinical values between that of the 8 mU group and the placebo group in most outcome measures.[3]

The patients in this study had baseline and yearly magnetic resonance imaging (MRI) scans which were analysed in blinded fashion at one study site. MRI activity was assessed by measuring new or enlarging lesions in a subset of 52 patients who had scans every six weeks for two years. MRI activity was reduced in the IFN-β 8 mU treatment group by 80 per cent compared to the placebo group ($p = 0.0062$). The rate of new lesions, active lesions and number of patients free of new lesions, all significantly favored the IFN-β 8 mU group. MRI lesion burden, measured on T_2 weighted images, was significantly less at two years in the treatment group ($p < 0.001$).[24]

By the time all enrolled patients completed three years on protocol, the total data set for the blinded, placebo-controlled study included patients with a median time on study of almost four years, including a few patients who completed five years. The analysis of the three year data and that for the entire data set (all patients, all time on study) shows a continued significant decrease in the relapse rate of about 30 percent ($p = 0.006$, pooled data, all patients, all time points on study). The same holds true for each individual year, although significance was achieved individually only for the first two years, probably due to loss of power from successive drop-outs in the later years. Progression of disease, assessed by the proportion of patients with a sustained worsening by one point on the EDSS, showed a trend, but not a significant difference, in favor of IFN-β. There are several explanations for this. The study was not powered to show a change in EDSS, but rather to assess change in relapse rate. The placebo group showed little change in the EDSS over the course of the study, thus limiting the ability of the study to discern a

difference in this population. The recognized issues of the sensitivity of the EDSS also need to be considered. The MRI data for all patients over the course of the study continued to show a dramatic effect from treatment with IFN-β, with no significant increase in lesion burden through year five. The placebo group increased their T_2 burden by about 10 per cent per year.[25]

A second, large, double-blind, placebo-controlled multicenter trial of IFN-β, utilizing recombinant IFN β-1a, reported results in March 1996. This form of IFN-β is glycosylated and more closely resembles the natural occurring molecule. The study differed from the IFN-β-1b study in several important ways. The drug was administered intramuscularly, weekly at a dose of 6 mU. The inclusion criteria were relapsing–remitting MS, EDSS scores of 1.0 to 3.5, and two or more exacerbations in the previous three years. The primary outcome measure was time to onset of sustained increase in disability, as measured by a worsening of the Kurtzke EDSS score by at least one point. The study demonstrated a significant effect of IFN-β on delaying disability ($p = 0.02$). Also seen were significantly fewer exacerbations ($p = 0.03$) and significant reduction in MRI activity in patients receiving IFN-β, as measured by the number and volume of gadolinium-enhancing lesions on MRI scans. The effect on T2 burden was not as impressive, a significant difference at the end of one year, but no significant difference at two years.[26]

Both large studies of IFN-β demonstrated that the agents were well tolerated and safe. Patients receiving IFN-β may develop a 'flu-like syndrome of fever, chills, myalgias, headache, which tend to resolve over time and also respond to antipyretic–analgesic medications. IFN-β-1b recipients, who received the drug subcutaneously, had frequent skin reactions, primarily redness at the injection site and rarely necrosis. Also seen in the IFN-β-1b study were elevations of hepatic transaminases, but no liver disease, and rarely suicidal behavior. Clinical experience with IFN-β-1b in the US over the past three years, in over 40,000 patients, has confirmed the safety profile of this agent, without the appearance of any new side effects or complications.[27]

Additional evidence for the effectiveness of IFN-β comes from studies of its effect on gadolinium-enhanced MRI scans, where IFN-β produced a marked reduction in the number of enhancing lesions,[28] suggesting an effect on the breakdown of the blood–brain barrier (BBB) which occurs as an early manifestation of new lesions in MS.[29] Further supportive data comes from studies of the other type 1 interferon, IFN-α. A smaller, but well controlled and designed study demonstrated that IFN-α had beneficial effects on both relapse rate and MRI activity.[30]

In viewing the combined results of these studies of IFN-β, there can be little doubt as to the effectiveness of this agent. IFN-β reduced the frequency of exacerbations, slowed accrual of disability and dramatically reduced MRI activity in patients with MS. Direct comparison of IFN-β-1a to 1b is not possible due to differences in study design, populations and dosages. While there are a number of potential criticisms of each of the major IFN-β studies, they support the conclusions of each study and provide considerable evidence for consistency of effect. Analysis of the drop-outs from the IFN-β-1b study reveals that the more severely affected placebo patients were in the drop-out group, thus strengthening the study's conclusions. Further, the long-term results of the IFN-β-1b study strongly suggest a persistence of effect.[25]

However, the usefulness of IFN-β may be mitigated by the development of neutralizing antibodies. Although these antibodies were found in patients in both IFN-β studies, a detailed analysis has only been published for the IFN-β-1b population.[31] This analysis revealed that 35 per cent of patients treated with IFN-β developed neutralizing antibodies after three years' exposure, the vast majority by the end of the first year. In those patients developing neutralizing antibodies, the relapse rate approximated that seen in placebo patients, suggesting a loss of efficacy. Conversely, in the 65 per cent of treated patients who did not develop these antibodies, the relapse rate reduction was approximately 50 per cent, strengthening the evidence for the clinical efficacy of IFN-β. Guidelines for the use of antibody determination in patients receiving IFN-β have been published,[32] but additional analysis of the study data is underway to determine the long-term effect of the antibodies and their persistence. Not all patients who developed antibodies lost efficacy. Further, in both IFN-β studies, patients who developed antibodies tended to have less progression of disease as measured by change in EDSS than those without antibodies. Clearly, more data will be needed to better understand the full implications of this phenomenon.

Another mitigating factor for long-term usage of IFN-β is patient or physician directed discontinuation of therapy. For IFN-β-1b, the drop-out rate has been about 25 per cent. This rate tends to be greater in individual practitioner's practices and lower at dedicated MS centers. The initiation of a relatively complicated parenteral therapy is time consuming and puts a considerable burden on the busy practitioner, most of whom do not have trained nurses available. The potential side effects, especially early in the course of therapy, can lead to increased time on the telephone or in the office. These strains on the physician's resources could lead to early termination of therapy. Patients will need to be supported through the initial treatment period and also well into therapy to avoid discontinuation of an effective therapy. Central to patient compliance is careful education on the handling and administration of the drug, the potential side effects and the realistic expectations of treatment with IFN-β. Discontinuation early in therapy usually is secondary to side effects, primarily the 'flu-like syndrome, although a rare patient will develop marked increases in hepatic enzymes, necessitating cessation. Late discontinuation may be due to the small percentage of patients who have persistent 'flu-like symptoms, but more commonly results from the unrealistic expectation that IFN-β will produce noticeable improvement in their disease.[27] Despite our best attempts at education, some patients, with the aid of the non-scientific media, expect treatment with IFN-β to produce a reduction in clinical deficits. Further challenging our ability to maintain patients on therapy is the lack of a truly tangible benefit to therapy with IFN-β. The clinical trials demonstrate fewer and less severe exacerbations and slower accumulation of disability. However, these effects are not discernible to the individual patient who has no way of knowing what their particular course would be during any given period of time. Thus, the individual who remains completely stable, unchanged and without exacerbation, after a year on therapy with IFN-β may not be overly impressed with the result of frequently injecting himself for the past year. To the contrary, such an individual might view more negatively a mild exacerbation which occurs while on IFN-β therapy than they might have prior to therapy. This situation serves to highlight the difficulty of translating the results of the required population-based studies into a context which our patients, as individuals, can appreciate.

Another concern raised by the marketing of IFN-β is the cost. Currently, both available agents are exceedingly expensive, costing approximately US$10,000 yearly, in the US and even more in Europe. Such an expensive therapy has considerable effects on the ability of patients to obtain and maintain therapy and puts enormous strain on the already over-burdened health care budgets of individuals, insurers and government-sponsored programs. One would hope that competition in the marketplace would lessen the costs, but that has not yet occurred. However, there are no alternative therapies available which match the clinically proven efficacy of IFN-β. It is unfair to patients and to society in general to limit the availability of this therapy to patients under the guise of cost effectiveness, until and unless a less expensive, equally (or hopefully more) efficacious therapy is available. As of this writing, the cost for copolymer 1, a non-interferon injectable with efficacy similar to IFN-β, is expected to be similar to IFN-β.[33]

There remain many unanswered questions regarding the use of IFN-β in MS. Will IFN-β be effective for progressive forms of MS? The available information includes data on the relapsing form of MS. Several clinical trials are currently underway to see if patients with the secondary progressive form of MS will benefit from IFN-β. What is the optimal dose of IFN-β? In the IFN-β-1b trial, two doses were tested and a dose response effect favoring the higher dose was seen. This would suggest that a dose above the currently utilized 8 mU should be tested. With IFN-β-1a, the dose would appear to be much lower, as measured in units of protein administered and the reduced side effect profile (apparently, the two agents use different measures of activity so their dosage in mU is not comparable). The difference may relate to the slight differences in the two molecules, but there is little evidence to suggest that they are biologically dissimilar. The optimal method of dosing needs to be determined. Subcutaneous dosing is more convenient, but intramuscular dosing may provide longer biological activity. Might there be a role for oral administration, as seen in animal studies?[34] Although no significant new side effects of IFN-β have surfaced since the agent became commercially available, our experience is still limited. Similarly, we do not know if there will be a persistence of beneficial effect of IFN-β. The data from the IFN-β-1b study suggests a continued effect, both clinically and on MRI, into later years,[25] but more experience is needed. Will IFN-β provide the starting point for combination therapy with additional agents to produce an enhanced clinical response?

Summary

The clinical effects of IFN-β are difficult to ignore. Two forms of IFN-β have been tested and found to be efficacious. Taken together, the clinical trials demonstrate that IFN-β reduces the frequency and severity of exacerbations, slows the accumulation of disability and suppresses MRI activity and lesion accrual. While these results are not overwhelming, and are thought by some to be little more than modest, they represent the best available therapies (see Chapter 13 for another analysis of the IFN-β clinical trials). It is hoped that further study of interferons as well as newer, more specific agents will lead to increased clinical efficacy. The IFN-β clinical trials have assisted in the effort to find better therapies by demonstrating that well designed, controlled studies of treatment for MS can be performed, produce a clinically relevant result and lead to an economically viable preproduct for marketing. This has probably led to the current situation where there are more clinical trials for MS underway worldwide than ever before.

References

1. Noronha A, Toscas A, Jensen MA. Interferon beta decreases T cell activation and interferon gamma production in multiple sclerosis. *J Neuroimmunol* 1993; **46:** 145–153.
2. Rudick RA, Carpenter CS, Cookfair DL *et al.* In vitro and in vivo inhibition of mitogen-driven T-cell activation by recombinant interferon beta. *Neurology* 1993; **43:** 2080–2087.
3. The IFNB MS study group. Interferon beta-1b is effective in relapsing–remitting multiple sclerosis. I. Clinical results of a multicenter, randomized, double-blind, placebo-controlled trial. *Neurology* 1993; **43:** 655–661.
4. Hong-Tao L, Riley J, Babcock G *et al.* Interferon (IFN) beta acts downstream of IFN-gamma-induced class II transactivator messenger RNA accumulation to block major histocompatibility complex class II gene expression and requires the 48-kD DNA-binding protein, ISGF3-gamma. *J Exper Med* 1995; **182:** 1517–1525.
5. Panitch HS, Hirsch RL, Schindler J *et al.* Treatment of multiple sclerosis with gamma interferon: exacerbations associated with activation of the immune system. *Neurology* 1987; **37:** 1097–1102.
6. Brod SA, Marshall GD, Jr, Henninger EM *et al.* Interferon-beta 1b treatment decreases tumor necrosis factor-alpha and increases interleukin-6 production in multiple sclerosis. *Neurology* 1996; **46:** 1633–1638.
7. Porrini AM, Gambi D, Reder AT. Interferon effects on interleukin-10 secretion. Mononuclear cell response to interleukin-10 is normal in multiple sclerosis patients. *J Neuroimmunol* 1995; **61:** 27–34.
8. Noronha A, Toscas A, Jensen MA. Interferon beta augments suppressor cell function in multiple sclerosis. *Ann Neurol* 1990; **27:** 207–210.
9. Abreu SL, Tondreau J, Levine S *et al.* Inhibition of passive localized experimental allergic encephalomyelitis by interferon. *Int Arch Allergy Appl Immunol* 1983; **72:** 30–33.
10. Abreu SL. Suppression of experimental allergic encephalomyelitis by interferon. *Immunol Comm* 1982; **11:** 1–7.
11. Duong TT, Finkelman FD, Singh B *et al.* Effect of anti-interferon-gamma monoclonal antibody treatment on the development of experimental allergic encephalomyelitis in resistant mouse strains. *J Neuroimmunol* 1994; **53:** 101–107.
12. Lublin FD, Knobler RL, Kalman B *et al.* Monoclonal anti-gamma interferon antibodies enhance experimental allergic encephalomyelitis. *Autoimmunity* 1993; **16:** 267–274.
13. Duong TT, St Louis J, Gilbert JJ *et al.* Effect of anti-interferon-gamma and anti-interleukin-2 monoclonal antibody treatment on the development of actively and passively induced experimental allergic encephalomyelitis in the SJL/J mouse. *J Neuroimmunol* 1992; **36:** 105–115.
14. Billiau A, Heremans H, Vandekerckhove F *et al.* Enhancement of experimental allergic encephalomyelitis in mice by antibodies against IFN-gamma. *J Immunol* 1988; **140:** 1506–1510.
15. Voorthuis JA, Uitdehaag BM, de Groot CJ *et al.* Suppression of experimental allergic encephalomyelitis by intraventricular administration of interferon-gamma in Lewis rats. *Clin Exp Immunol* 1990; **81:** 183–188.
16. Kalman B, Knobler RL, Perreault M *et al.* Inhibition of EAE by intracerebral injection of interferon-gamma (IFN-gamma). *Neurology* 1992; **42** (suppl 3): 346 (abstract).
17. Camenga DL, Johnson KP, Alter M *et al.* Systemic recombinant alpha-2 interferon therapy in relapsing multiple sclerosis. *Arch Neurol* 1986; **43:** 1239–1246.
18. Knobler RL, Panitch HS, Braheny SL *et al.* Systemic alpha-interferon therapy of multiple sclerosis. *Neurology* 1984; **34:** 1273–1279.
19. Kastrukoff LF, Oger JJ, Hashimoto SA *et al.* Systemic lymphoblastoid interferon therapy in chronic progressive multiple sclerosis. *Neurology* 1990; **40:** 479–486.

20. Jacobs L, Salazar AM, Herndon R *et al*. Multicentre double-blind study of effect of intrathecally administered natural human fibroblast interferon on exacerbations of multiple sclerosis. *Lancet* 1986; **2**: 1411–1413.

21. Milanese C, Salmaggi A, La Mantia L *et al*. Double blind study of intrathecal beta-interferon in multiple sclerosis: clinical and laboratory results. *J Neurol Neurosurg Psychiatry* 1990; **53**: 554–557.

22. Abreu SL, Thampoe I, Kaplan P. Interferon in experimental autoimmune encephalomyelitis: intraventricular administration. *J Interferon Res* 1986; **6**: 627–632.

23. Knobler RL, Greenstein JI, Johnson KP *et al*. Systemic recombinant human interferon-beta treatment of relapsing–remitting multiple sclerosis: pilot study analysis and six-year follow-up. *J Interferon Res* 1993; **13**: 333–340.

24. Paty DW, Li DK, UBC MS/MRI Study Group *et al*. Interferon beta-1b is effective in relapsing–remitting multiple sclerosis. II. MRI analysis results of a multicenter, randomized, double-blind, placebo-controlled trial. *Neurology* 1993; **43**: 662–667.

25. The IFNB Multiple Sclerosis Study Group, The University of British Colombia MS/MRI Analysis Group. Interferon β-1b in the treatment of multiple sclerosis: final outcome of the randomized controlled trial. *Neurology* 1995; **45**: 1277–1285.

26. Jacobs LD, Cookfair DL, Rudick RA *et al*. Intramuscular interferon beta-1a for disease progression in relapsing multiple sclerosis. *Ann Neurol* 1996; **39**: 285–294.

27. Lublin FD, Whitaker JN, Eidelman BH *et al*. Management of patients receiving interferon beta-1b for multiple sclerosis: report of a consensus conference. *Neurology* 1996; **46**: 12–18.

28. Stone LA, Frank JA, Albert PS *et al*. The effect of interferon-beta on blood-brain barrier disruptions demonstrated by contrast-enhanced magnetic resonance imaging in relapsing–remitting multiple sclerosis. *Ann Neurol* 1995; **37**: 611–619.

29. Kermode AG, Thompson AJ, Tofts P *et al*. Breakdown of the blood-brain barrier precedes symptoms and other MRI signs of new lesions in multiple sclerosis. Pathogenetic and clinical implications. *Brain* 1990; **113**: 1477–1489.

30. Durelli L, Bongioanni MR, Cavallo R *et al*. Chronic systemic high-dose recombinant interferon alfa-2a reduces exacerbation rate, MRI signs of disease activity, and lymphocyte interferon gamma production in relapsing–remitting multiple sclerosis. *Neurology* 1994; **44**: 406–413.

31. The IFNB Multiple Sclerosis Study Group, The University of British Columbia MS/MRI Analysis Group. Neutralizing antibodies during treatment of multiple sclerosis with interferon β-1b: experience during the first three years. *Neurology* 1996; **47**: 889–894.

32. Paty DW, Goodkin DE, Thompson A *et al*. Guidelines for physicians with patients on IFNB-1b: the use of an assay for neutralizing antibodies (NAB). *Neurology* 1996; **47**: 865–866.

33. Johnson KP, Brooks BR, Cohen JA *et al*. Copolymer 1 reduces relapse rate and improves disability in relapsing–remitting multiple sclerosis: results of a phase III multicenter, double-blind placebo-controlled trial. *Neurology* 1995; **45**: 1268–1276.

34. Brod SA, Khan M, Kerman RH *et al*. Oral administration of human or murine interferon alpha suppresses relapses and modifies adoptive transfer in experimental autoimmune encephalomyelitis. *J Neuroimmunol* 1995; **58**: 61–69.

13

Are placebo-controlled clinical trials still ethical in multiple sclerosis?

John H Noseworthy

Introduction

The last decade has seen a proliferation of pilot, preliminary and randomized placebo-controlled clinical trials (RCTs) designed to determine whether it is possible to alter the natural history of multiple sclerosis (MS). In addition, there has been a noticeable improvement in the methodology underlying the design of these studies. Advances in the understanding of humoral and cellular immunology, transplantation immunotherapy and molecular biology have yielded a number of potentially effective therapeutic strategies for down-regulating the immune-mediated injury which is thought to be responsible for the MS lesion. Advanced magnetic resonance imaging (MRI) techniques (particularly serial MRI and improved automated methods for following changes in MRI-detected lesion burden), have provided convincing imaging evidence that it is possible to reduce the frequency and degree of blood–brain barrier (BBB) disruption and the steady accumulation of MRI-detected lesions with a variety of experimental treatments. Phase 3 RCTs have now provided support that patients treated with either interferon (IFN)-β-1b[1–3] (Betaseron), IFN-β-1a (Avonex),[4] or copolymer-1 (glatiramer acetate) (Copaxone)[5] fare better than placebo-treated patients in terms of relapse frequency (all three agents), MRI activity (both interferons), and possibly the rate of clinically-determined disability progression (IFN-β-1a). Hundreds of patients are now enrolled in phase 2 and phase 3 placebo-controlled clinical trials of these and other agents to extend and confirm these findings.

IFN-β-1b (Betaseron, Betaferon) is now widely available in North America and Europe, and IFN-β-1a (Avonex) and copolymer-1 (glatiramer acetate) (Copaxone) are becoming increasingly available for widespread clinical use. Each of these agents could be employed as the control limb in future trials. It is appropriate at this point to reflect on these promising early results, and to re-evaluate whether current and future clinical trials still require a control group of patients randomized to receive an inactive placebo. To address this question, we will briefly review the charge of institutional review boards (IRBs, equivalent to ethics committees), the rationale for including placebos as the control agent in contemporary MS trial design, the strength of the evidence that current treatments favorably alter the natural history of MS, the types of patients to whom these findings apply, and describe one person's perspective on this issue of the future of placebos in evaluating MS therapies.

The ethics of controlled clinical trial research: placebos

Investigators designing and conducting RCTs are motivated to do what is best for individual patients and, whenever possible, to advance knowledge to enhance the care of future patients. The ethics relevant to the design of an RCT are considered not only by the investigator and his/her colleagues, but also by funding agencies, IRBs, health licensing bodies (e.g. the Food and Drug Administration or equivalent agency) and, of course, by patients and their families. Practically speaking, the ethics of each trial is initially addressed at each center by IRBs. The trialist needs to be aware of the principles used by IRBs to guide their decisions about what is acceptable from an ethical standpoint.[6] Following the publication of the Nuremberg Code (1949) and the Declaration of Helsinki (1964), medical institutions were required to state the principles they would use to protect the rights and welfare of humans participating in medical and behavioral research. Most accepted the Declaration of Helsinki. In 1975, this statement was revised and included the recommendation that experimental protocols were to be reviewed by independent committees 'for consideration, comment and guidance'.

In the US, the National Commission for the Protection of Human Subjects of Biomedical and Behavioral Research guided federal policy making. Throughout its deliberations, the Commission followed three equal, fundamental ethical principles:

- Justice: e.g. each person must be treated fairly and should receive what he is owed
- Respect for persons: e.g. persons are never to be considered a means to an end; all persons are autonomous and when they are unable to act independently, others must be appointed to act for them
- Beneficence: e.g. physicians must aim to do no harm, maximize the potential benefits to their patients and promote good in their efforts to advance societal benefit by their investigations.

The third principle (beneficence) presents the greatest challenge to those designing RCTs. In what way have new treatments been shown to 'maximize benefit' for patients with MS? Are these advances of sufficient magnitude and free of significant 'harm' that they should be offered to all study subjects as the control limb against which future therapies are to be measured? Investigators must answer these questions and then provide this information to patients (informed consent) and to their IRBs before proceeding further. MS clinical trials at all stages (phase 1, 2 and 3) are subject to IRB review to ensure that they are scientifically sound and that the needs of patients are protected. An understanding of the positive results of recent trials, and the limitations of these results, will determine what constitutes ethical MS trial design.

Why have placebo controls been necessary in MS clinical trials?

In the past, the need for placebo controls in MS trials has been questioned. In parts of Europe, it was difficult for several decades to conduct placebo-controlled trials due to a sense amongst physicians that azathioprine significantly impacts the long-term clinical course of progressive MS. This perception may have been lessened somewhat after the publication of a meta-analysis of published azathioprine trials.[7] A decade ago, others questioned whether placebos could or should be used in the evaluation of treatments for progressive MS after the initial publications of the studies of induction and pulse 'booster' cyclophosphamide administration.[8] The results of subsequent placebo-controlled trials[9–11] and the passage of time have replaced this sentiment with the sense that placebo controls are essential in this clinical setting (see below).

Few chronic illnesses are less predictable than MS. The etiology, pathogenesis, and factors which determine MS susceptibility and prognosis are unknown. As reviewed by others in this monograph, extensive human and experimental evidence suggests that both genetic and environmental factors are instrumental in determining susceptibility, but there remains little understanding of why the clinical course is so variable. Most feel that the benign and more aggressive forms of relapsing–remitting and secondary progressive MS probably share a common etiology (etiologies?). Patients may remain well for long periods of time without treatment, whereas others progress rapidly to a moderate or severe disability despite all efforts to slow the disease course.

Several major clinical trials have shown that the clinical behavior of patients selected for enrolment in phase 3 trials often 'regress to the mean' shortly thereafter.[1,3–5,10,11] This apparent stabilization in the clinical course of placebo-treated patients reduces the ability of the trial to demonstrate a therapeutic benefit (reduced statistical power). In several studies, however, serial MRI scanning has demonstrated that this apparent, often temporary, clinical stabilization is not accompanied by MRI evidence of remission.[2–4] Each of these developments significantly impact on the ability of the clinical trialist to be confident that apparent short-term clinical stability (or even improvement) can be attributed to the putative treatment with confidence. These confounding

tendencies were largely unrecognized until recently. This naiveté presumably explains, in part, why many uncontrolled or incompletely controlled MS trials during the 1950s to the 1980s reported positive results, findings which were not confirmed subsequently by more carefully controlled studies (type I error; false positive).[12]

Landmark natural history studies and recent work using serial MRI techniques underscore the unpredictability of this illness. It is widely agreed that clinical measures of disease activity (e.g. relapse rate, progression of disability measured by clinical rating scales, need for corticosteroid intervention, temporal changes in the neurologic examination, etc.) grossly underestimate the biological activity of MS. Serial MRI studies have shown that there can be dramatic, clinically unsuspected month-to-month variability in the number and size of new lesions, particularly in patients with relapsing–remitting disease.[13,14] Similarly, the cross-sectional area of MRI-detected change may increase by as much as 10 per cent per year in relapsing–remitting patients treated with placebo, despite little or no change in the neurologic examination.[2,3]

Better measures are clearly needed to distinguish patients destined to have a benign prognosis (up to 20 per cent may have little disability 10–20 years after the onset of the illness) from those who develop irreversible or progressive neurological handicap within 5–15 years of diagnosis. In addition to poor sensitivity (ability to detect change), current clinical measures suffer from subjectivity and problems with reproducibility and validity. Patients and neurologists may have difficulty agreeing on what entails a 'relapse'. There is considerable inter- and intra-rater variability in the scoring of the most frequently used rating scale (Expanded Disability Status Scale – EDSS – score of Kurtzke).[15] This scale is non-linear and is difficult to use in a reliable fashion. It largely ignores changes in upper limb function, it is insensitive to changes in behavior and cognition, it is excessively ambulation-dependent, and it is an imperfect measure of disease activity and MRI-detected disease burden.[16] In its defense, the EDSS was not designed to determine short-term changes in disease activity, but it has assumed the pre-eminent position as the primary clinical outcome measure in many definitive trials.

Additional evidence that the EDSS is a fragile measure of treatment efficacy was found in the secondary analysis of the Canadian cooperative study of cyclophosphamide and plasma exchange in patients with progressive disease. In this analysis, it was shown that the presence or absence of evaluator blinding resulted in such important differences in EDSS rating that the primary interpretation of the trial data would have been reversed if unblinded evaluations were used to rate clinical changes.[17]

The need for a surrogate marker of disease activity in MS

Many of these important limitations in our ability to detect disease activity and treatment benefit would be overcome if there were a validated, sensitive surrogate outcome measure. Valid surrogate markers predict rare or distant outcomes.[18] As is the case with other chronic diseases (e.g. atherosclerosis, diabetes, cancer, AIDS, etc.), MS clinical trialists are aggressively seeking a surrogate measure which could significantly shorten the time for drug development and reduce both the numbers of patients and duration of follow-up needed to conduct definitive phase 3 RCTs. Three of the

most important requirements for an adequate surrogate marker in a clinical trial are that the surrogate measurement occurs more often than the primary clinical outcome, the surrogate should be qualitatively and quantitatively related to the primary outcome, and an effect of treatment on the surrogate must ultimately be associated with an effect on the primary outcome (e.g. irreversible disability in MS).

It currently appears most likely that some form of MRI technique will meet the rigorous requirements for a valid surrogate outcome measure. Serial MR studies already fulfil a number of the requirements for a surrogate measure in that MRI changes typically occur both more often and more quickly in the disease course than do clinical measures. MRI studies are quantitative, objective, reproducible, subject to standardization, biologically plausible, and seem to be sufficiently sensitive to disease activity to reduce the likelihood of a false negative trial result (type 2 error).

Unfortunately, however, changes in MRI behavior have not yet been convincingly shown to be sufficiently specific or predictive of disease progression to allow clinicians to feel confident that a short-term change in MRI behavior will accurately predict an important later change in clinically identifiable disease progression. As was clearly demonstrated in the North American IFN-β-1b (Betaseron) trial, serial MRI changes paralleled clinical response and were more sensitive than clinical measures in identifying a benefit from treatment.[2,3] On the other hand, statistical correlations between MRI and clinical behavior were modest at best.[3] In addition, there was an important discrepancy between the clinical and MRI behavior of the patients receiving 1.6 mIU of IFN-β-1b (Betaseron) which still has not been adequately explained. These patients derived significant MRI benefit (reduction in MRI 'activity' in the cohort of patients scanned frequently), yet progressed to the point of 'confirmed clinical worsening' (increase of ≥ 1.0 EDSS points on two consecutive evaluations separated by at least three months) sooner than placebo-treated patients (3.49 versus 4.18 years).[3] Is this paradoxical observation explained by a problem with the EDSS, with the clinical relevance of MRI or with some incompletely understood effect of low dose IFN-β-1b (Betaseron) on clinical-MRI interaction? The relationship between MRI change and long-term disability needs to be understood before serial measurements of MRI activity can be considered a valid surrogate measure. At present, several hundred patients are involved in a series of definitive phase 3 trials, each of which are investigating a variety of primary and secondary MRI measures (*Table 13.1*). It is hoped that the information resulting from these studies will provide compelling evidence that MRI can be used in the future as a surrogate measure in MS trials.

Equipoise

Randomized, controlled, clinical trials cannot be conducted unless there is agreement amongst experts in the field that there is a chance that a putative experimental treatment may be equally effective or more effective than 'standard therapy'. In the current era, placebos have replaced 'no treatment' in this setting in order to permit blinding to the treatment assignment. There is not an extensive literature confirming that 'no treatment' and placebos are comparable, but few investigators have been willing to accept the complexity of adding another treatment arm (e.g. 'no treatment') to placebo-controlled trials.

In 1987, Freedman introduced the concept of 'equipoise'.[19] This concept dictates that there should be genuine uncertainty (called by Freedman an 'honest null hypothesis') whether treatment A or treatment B is preferable. As such, the investigator should be 'equally poised' with respect to his preference for either treatment. If these two treatments (one of which is the control therapy, possibly a placebo) are not equivalent, ethical practice requires that the superior treatment be given. If equipoise is significantly disturbed, the trial should either not be started or should be terminated or changed to restore equipoise. In practice, however, it is rare that there is a pure $50:50$ split with respect to the advantages and disadvantages of such therapies, either from the individual's perspective (theoretical equipoise) or for the collective opinion (clinical equipoise). Johnson *et al.*[20] performed a study to determine the level of collective equipoise at which a clinical trial is no longer ethical. In a survey of 113 persons (lay persons and physicians), they determined that a higher level of collective equipoise (e.g. at or close to $50:50$) is required for a highly emotionally charged clinical research program (e.g. when infants and children are the subjects of research, life-threatening conditions, etc.). Those surveyed felt that a greater disparity of opinion (e.g. lower level of equipoise: e.g. $70:30$ preference) was ethically acceptable if the condition to be studied involved animals, symptomatic treatments, or if the condition was a reversible, low risk illness. Fifty per cent of the lay subjects surveyed felt that it was unethical to proceed with a clinical trial if equipoise was disturbed beyond $70:30$, and only 3 per cent accepted that a trial should be performed if equipoise was disturbed beyond $80:20$. Using these principles, there should be a higher level of collective equipoise when one is initiating a prolonged clinical trial designed to determine whether treatment A is better than treatment B in

Trial (sponsor; yr. completion)	MS Type (n)	Design	Comments
15-Deoxyspergualine (Behringwerke AG; 1996)	RR and SP (236)	R, DB, PC	Interim analysis suggests disappointing results
Sulfasalazine (Upjohn-Pharmacia; 1997)	RR and SP (199)	R, DB, PC	Primary outcome – EDSS change 9 USA and Canadian centers
2-Chlorodeoxyadenosine (CdA; 1996)	RR (52)	R, DB, PC	CdA sc (5d/month × 6) × Plb
2-Chlorodeoxyadenosine (RW Johnson; 1997)	Chronic progressive (150)	R, DB, PC	6 North American centers 2 doses (sc) × Plb
Oral myelin (Autoimmune Inc; 1997)	RR (514)	R, DB, PC	13 North American centers
IVIg in MS (NIH; 1998)	Permanent motor deficit (76)	R, DB, PC	Does IVIg reverse permanent weakness?
IVIg in ON (NIH; 1997)	Permanent visual loss (60)	R, DB, PC	Does IVIg reverse permanent visual loss?
Linomide (Upjohn-Pharmacia; 1999)*	RR and SP (700)	R, DB, PC	Primary outcome – EDSS change 27 North American centers 3 active doses × Plb
Linomide (Upjohn-Pharmacia; 1999)*	RR and SP (350)	R, DB, PC	Primary outcome – EDSS change European and Australian Multicenter Study 2 active doses × Plb
Linomide (Upjohn-Pharmacia; 1999)*	RR (501)	R, DB, PC	Multicenter Study – Europe, Australia, and Canada 2 active doses × Plb
IFN-β-1b (Berlex; 1999)	SP (900)	R, DB, PC	Multicenter North American Study 2 active doses × Plb
IFN-β-1b (Schering; 1999)	SP (700+)	R, DB, PC	30 European centers
IFN-β-1a (Ares-Serono; 1997–98)	RR and SP (2 trials, >500 pt each)	R, DB, PC	15 centers in Canada, Europe and Australia; 2 IFN doses × Plb
IFN-β-1a (Biogen; 1999)	RR and SP (808)	R, DB, PC	Multicenter European Study 2 IFN doses × Plb
IFN-β-1a (Biogen; 1999)	Monosymptomatic (380)	R, DB, PC	Multicenter North American Study; Does IFN-β-1a delay conversion to clinically definite MS?
IFN-β-1a (Ares-Serono; 1999)	Monosymptomatic (250)	R, DB, PC	European Study Does IFN-β-1b delay conversion to clinically definite MS?

Abbreviations: RR = relapsing–remitting; SP = secondary progressive; R = randomized; DB = double blind; PC = placebo controlled; ON = optic neuritis; Plb = placebo
*Discontinued due to unexpected side effects

Table 13.1
Ongoing phase 2 and 3 MS therapeutic trials.

preventing irreversible disability, than would be required for a study of a symptomatic treatment for MS, or for a short term trial designed to reverse recently acquired, yet apparently permanent neurologic deficits.

In the 'modern era' of MS trials, one survey suggested that there was equipoise for this need for placebos in pivotal trials;[21] perhaps such a survey should now be repeated in the wake of the interferon and copolymer studies.

Status of definitive therapy in each of the major MS clinical scenarios

Has the natural history of MS been altered by treatment in a meaningful way? As reviewed below, the answer to this question is unfortunately 'no' for at least several of the situations in which MS patients find themselves (e.g. first episode of disease, acute relapse, catastrophic steroid-unresponsive relapse, patients with an apparently irreversible 'fixed neurological deficit', and primary progressive MS). The situation is less clear for patients with 'relapsing' MS.

Relapsing–remitting and 'relapsing' MS

By way of introduction, it appears that IFN-β-1b (Betaseron),[1–3] IFN-β-1a (Avonex),[4] and copolymer-1 (glatiramer acetate) (Copaxone)[5] all reduce relapse rate beyond the apparent tendency for relapses to diminish after enrollment into an RCT (natural history and 'regression to the mean'). Both interferons seem to have a marked (IFN-β-1b) or moderate (IFN-β-1a) impact on cranial MRI behavior. Studies performed after the pivotal IFN-β-1b trial have shown convincingly that this agent dramatically reduces gadolinium enhancements in serial studies of relapsing–remitting patients. I

will review the pertinent findings from the three recent pivotal trials which relate to whether each agent might replace placebos as standard therapy (e.g. control group) in RCTs.

IFN-β-1b

Three years ago, the US Food and Drug Administration (FDA) licensed Betaseron for use in ambulatory relapsing–remitting MS patients. Analysis of the extension limb of this trial provided additional supportive evidence that IFN-β-1b (Betaseron)-treated relapsing–remitting patients had fewer clinical relapses, need for steroid intervention, hospitalizations, and MRI evidence of ongoing disease activity than placebo-treated patients.[3] Regrettably, however, there was no convincing effect on clinical evidence of disability progression (e.g. EDSS). With this evidence that IFN-β-1b alters the natural history of MS, what are the major factors which limit IFN-β-1b replacing placebos in trial design?

Failure to demonstrate impact on EDSS progression Although there was a trend for high dose IFN-β-1b patients to show favorable slowing of EDSS progression, these findings did not reach statistical significance. In addition, patients receiving the low dose reached 'confirmed' clinical failure (worsening of ≥1.0 EDSS points on two consecutive visits separated by at least three months) earlier than placebo-treated patients, despite an apparent beneficial MRI response to treatment.[3,14]

Neutralizing antibodies The analysis of the extension trial revealed the vexing problem of neutralizing antibody formation in IFN-β-1b (Betaseron) treated patients. Thirty-eight per cent of patients receiving alternate day 8 mIU s.c. IFN-β-1b (Betaseron) developed neutralizing antibodies.[3] Most patients 'converted' within the first 12 months and, with the development of these antibodies, the clinical benefit of the treatment on relapse rate was lost.

These two findings (lack of convincing effect on EDSS progression and neutralizing antibody formation), together with limitations in clinical-MRI correlation (reviewed above), the high cost of treatment and the high frequency of mild-to-moderate interferon-related adverse events[1,3] have limited the enthusiasm for clinical trialists to use IFN-β-1b (Betaseron) in place of placebos for the control group in ongoing phase 2 and phase 3 clinical trials. General discussion amongst MS trialists, however, suggests that opinion may still be divided within the field about whether IFN-β-1b (Betaseron) might impact disability progression. Proponents of IFN-β-1b (Betaseron) argue that preferential 'dropping-out' by placebo-treated, 'failing' patients and the insensitivity of the EDSS to change both contributed to the inability of the study to show an impact on disability. The opportunity to clarify this has now, of course, been lost by the widespread availability of IFN-β-1b (Betaseron), although a partial answer may be forthcoming from the placebo-controlled, phase 3 study in patients with secondary-progressive disease (*Table 13.1*). The important clinical[1,3] and MRI benefits[2,3,14] demonstrated with IFN-β-1b (Betaseron), however, have mandated at the very least that consent forms for ongoing placebo-controlled clinical trials reflect this important advance in therapy for MS patients.

IFN-β-1a (Avonex)

Perhaps the greatest challenge to the concept that placebos are needed in phase 3 MS trials arises from the results of the IFN-β-1a (Avonex)[4] trial and the subsequent approval of this drug by the FDA for the indications of reducing both relapse rate and disability progression in 'relapsing MS'. As such, I will review a couple of issues relating to this trial which may be pertinent to this discussion point. Specifically, what are the factors that limit IFN-β-1b replacing placebos in trial design?

What is 'relapsing' MS? In the publication of the IFN-β-1a (Avonex)[4] study results, the authors state that mildly disabled patients with 'relapsing' MS were randomized to receive either weekly i.m. injection of IFN-β-1a (Avonex) or placebo. The use of the term 'relapsing' MS was not anticipated by non-participants in the trial in that the study was alleged to be evaluating whether IFN-β-1a (Avonex) altered the natural history of relapsing–remitting MS. The recent consensus statement describing definitions of the clinical course of MS by Lublin *et al.*[22] unfortunately came too late to clarify the nature of the pre-enrollment clinical course experienced by the patients enrolled in this trial and does not define 'relapsing' MS *per se*.

One crucial question is whether there was an equal distribution of relapsing–remitting and relapsing–progressive (now called secondary progressive) patients in each treatment arm. Evidently this important question cannot be answered retrospectively. Clearly, an unequal distribution of these two varieties of 'relapsing' MS could have significantly influenced the results of the study in either direction. Sceptics will wonder whether a greater proportion of relapsing (secondary) progressive patients may have been randomized to the placebo group, a catastrophic accident of randomization which could have led to an important type 1 error (false positive result). Given the mild EDSS range (1.0 to 3.5), and the authors' description of the eligibility requirements, however, it seems improbable that a large number of secondary progressive patients were enrolled. This being the case, however, it is equally certain that we cannot conclude that IFN-β-1a (Avonex) has been adequately tested in 'relapsing' (secondary) progressive MS.

Relapse rate reduction Although patients treated for two years (57 per cent of randomized patients) enjoyed a relapse rate reduction of 32 per cent, the magnitude of the effect on relapse rate was considerably less for all enrolled patients. As illustrated in Table 5 of their report,[4] the annualized relapse rate reduction was 18 per cent for all randomized patients. This is less than the 34 per cent annualized relapse rate reduction seen at two years in the patients treated with IFN-β-1b (Betaseron).[1,3]

What is the meaning of EDSS change within the mild range of the scale? Critics of the EDSS have previously pointed out the uncertainty of 0.5 or even 1.0 point changes within the range of the EDSS examined by the IFN-β-1a (Avonex) study. The investigators' use of confirmed verification of EDSS worsening over a six-month period, however, significantly strengthened the observations made in this study. As such, it appears that IFN-β-1a (Avonex)-treated patients were less likely to show confirmed EDSS worsening than were placebo-treated patients. It is unclear, however, how attack-related worsening was handled by the investigators. Additional analysis of these data will probably clarify this concern.

Is IFN-β-1a significantly better than INF-β-1b at slowing disability progression in MS patients? The FDA has required that EDSS progression (and not MRI evidence of disease progression, alone) must be favorably influenced by treatment to infer slowing of disease progression. In doing so, the FDA has ruled that IFN-β-1a (Avonex) does affect the development of clinical disability in the short term for patients with 'relapsing MS'. The FDA decided that IFN-β-1b (Betaseron) does not alter the likelihood of later disability and an advisory committee to the FDS opined that neither does copolymer-1 (glatiramer acetate) (Copaxone; see later).

If one accepts the results as published, it would appear that there is a difference in these two trials. In critically reviewing these papers, however, the differences in the behavior of the two placebo-control groups is troubling. Clearly, differences in eligibility criteria and in the guidelines used to measure disability make a direct comparison of the two trials risky. The IFN-β-1a investigators redefined the guidelines for scoring the functional systems (they refined the definitions of pyramidal dysfunction to help distinguish patients with mild and moderate weakness, for example).[23,24] Nonetheless, when these comparisons are made, one is struck that the one year 'confirmed progression' rates were similar for patients randomized to receive IFN-β-1a, IFN-β-1b and IFN-β-1b placebo (11 to 13 per cent), whereas the IFN-β-1a placebo patients did markedly less well (22 per cent of the IFN-β-1a placebo group reached 'confirmed progression' at one year). At two years, the 'confirmed progression' rate was similar between the two active interferon groups (approximately 19 per cent for IFN-β-1b and 21.9 per cent for IFN-β-1a patients), whereas the IFN-β-1a placebo patients were much more likely to have reached confirmed progression (34.9 per cent) compared with the placebo group in the IFN-β-1b trial (28 per cent). This issue has not been adequately debated in a peer-reviewed forum to this point.

Limited follow-up Prior to the publication of the IFN-β-1a (Avonex) trial, few would have thought it possible to show an impact on disease progression with a trial of such limited duration (only 57 per cent of enrolled patients were followed for two years; 77 per cent were followed for 18 months). Indeed, those who designed the trial anticipated the need for a longer period of observation but, with fewer drop-outs than anticipated, a decision was made to end the study 'earlier than originally planned ... without knowledge of any interim efficacy results'.[4] Longer and more complete follow-up (if positive) would have provided more convincing evidence that there was an important impact on disability progression. This opportunity is now irrevocably lost.

Neutralizing antibodies Neutralizing antibodies occurred less frequently than with IFN-β-1b (12 months: 14 versus 21 per cent, 18 months: 21 versus 36 per cent and 24 months: 22 versus 38 per cent). Further work is needed, however, to determine the true prevalence and clinical significance of neutralizing antibody formation to IFN-β-1a (Avonex) as neutralizing antibodies developed primarily in the first three years after initiating IFN-β-1b, and only 57 per cent of IFN-β-1a patients were followed for two years. In addition, different assays were used and no comparison studies have yet been performed to show convincingly that IFN-β-1a is less likely than IFN-β-1b to initiate neutralizing antibody formation. Indeed, evidence from the interferon literature suggests that it is likely that neutralizing antibody formation will continue to be a vexing problem for this and future interferon studies.

MRI findings less conclusive than INF-β-1b results The MRI findings provide support for a treatment effect but are less convincing than the results of the IFN-β-1b (Betaseron trial). Of particular concern is the observation that cumulative MRI burden did not significantly increase in the placebo-treated patients during the short period of follow-up.

Copolymer-1 (glatiramer acetate) (Copaxone)

The phase 3 North American copolymer 1 trial in relapsing–remitting MS reported a reduction of clinical relapse rate similar to, but less than, that experienced with IFN-β-1b (29 per cent versus 34 per cent).[5] Again, however, no con-

vincing reduction of disability progression was shown by the study. Regrettably, insufficient MRI data were collected to determine whether copolymer-1 (glatiramer acetate) favorably influences MRI behavior in patients with mild, relapsing–remitting MS. At the time of this writing, an advisory panel has recommended that the FDA approve copolymer-1 (glatiramer acetate) (Copaxone) for use in relapsing–remitting patients to reduce attack rate. The action of the FDA is anxiously awaited.

IFN-β-1b (Betaseron), IFN-β-1a (Avonex), and copolymer-1 (glatiramer acetate) (Copaxone): general discussion

At first glance, as outlined above, one might feel that each of these agents offers an advantage over placebo to patients in relapsing–remitting RCTs (*Table 13.2*). Certainly placebos do not offer the same degree of relapse rate reduction as any of the three agents and the interferons have a convincing MRI effect not seen in placebo-treated patients.

Conversely, both interferons (and to a lesser degree, copolymer-1 (glatiramer acetate) (Copaxone) offer some significant disadvantages as control groups. Each of these treatments are associated with either mild (copolymer/glatiramer acetate), moderate (IFN-β-1a) or moderate-to-marked (IFN-β-1b) side effects, inconvenience and cost. Perhaps of greater concern, however, is the development of neutralizing antibodies, discussed above. Much remains to be learned about the clinical importance of these antibodies, their possible cross reactivity with both exogenous and endogenous interferons, the potential long-term consequence to the patient's health, and, of course, the need to develop strategies to reduce their development.[25,26] Perhaps more than any other factor (modest clinical benefit, uncertain impact on disability, cost and inconvenience), the neutralizing antibody issue has

Agent	Advantages	Disadvantages	
		Features common to all three agents	Treatment specific
Copolymer-1 (Glatiramer acetate) (Copaxone)	↓ relapse rate	Feasibility: Industry co-operation in trial design Increased sample size (partially effective therapies) Relative inconvenient route, drug costs and adverse event profiles	No ↓ EDSS progression MRI effect unknown
IFN-β-1b (Betaseron)	↓ relapse rate MRI benefit		No ↓ EDSS progression MRI-clinical correlation uncertain Neutralizing Abs
IFN-β-1b (Avonex)	↓ relapse rate ↓ EDSS progression MRI benefit		MRI effect less than IFN-β-1b Neutralizing Abs

Table 13.2
Advantages and disadvantages of active MS therapies compared with placebo treatment.

influenced me to be cautious about initiating interferon therapy in patients who have infrequent or self-limiting relapses, particularly if they have only a mild disability.

Eliminating the placebo group from clinical trials significantly complicates trial design in a number of ways. The decision to mandate that all patients receive an active, parenteral drug (interferon or copolymer/glatiramer acetate), would make trial design cumbersome, particularly if the putative experimental agent is also a parenteral agent (e.g. two separate injection programs). In an effort to determine whether a putative agent is more effective than a partially effective therapy, sample size must be increased between 30 and 40 per cent to detect a treatment effect.[27] Trial costs will be magnified tremendously and issues of co-operation between various funding agencies (possibly involving two or more pharmaceutical compa-nies) will present a considerable confounding factor. Not all eligible patients will want to be started on interferons and, doubtless, others will decide against copolymer/glatiramer acetate because of either an aversion to administering parenteral medications or from concerns about the uncommon and poorly understood 'systemic reaction' reported with its use.[5] In addition, many patients have discontinued IFN-β-1b either because of perceived lack of efficacy or intolerance to the adverse effects, and these patients may seek enrolment in future clinical trials. Clearly, in considering eligibility for future trials, investigators will need to consider whether such patients will be eligible for enrolment, their neutralizing antibody status will need to be determined, and stratification strategies will need to be employed to balance treatment groups with respect to previous exposure to interferons.

Currently, practitioners and patients ponder the results of these three pivotal trials on a daily basis in deciding how to treat their patients. All three agents will probably be available shortly for widespread use in the USA. In other countries, this may soon exist to a similar degree, although the UK, Australia and a number of European countries have been more selective in approving MS therapies. Clearly, IFN-β-1a and copolymer-1/ glatiramer acetate will not replace placebos in countries where they are not widely available. As illustrated in *Table 13.1*, a number of placebo-controlled RCTs will be completed in the near future. Will one or more of these show unequivocal evidence that clinical disease progression can be significantly slowed or halted? If so, will that evidence be sufficient to obviate the need for future placebo control groups? Will this decision be made by the collective community of MS clinical trial design experts, or will they defer to the FDA and other drug licensing boards worldwide?

Consensus amongst MS trialists and, thereafter, guidelines for the next wave of clinical trial research awaits additional editorial review of the IFN-β-1a (Avonex) data and further data analysis by the IFN-β-1a (Avonex) investigators. The clinical trialists who are conducting the major phase 2 and 3 trials currently underway (*Table 13.1*) have not abandoned their placebo design. I am in full agreement with this decision. Once again, the uncertainty of what types of patient comprise the 'relapsing MS' population in the IFN-β-1a (Avonex) trial and the minimal disability of the patients in this trial presumably has influenced these decisions to proceed with the original design. This collective group of MS experts by this action has suggested that neither the interferons nor copolymer-1 (glatiramer acetate) have been shown convincingly to slow clinical disease progression, to the

point that placebos should be considered unethical in patients with relapsing–remitting and secondary progressive MS.

Primary progressive MS

It is less certain that primary progressive MS (PPMS) is, indeed, the same disease as relapsing–remitting and secondary progressive MS. Until this is clarified, however, these various forms of human demyelinating disease will be considered by most experts to be varieties of a single, enigmatic illness. Most MS patients presenting with slowly progressive ('primary progressive') MS never suffer from a clinically recognized exacerbation. Patients typically worsen slowly with variable periods of apparent stabilization. This clinical phenotype appears to be made up of two subcategories defined by MRI. The first of these (for the purposes of this discussion called 'true' PPMS), characteristically have minimal MRI disease burden. Cerebral MRI scans show few areas of T_2 signal abnormality and gadolinium enhancements occur infrequently in serial studies.[28,29] Patients may have a small number of MRI signal changes on spinal imaging, but in most these changes are minor, as well. With time, there is MRI evidence of spinal cord atrophy. In the second category, serial MRI studies parallel the changes seen in patients with secondary progressive MS. As such, there may be widespread T_2 signal change in the cerebral hemispheres and spinal cord, and gadolinium enhancements are not infrequent. To this point, there is no adequate explanation why this group of patients have few (or no) recognizable clinical exacerbations other than the apparent sparing of eloquent motor and sensory tracts by these MRI-identified episodes of apparent inflammatory demyelination.

There is currently no evidence that available therapies significantly impact the clinical course of PPMS. Indeed, this subset of MS patients is usually excluded from participation in clinical trials as it is difficult to determine efficacy given the very slow disease progression (years). Clearly, at least until a validated surrogate outcome is identified which will shorten the time to determine possible efficacy, future RCTs in PPMS will need to be placebo-controlled.

Acute MS attacks

A number of clinical and MRI imaging studies have shown that ACTH and corticosteroids (oral and parenteral) favorably influence the short-term natural history of MS exacerbations. Computed tomography (CT) and MRI studies have shown that steroids temporarily reverse the BBB disruption which accompanies these attacks, although follow-up studies show that this effect is short-lived (weeks).[30] The optimal treatment of MS relapses is unknown, although many physicians and patients hold strong personal preferences. In recent years, intravenous methylprednisolone (either alone or followed by a short tapering course of oral prednisone) has become widely used and, in many centers, has replaced the more traditional use of either parenteral ACTH or oral prednisone for the treatment of clinically significant MS attacks. Although steroids are widely used in North America, certain prominent MS centers worldwide rarely, if ever, prescribe steroids in this setting. The issue of steroid use in acute MS attacks has not been adequately studied by properly designed, blinded and placebo-controlled trials, and there seems little current likelihood that this trend will be reversed, presumably because most feel that whatever effect steroids bring, their benefit is likely to be limited in scope and duration.

The question of whether placebo-controlled studies are ethical in this setting is now partic-

ularly relevant as a wide array of therapeutic agents which influence BBB integrity, T-cell trafficking and immune activation are becoming available for study to determine whether they may influence the natural history of acute MS exacerbations. The issue facing the clinical trialist designing such studies is the same for each of these agents, namely is it ethical to do a placebo-controlled trial or must all patients receive steroids? This scenario has not been tested by modern phase 1–3 RCTs. One option for a phase 1 trial would be to delay steroid use for several days awaiting clinical or MRI evidence of apparent benefit while providing physicians and patients with the option to follow-up with a course of steroids ('rescue') if patients continue to worsen or fail to improve. A second option would be to use a double-blind, placebo-controlled, cross-over design, with recovered patients not crossing over. Clearly, these designs would need to be approved by IRBs and patients (informed consent).

First attack of possible MS

Recently published longitudinal studies from the Queen Square MRI Unit in London illustrated the pivotal importance of baseline MRI studies in patients with first episodes of central nervous system (CNS) demyelinating disease.[31] Specifically, patients with little or no cranial MRI evidence of MS at onset (<3 discrete lesions) appear to have a low five-year risk of developing clinically definite MS after a single episode of optic neuritis, isolated brain stem, or partial spinal cord presentations of inflammatory demyelinating disease (approximately 7 per cent). Conversely, the risk of converting to clinically definite MS approaches 80 per cent if the initial event is accompanied by three or more cranial MRI-detected lesions.

Is it possible to delay or prevent the development of clinically definite MS in patients who suffer a single episode of inflammatory demyelinating CNS injury? This important question surfaced with the *post hoc* analysis of the Optic Neuritis Treatment Trial (ONTT).[32] Intravenous methylprednisolone and oral prednisone, administered consecutively, appeared to reduce the two-year risk of developing clinically definite MS (7.5 per cent risk versus 16.7 per cent for placebo-treated patients). This observation inspired two large phase three multicenter trials designed to determine whether interferons provide an additional or protective effect in steroid-treated, high-risk (e.g. ≥3 cranial MRI abnormalities) patients presenting with their first episode of possible MS (*Table 13.1*).

Currently, there are no trials being designed or conducted to determine whether this retrospectively identified apparent steroid benefit can be confirmed. It appears unlikely that such a trial will be launched in the near future; the two studies summarized in *Table 13.1* will be extraordinarily difficult to perform given the limited number of patients and the difficulty in identifying and enrolling these patients within one month of presentation. There seems little likelihood of launching, in addition, a placebo-controlled trial to confirm the original steroid observation.

'Catastrophic' MS attacks

A minority of patients experience severe or life-threatening MS attacks rendering them comatose, aphasic, quadriplegic, or paraplegic. In this setting, most clinicians would use high-dose corticosteroids, and at least partial recovery is seen in the majority of patients. Occasionally, however, catastrophic MS attacks appear to be steroid-resistant. One small, open-label series[33] and a number of isolated case reports have suggested that plasma exchange (PE) may be followed by moderate or dramatic recovery in apparently steroid-

resistant cases. Having made the original observation that PE might be beneficial in such cases, our group was unwilling to design a pure placebo-controlled trial to answer this question. Instead, under the direction of Drs B Weinshenker and M Rodriguez, we are exploring whether PE may reverse such catastrophic injury in an NIH-funded, sham PE-controlled, cross-over trial design in patients who have failed high-dose intravenous methylprednisolone therapy. Results are expected by late 1997.

'Fixed neurological deficits'

Most patients recover partially or fully from early attacks. As shown in the ONTT, more than 70 per cent of patients recover to at least 20/40 (6/12 Europe) vision within six months of their first episode of inflammatory optic neuritis.[34] In 1973, Kurtzke *et al.* demonstrated that only 8.7 per cent of patients unrecovered after 16 weeks improved significantly.[35] Is it possible to reverse a recently acquired but apparently permanent deficit in MS? In the experimental literature, Rodriguez and colleagues have shown that it is possible to induce abundant spinal cord remyelination, in the setting of chronic Theiler's virus infection, by the administration of either pooled polyclonal mouse immunoglobulin(Ig), purified IgG directed against spinal cord antigens, or with the administration of one of several monoclonal antibodies of the IgM class.[36,37] Van Engelen and colleagues reported that IVIg administration may be followed by significant recovery of visual function in patients with steroid-unresponsive, long-standing, inflammatory optic neuritis.[38] These and other clinical and experimental studies have inspired our group to initiate 2 NIH-funded placebo-controlled, double-blind trials designed to determine whether IVIg administration is followed by recovery of either muscle weakness in MS or visual function in patients with irreversible, moderately severe visual loss from inflammatory optic neuritis.[39] Results of these studies are anticipated within the next 18 months.

Summary

Placebo-controlled trials are not only ethical but urgently needed to define whether it is possible to alter the natural history of primary progressive MS and to identify whether one can induce recovery in the setting of either steroid-unresponsive, catastrophic worsening or apparently irreversible, long-standing fixed neurological deficits. The important, and as yet unexplored, setting of altering recovery from an acute MS exacerbation probably requires a 'steroid rescue' escape clause or a cross-over design with a steroid limb for patients who either continue to worsen or appear to be non-responsive to new therapies. Neither IFN-β-1b (Betaseron, Betaferon) nor copolymer-1 (glatiramer acetate) (Copaxone) have been convincingly shown to impact disability progression. As such, neither one of these agents should be used to replace a convincing placebo in trials designed to slow disability progression. Of the many agents which have been studied and are currently under investigation, IFN-β-1a (Avonex) is the only therapy which currently merits serious consideration as the 'standard effective therapy' to replace a placebo-control group. At the time of writing, the results of the extensive and, hopefully definitive, trials of an identical agent (IFN-β-1a; Rebif (Ares Serono); *Table 13.1*) are unknown. If these trials provide convincing additional supportive evidence that disease progression can be significantly impacted by IFN-β-1a, MS trialists will need to regroup and decide whether placebos are obsolete for patients with relapsing–remitting and secondary-progressive MS. Whether there will be consensus that 'relapsing MS' includes both relapsing–remitting and secondary-progressive MS patients (and, by that decision, perhaps implying that all patients with relapsing forms of this disease should be offered IFN-β-1a in the setting of a definitive trial) will presumably be decided within the next 2–3 years. It remains highly likely, however, that placebo-controlled trials will be with us for some time to deal with patients who refuse parenteral interferons and for those who have developed either neutralizing antibodies to them or who have apparently failed to respond to this class of agents.

Acknowledgements

I thank Mrs Laura Irlbeck for preparing the manuscript.

References

1. IFNB Multiple Sclerosis Study Group. Interferon beta-1b is effective in relapsing–remitting multiple sclerosis. I. Clinical results of a multicenter, randomized, double-blind, placebo-controlled trial. *Neurology* 1993; **43**: 655–661.

2. Paty DW, Li DKB, the UBC MS/MRI Study Group *et al*. Interferon beta-1b is effective in relapsing–remitting multiple sclerosis. II. MRI analysis results of a multicenter, randomized, double-blind, placebo-controlled trial. *Neurology* 1993; **43**: 662–667.

3. IFNB Multiple Sclerosis Study Group, University of British Columbia MS/MRI Analysis Group. Interferon beta-1b in the treatment of MS: Final outcome of the randomized controlled trial. *Neurology* 1995; **45**: 1277–1285.

4. Jacobs LD, Cookfair DL, Rudick RA *et al*. Intramuscular interferon beta-1a for disease progression in relapsing multiple sclerosis. The Multiple Sclerosis Collaborative Research Group (MSCRG). *Ann Neurol* 1996; **39**: 285–294.

5. Johnson KP, Brooks BR, Cohen JA *et al*. Copolymer 1 reduces relapse rate and improves disability in relapsing–remitting multiple sclerosis: results of a phase III multicenter, double-blind placebo-controlled trial. The Copolymer 1 Multiple Sclerosis Study Group. *Neurology* 1995; **45**: 1268–1276.

6. Levine RJ. *Ethics and Regulation of Clinic Research*, 2nd edn. New Haven: Yale University Press 1988.

7. Yudkin PL, Ellison GW, Ghezzi A *et al*. Overview of azathioprine treatment in multiple sclerosis. *Lancet* 1991; **338**: 1051–1055.

8. Weiner HL. An assessment of plasma exchange in progressive multiple sclerosis. *Neurology* 1985; **35**: 320–322.

9. Noseworthy JH, Vandervoort MK, Ebers GC. Acceptance of placebo-control trial design by progressive multiple sclerosis patients. The Canadian Cooperative Multiple Sclerosis Study Group. *Neurology* 1989; **39**: 606–607.

10. The Canadian Cooperative Multiple Sclerosis Study Group. The Canadian cooperative trial of cyclophosphamide and plasma exchange in progressive multiple sclerosis. *Lancet* 1991; **337**: 441–446.

11. Likosky WH. Experience with cyclophosphamide in multiple sclerosis: the cons. *Neurology* 1988; **38**: 14–18.

12. Sibley WA. *Therapeutic Claims in Multiple Sclerosis*, 3rd edn. New York: Demos 1992.

13. McFarland HF, Frank JA, Albert PS *et al*. Using gadolinium-enhanced magnetic resonance imaging lesions to monitor disease activity in multiple sclerosis. *Ann Neurol* 1992; **32**: 758–766.

14. Stone LA, Frank JA, Albert PS *et al*. The effect of interferon-beta on blood-brain barrier disruptions demonstrated by contrast-enhanced magnetic resonance imaging in relapsing–remitting multiple sclerosis. *Ann Neurol* 1995; **37**: 611–619.

15. Noseworthy JH, Vandervoort MK, Wong CJ *et al*. Interrater variability with the Expanded Disability Status Scale (EDSS) and Functional Systems (FS) in a multiple sclerosis clinical trial. *Neurology* 1990; **40**: 971–975.

16. Willoughby EW, Paty DW. Scales for rating impairment in multiple sclerosis: a critique. *Neurology* 1988; **38**: 1793–1798.

17. Noseworthy JH, Ebers GC, Vandervoort MK *et al*. The impact of blinding on the results of a randomized, placebo-controlled multiple sclerosis clinical trial. *Neurology* 1994; **44**: 16–20.

18. Prentice RL. Surrogate endpoints in clinical trials: definition and operational criteria. *Stat Med* 1989; **8**: 431–440.

19. Freedman B. Equipoise and the ethics of clinical research. *N Engl J Med* 1987; **317**: 141–145.

20. Johnson N, Lilford RJ, Brazier W. At what level of collective equipoise does a clinical trial become ethical? *J Med Ethics* 1991; **17**: 30–34.

21. Noseworthy JH, Vandervoort MK, Hopkins M *et al*. A referendum on clinical trial research in multiple sclerosis: the opinion of the partici-

pants at the Jekyll Island workshop. *Neurology* 1989; **39**: 977–981.

22. Lublin FD, Reingold SC. National Multiple Sclerosis Society (USA) Advisory Committee on Clinical Trials of New Agents in Multiple Sclerosis. Defining the clinical course of multiple sclerosis: Results of an international survey. *Neurology* 1996; **46**: 907–911.

23. Goodkin DE. MS clinical trial design for the future. *Multiple Sclerosis* 1996; **1**: 393–399.

24. Kurtzke JF. Rating neurologic impairment in multiple sclerosis: An expanded disability status scale (EDSS). *Neurology* 1983; **33**: 1444–1452.

25. IFNB Multiple Sclerosis Study Group and the University of British Columbia MS/MRI Analysis Group. Neutralizing antibodies during treatment of multiple sclerosis with interferon beta-1b: Experience during the first three years. *Neurology* 1996; **47**: 889–894.

26. Paty DW, Goodkin D, Thompson A *et al.* Guidelines for physicians with patients on IFNb-1b: The use of an assay for neutralizing antibodies (NAB). *Neurology* 1996; **47**: 865–866.

27. Rudick R, Antel J, Confavreux C *et al.* Clinical outcomes assessment in multiple sclerosis. *Ann Neurol* 1996; **40**: 469–479.

28. Thompson AJ, Kermode AG, MacManus DG *et al.* Patterns of disease activity in multiple sclerosis: clinical and magnetic resonance imaging study. *Br Med J* 1990; **300**: 631–634.

29. Thompson AJ, Kermode AG, Wicks D *et al.* Major differences in the dynamics of primary and secondary progressive multiple sclerosis. *Ann Neurol* 1991; **29**: 5362.

30. Barkhof F, Tas MW, Frequin ST *et al.* Limited duration of the effect of methylprednisolone on changes on MRI in multiple sclerosis. *Neuroradiology* 1994; **36**: 382–387.

31. Morrissey SP, Miller DH, Kendall BE *et al.* The significance of brain magnetic resonance imaging abnormalities at presentation with clinically isolated syndromes suggestive of multiple sclerosis. *Brain* 1993; **116**: 135–146.

32. Beck RW, Cleary PA, Trobe JD *et al.* The effect of corticosteroid for acute optic neuritis on the subsequent development of multiple sclerosis. *N Engl J Med* 1993; **329**: 1764–1769.

33. Rodriguez M, Karnes WE, Bartleson JD *et al.* Plasmapharesis in acute episodes of fulminant CNS inflammatory demyelination. *Neurology* 1993; **43**: 1100–1104.

34. Beck RW, Cleary PA, Anderson MM, Jr *et al.* A randomized, controlled trial of corticosteroids in the treatment of acute optic neuritis. The Optic Neuritis Study Group. *N Engl J Med* 1992; **326**: 581–588.

35. Kurtzke JF, Beebe GW, Nagler B *et al.* Studies on the natural history of multiple sclerosis. 7. Correlates of clinical change in an early bout. *Acta Neurol Scand* 1973; **49**: 379–395.

36. Rodriguez M, Lennon VA. Immunoglobulins promote remyelination in the central nervous system. *Ann Neurol* 1990; **27**: 12–17.

37. Miller DJ, Sanborn KS, Katzman JA *et al.* Monoclonal autoantibodies promote central nervous system repair in an animal model of multiple sclerosis. *J Neurosci* 1994; **14**: 6230–6238

38. van Engelen BG, Hommes OR, Pinckers A *et al.* Improved vision after intravenous immunoglobulin in stable demyelinating optic neuritis. *Ann Neurol* 1992; **32**: 834–835.

39. Noseworthy JH, O'Brien PC, van Engelen BGM *et al.* Intravenous immunoglobulin therapy in multiple sclerosis: Progress from the Theiler's virus model to a randomized, double-blinded, placebo-controlled clinical trial. *J Neurol Neurosurg Psychiatry* 1994; **57** (suppl): 11–14.

14

Has magnetic resonance imaging become a surrogate marker in multiple sclerosis?

David H Miller

Introduction

The recent trials of beta interferons (IFN-βs)[1,2] and copolymer-1[3] have for the first time led to a widespread conviction that it may soon be possible to effectively modify the long-term course of multiple sclerosis (MS). At the same time, the trial results have raised many contentious questions. For example, what is the best way of quantifying relapses? Is relapse rate really a valid outcome when patient blinding is difficult to achieve because of side effects and when the relationship between relapse rate and long-term disability is far from clear?[4] Why have all three trials shown a significant effect on relapse rate yet only one has reported an effect on confirmed increase in disability? How meaningful are the results for predicting the long-term outcome for patients; is a two-year study long enough to draw firm conclusions?

Implicit in such questions is the widespread recognition that there are formidable problems in conducting treatment trials with clinical endpoints, such as relapse rate or progression in disability. The highly variable and unpredictable natural history of MS requires very large studies (usually involving hundreds of patients) of long duration (usually 2–3 years). It is not surprising, therefore, that there has been much emphasis on the use of alternative laboratory markers of disease activity to moni-

tor treatment efficacy. In this setting, the term 'surrogate marker' has become popular. A surrogate is something used in the place of, or as a substitute for, something else. To be an effective replacement of clinical outcomes the surrogate measure of disease activity needs to be objective, sensitive, accurate, reproducible, cost effective and, most importantly, predictive of clinical outcome. Magnetic resonance imaging (MRI) is currently the only serious candidate as an adequate surrogate. This chapter reviews its status.

Objectivity

In measuring clinical outcomes, objectivity is very difficult to achieve. Blinding may be broken for patients who experience treatment-related side effects, and for investigators by observation of overt side effects or indiscreet discussion of the patient's symptoms. MRI can totally avoid the bias which comes with unblinding. The radiologist who analyses the scans can be totally separate from the patient, and completely blinded to treatment status in a parallel group study design. Even in a baseline crossover design, where all patients are treated after a baseline period of scanning without treatment, blinding is maintained when the total number of enhancing lesions is counted and scans are analysed in a random order.

Could the placebo effect influence MRI activity? This is a theoretical possibility, but it seems unlikely to be of practical importance. It nevertheless needs to be formally assessed in a study comparing patients who received placebo in a double-blind study and a group of appropriately matched untreated patients who underwent the same MRI protocol as part of a natural history study.

Sensitivity

Given the relative insensitivity of clinical endpoints, it is of paramount importance that a surrogate marker should be more sensitive, allowing treatment effects to be seen more rapidly and in a smaller number of patients. In early relapsing–remitting (RR) MS (disease duration less than ten years), monthly T_2-weighted and standard dose gadolinium (0.1 mmol/kg) enhanced T_1-weighted brain MRI reveals about ten active (i.e. new and/or enhancing) lesions for every clinical relapse.[5–7] Similar levels of activity have been reported in secondary-progressive (SP) MS,[8,9] but the amount of MRI activity is a quantum less in those with primary-progressive (PP) disease.[8,9] Therapy-induced reductions in the number of active lesions have been demonstrated in as few as seven patients with RR or SP MS studied for only 6–9 months.[10] MRI activity does vary substantially between and within patients over time and interpatient variability is greater than intrapatient variability. Thus, crossover designs are more powerful than parallel group studies, although the latter provide a more robust assessment of therapeutic efficacy.[11,12] Limitations of a baseline crossover design (a period of run-in followed by a period of treatment) are the potential for regression to the mean due to case selection/entry criteria bias; the double crossover design may be contaminated by a carry-over effect of treatment from the first to the second phase. Nevertheless, successful trials using all three designs (baseline crossover, double crossover, and parallel groups) have been performed (see *Table 14.1*).[2,10,13–21]

Clinical subgroups

Although broadly similar levels of activity have been reported in small cohorts with early RR or SP MS, on closer inspection of the SP cohorts some differences emerge. SP patients who continue to have relapses have more MRI activity than those who do not,[9] and, compared to early RR MS, a rather higher proportion of SP patients have low levels of MRI activity. Recent sample size calculations, based on natural history studies of 31 RR and 28 SP patients, found that larger sample sizes are needed to show a given MRI treatment effect in the SP group.[22] It also showed that in a parallel-group design, there is a substantial improvement in power in both groups by obtaining two pre-treatment baseline scans one month apart (rather than a single scan immediately before starting treatment).

Patients with benign MS (RR disease with minimal disability after ten or more years of disease) have much less MRI activity on serial studies,[6,23] but are rarely considered suitable for inclusion in treatment trials on clinical grounds. The most vexing group are those with PP disease. Serial MRI shows new lesions with about one tenth of the frequency seen in early RR disease, and few of these display gadolinium enhancement.[8,9] The low sensitivity of conventional MRI in PP MS precludes its use in pilot studies. Even triple dose gadolinium (see next section) adds little[24] or nothing[25] in the PP subgroup.

Strategies to improve sensitivity

New enhancing lesions are seen twice as often as new T_2 lesions on monthly brain MRI in

Therapy	Design	Effect (%)	Reference
Beta interferon 1b	Parallel groups (RR)	60–75	13
Beta interferon 1b	Baseline crossover (RR)	75	14
Beta interferon 1a	Parallel groups (RR)	50	2
Beta interferon 1a	Baseline crossover (RR)	64	15
Campath-1H	Baseline crossover (SP)	90	10
Mitoxantrone	Parallel groups (RR/SP)	80	16
Linomide*	Parallel groups (RR)	70	17
Linomide*	Parallel groups (SP)	55	18
IVIg	Double crossover (RR)	70	19
Alpha interferon	Parallel groups (RR)	95	20
Copolymer-1	Baseline crossover (RR)	60	21

*Discontinued due to unexpected side effects

Table 14.1
Studies showing a reduction in MRI activity.

RR or SP MS.[26] Weekly scanning[27] and spinal imaging[28] give only modest increases (about 10–15 per cent) but more substantial gains are apparent using a variety of techniques to improve the detection of enhancing lesions: triple-dose gadolinium (0.3 mmol/kg),[29] magnetization transfer T_1-weighted sequences,[25,30] delayed scanning,[25] and thinner slices (down to 1 mm with volume acquisition sequences[31]). Of these, triple dose adds the most: there is a 70 per cent increase in the number of enhancing lesions compared with single dose.[29] With a combination of triple dose, MT sequences and a delay post gadolinium injection of 20–40 minutes, the increase is 120 per cent,[25] which is the largest gain reported to date. Serial studies are being performed to determine the sample size benefits of triple dose gadolinium (M Filippi, personal communication). It is not inevitable that the gain in sensitivity will markedly reduce sample size; should there be an increase in variability of activity between patients, sample sizes could actually increase.

With respect to unenhanced imaging, strategies to increase sensitivity for small lesions (compared to the standard proton density PD/T_2-weighted sequences) include thinner slices,[32] fast FLAIR[33,34] and 3D fast spin echo which provides T_2-weighted images with 1–1.5 mm thick slices (*Fig. 14.1*). Preliminary data at 4 Tesla (compared to the standard 0.5–1.5 Tesla systems) suggest that resolution of small lesions is much improved (R Grossman, personal communication). The role of all these approaches in monitoring therapy is yet to be defined.

Accuracy

The gold standard for evaluating the accuracy of MRI is the pathology itself. An accurate technique should visualize all the macroscopic plaques, and also be able to quantify the microscopic lesions which are known to occur in the normal appearing white matter. T_2-weighted imaging of post mortem brain correlates quite well with macroscopic pathological findings,[35,36] suggesting that this sequence is fairly accurate in detecting plaques. Resolution of course limits detection of smaller lesions. The usual slice thickness in MR studies is 5 mm, and small lesions are undoubtedly missed: in one study, there was a 9 per cent increase in lesion load when slice thickness was reduced to 3 mm, and it was estimated that the increase would be 20 per cent had it been possible to go down to 1 mm.[32] Experience with fast FLAIR has emphasized that T_2-weighted imaging fails to detect some lesions, especially those in a subcortical/cortical location.[33,34] So it is clear that the current sequences provide only an approximate estimate of the load of lesions. Nevertheless, it is still adequate for therapeutic assessments.

A critical question is how accurate are computer assisted techniques at segmenting visible MS lesions? The validation issue here requires a comparison of the new technique with the observations of an experienced observer as to what is or is not a lesion. The measurement of lesion load by manual outlining on a computer screen by an experienced rater of lesions previously identified by an experienced observer (usually a clinician) can be considered as a gold standard, albeit an imperfect one, for accuracy. Automated techniques, in which a computer generated algorithm performs the lesion segmentation, have the attraction of being faster and more reproducible than manual outlining, but are not necessarily as accurate. An expert is still required to evaluate the result and where there are clearly inaccuracies (false positive or negative), manual editing may be necessary. If inaccuracies are exactly the same on all serial scans of an individual, they will not be a problem, because true biological changes should still be apparent. But if the inaccuracies vary from scan to scan, completely spurious results may be obtained. Standardization of the MRI data acquisition over time on the same scanner, let alone different scanners, is hard to achieve: changes in factors such as gradient performance, magnetic field homogeneity, image uniformity and coil loading will all affect the degree of inaccuracy. For the present, a semi-automated approach seems wise: i.e. the application of an automated method with manual editing of obvious inaccuracies.

Reproducibility

It is important that the MRI outcome measure should have a high degree of reproducibility. If not, changes over time might be attributable to measurement error rather than to biological events. The two main outcomes used in trials to date are counting the number of active (usually enhancing) lesions in pilot studies,

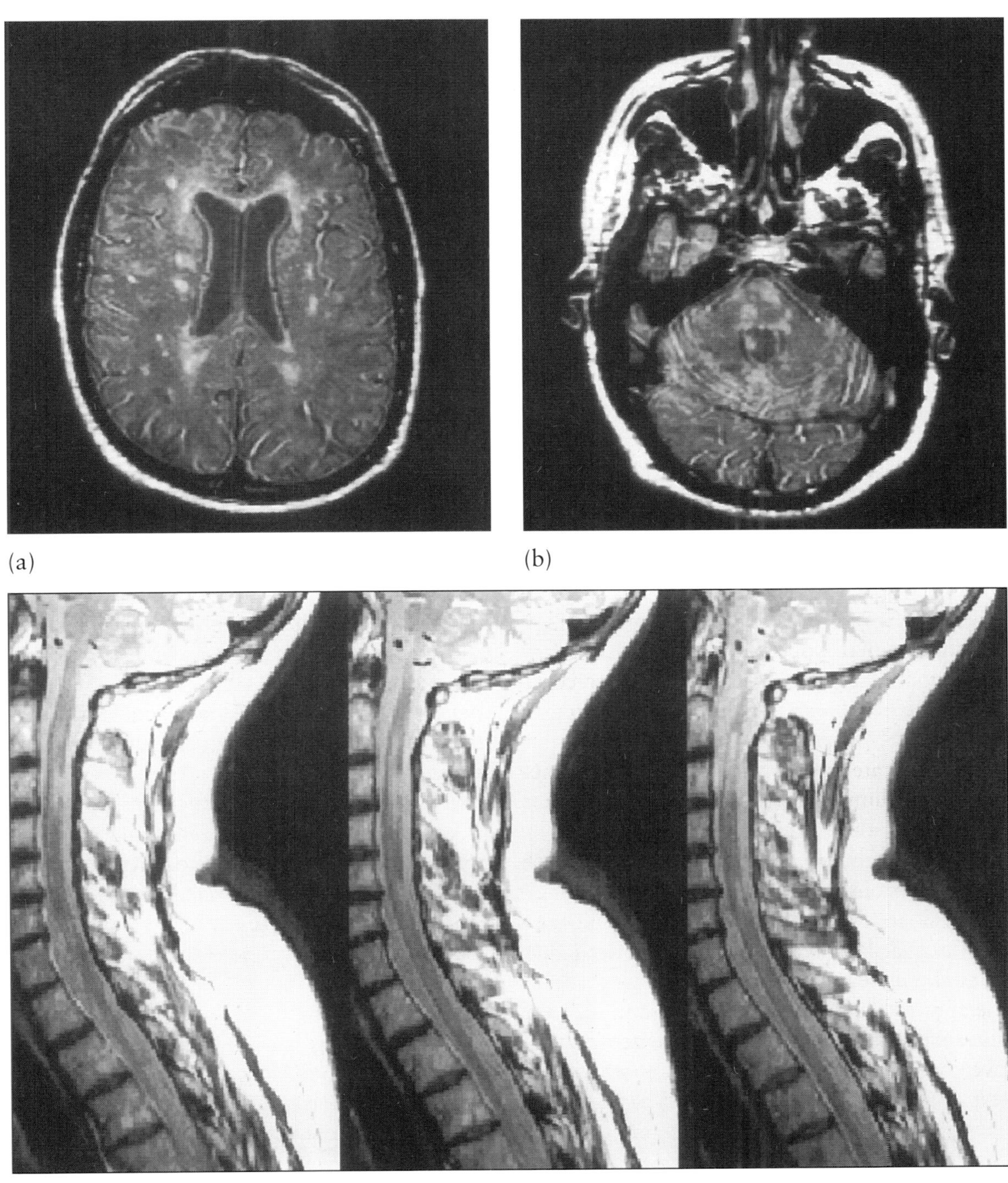

(a)

(b)

(c)

Fig. 14.1
T_2-weighted 3D fast spin echo sequence with 1.5 mm thick slices through the lateral ventricles (a), posterior fossa (b) and spinal cord (c) in patients with MS. There are multifocal high signal lesions in all regions.

and measuring the total T_2 lesion load in phase 3 studies. Standardization between observers in the definition of enhancing lesions has been attempted in an EC-funded network for optimizing MR techniques for monitoring the disabling pathology in MS (MAGNIMS). Without rules experienced observers have a good inter-rater reproducibility in defining enhancing lesions,[37] but less experienced observers do not. With rules, even less experienced observers show a good reproducibility. This emphasizes the need for training and experience for investigators who will be analysing MRI lesion activity in MS trials. The reproducibility of counting new T_2 lesions is the subject of an ongoing MAGNIMS study.

Turning to T_2 lesion load, manual outlining has only a modest reproducibility: intra-rater variabilities of 6–10 per cent are reported,[38] with even higher inter-rater variabilities. Given that the mean increase in T_2 lesion load in a population of relapsing–remitting patients is 5–10 per cent per year, such measurement errors might potentially obscure a moderate treatment effect (a large treatment effect can still be shown).[13] More automated methods can certainly improve reproducibility, but this should not be achieved at the expense of introducing inaccuracies which vary from one scan to the next. For example, application of a single global threshold to T_2-weighted images is fast and reproducible, provided the same threshold is applied to the same image,[39] but it is liable to be very inaccurate: lower thresholds include a good deal of normal cortex, and higher thresholds miss lesion areas which are only mildly hyperintense with respect to normal white matter. Other automated approaches, such as cluster analysis using multiparametric data, or 3D fuzzy connectivity, are more promising, although large scale validation studies are lacking.[40] At present, my preference is to use a semi-automated local

thresholding technique. In this case, the expert identifies lesions and the computer programme delineates them using a local thresholding algorithm called Contour (developed by D Plummer, UCL Department of Medical Physics). We have found that this is appreciably more reproducible than manual outlining, with intra-rater variabilities of 2–4 per cent (versus 6–10 per cent for manual).[38] In future, the ideal technique should be faster and more automated while maintaining or improving the high degree of accuracy and reproducibility now achieved with Contour.

Cost effectiveness

MRI is expensive, but only relatively so – an MRI study which can show a treatment effect in a small number of patients within a few months will cost much less than a large-scale, long-term, clinical outcome study. Such an approach also reduces the number of patients exposed to potential side effects from new therapies. So MRI *is* cost effective in the setting of pilot studies to evaluate new therapies. If such a study is positive, there is a rational basis for proceeding to the expensive large-scale clinical trial; if it is negative, there is a good case for not investigating the therapy further.

Clinical predictive value

The most important requirement of all for a good surrogate is that its findings are predictive of future clinical outcome. In MS, the two common clinical outcomes are relapse rate and sustained progression in disability. Of these the latter is the more important. Relapse rate *per se* is a poor predictor of future disability[4] – by and large patients recover from relapses. This section will concentrate mainly on the MRI–disability relationship but will also discuss the MRI–relapse correlates.

There are multiple factors which impinge on the MR–clinical relationship. These include clinical issues such as the scales to quantify relapses or disability, and MRI factors including the extent, site and pathological nature of lesions, microscopic pathology in the normal appearing white matter, and cortical re-adaptation mechanisms which can now be explored using functional MRI.[41]

Clinical scales

Inadequacies of the commonly-used clinical scales are a major issue in their own right (see Hobart, Chapter 15). The problems of subjectivity, poor reproducibility, lack of representation of all facets of functional impairment, and insensitivity to change, are well recognized;[42] 'noise' in such scales may contribute as much to the uncertain clinical–MRI relationship as do factors related to MRI. An improvement in MR measures must go hand in hand with optimizing clinical outcomes.

Lesion extent

Established MS

PD-(long TR and short TE) and T_2-weighted (long TR, long TE) conventional spin echo sequences have been the most widely used method for depicting MS lesions. A high sensitivity in detecting plaques was demonstrated early on in correlative post mortem studies.[35,36] It was also rapidly apparent that the total extent of lesions correlates only weakly with disability measured using the Expanded Disability Status Scale (EDSS).[43] Longitudinal studies have confirmed that changes in PD/T_2 lesion load correlate only modestly, if at all, with changes in EDSS.[44]

Most published studies have used 5 mm slice thickness. Reducing slice thickness increases lesion load by 9–20 per cent.[32] The additional small lesions detected may improve

correlations with disability, although I predict that any improvement will be modest.

Another sequence which detects more subcortical lesions is fast FLAIR. This uses an inversion recovery pulse with a long inversion time which suppresses cerebro-spinal fluid (CSF) signal; a long TE is then applied to give heavy T_2-weighting. This results in the detection of 20 per cent more lesions in subcortical white matter,[33,34] although significantly fewer lesions are seen in the posterior fossa.[34] Despite these differences, a recent study of 52 patients showed that the correlation of EDSS was no stronger with fast FLAIR lesion load (r = 0.44) than with T_2 lesion load (r = 0.49) (Gawne-Cain *et al.*, unpublished observations). In summary, current evidence in established MS suggests that the total extent of brain lesions correlates only modestly with locomotor disability.

Clinically isolated syndromes

Here the situation is very different. About 60 per cent of patients already have disseminated clinically silent brain lesions when they present with an isolated syndrome typical of MS, such as optic neuritis, brain stem or spinal cord syndromes.[45–48] There is a strong correlation between the presence and number of lesions and progression to clinically definite MS in the next 1–5 years.[49–56] MRI is therefore appropriately used to select patients for trials of therapy aimed at preventing conversion from an isolated syndrome to clinically definite MS.[57] We have recently completed a ten-year follow-up of our cohort at The National Hospital, who were first seen in the mid 1980s (J O'Riordan, unpublished observations). After ten years, over 85 per cent with two or more lesions have developed clinically definite MS, whereas only 11 per cent with a normal scan have. Moderate or severe disability (EDSS > 3) has developed in about 30 per cent with 1–10 lesions but in 72 per cent with more than ten lesions on the initial scan. Those entering the secondary progressive phase of the disease had a higher initial lesion number compared to those who have developed an RR course with minimal disability.

Lesion site

In established MS, the lack of relationship between brain lesion load and EDSS should not occasion much surprise – most cerebral hemisphere lesions are in locations which cannot *per se* result in locomotor disability. On the other hand, they might be expected to contribute to cognitive impairment, and indeed a correlation between brain lesion load and neuropsychological abnormalities has emerged, although only to a modest degree.[58,59] Most of the lesions leading to locomotor disability are in the spinal cord or posterior fossa. A higher posterior fossa lesion load has been reported in patients with progressive disease compared to benign MS in some[60,61] but not all[42] studies. The largest spinal MRI study involved 80 patients and used 3 mm thick contiguous sagittal slices and phased array coils which survey the entire cord in a single field of view. Although three quarters of patients had intrinsic focal cord lesions, their number and extent did not correlate with EDSS.[62] Another recent study has identified asymptomatic cord lesions in one third of patients with clinically isolated optic neuritis.[63] It is clear from these data that patients can have extensive MRI lesions in clinically eloquent pathways without functional consequences.

A recent study has reported diffuse signal changes on PD-weighted cord scans in patients with a progressive course.[64] The pathological basis of this interesting observation is uncertain; diffuse gliosis is one possibility.

The pathological nature of lesions

The pathological nature of lesions is likely to be critical in determining their functional effects. Acute MS lesions display inflammation (perivascular lymphocytes and diffuse macrophage infiltration), oedema, and active demyelination. Subacute lesions may show variable degrees of remyelination. Chronic plaques are usually completely demyelinated, with marked astrocytic gliosis and a variable degree of axonal loss.

Inflammation

Inflammation correlates well with gadolinium enhancement in both experimental allergic encephalomyelitis[65] and in MS.[66] Enhancement is consistently seen in new brain lesions in RR[6] and SP MS,[8] and usually lasts 2–6 weeks, similar to the duration of clinical relapses. Enhancing lesions in the brain are more common during relapse than remission,[67] although the great majority are asymptomatic: enhancing cord lesions are much more likely to result in clinical relapse.[28] Enhancement of the symptomatic optic nerve lesion has been correlated with acute visual loss and conduction block (reduced amplitude of the visual evoked potential) in acute optic neuritis.[68] This cumulative evidence suggests that gadolinium enhancement is a good surrogate marker for acute relapses. Currently available follow-up studies also indicate that the number of enhancing lesions on short-term MRI studies modestly predicts the risk for disability in the next 1–5 years.[69–71] There is not enough data to recommend short-term enhanced MRI as the definitive outcome of treatment efficacy, but the correlations which exist support its current role as the primary outcome measure in pilot studies.[57]

Demyelination and axonal loss
These are the key pathological substrates of functional impairment in MS. Conduction block results from demyelination, although is not necessarily permanent, as conduction can be restored by the insertion of sodium channels along the internodal membrane.[72] Axonal loss is undoubtedly the strongest candidate as the explanation for the irreversible and progressive disabilities often seen in the later years of the disease. Several MR methods have been proposed to monitor these pathologies.

Magnetization transfer (MT) imaging This method interrogates the pool of protons bound to macromolecules. Conventional MRI looks only at mobile protons, since bound ones have such a short T_2 relaxation time that they have already lost their nuclear magnetic resonance (NMR) signal by the time the data is acquired. However, there is a continuous exchange between the bound and mobile pools. In an MT imaging experiment, the conventional radiofrequency stimulation pulse is used with and without an off resonance (MT) pulse which saturates the bound pool. The difference in signal between the MT and non-MT images provides an indication of the number of bound protons and hence a measure of the amount of macromolecular structure in the tissue, which can be quantified as the MT ratio. Normal white matter has a high MT ratio because it is highly structured. Protons bound to myelin probably have a major impact on MT ratio and it follows that a major reduction probably indicates demyelination. Support for this view comes from several sources:

- acute experimental autoimmune encephalomyelitis (EAE), which is inflammatory but non-demyelinating, shows only a minor reduction in MT ratio[73]
- chronic EAE with demyelination is associated with a large reduction in MT ratio[74]

- lysolecithin-induced demyelination markedly reduces MT ratio[75]
- the lesions of progressive multifocal leucoencephalopathy and central pontine myelinolysis, disorders in which demyelination is the pathological hallmark, have low MT ratios[76,77]
- the observation of a graded relationship between visual evoked potential latency and MT ratio in the optic nerve following an episode of optic neuritis suggests that demyelination contributes to the MT ratio abnormalities.[78]

It is encouraging that there is a stronger correlation of EDSS with lesion MT ratio than with T_2 lesion load,[79] and follow-up after 18 months has revealed that new lesions in secondary progressive MS have significantly lower MT ratios than in benign disease.[80] Acute gadolinium-enhancing lesions often have a markedly reduced MT ratio consistent with demyelination, but may show recovery towards normal at follow-up.[81] This evolution may be due to resolution of oedema, remyelination or gliosis. Techniques for MT imaging in the cord have recently been developed,[82] and this will allow a more direct correlation between symptoms and MT changes. Whether MT ratios distinguish demyelination alone from that associated with axonal loss is uncertain, and requires exploration in appropriate experimental studies.

T_1 hypointense lesions About 20–30 per cent of lesions seen on T_2-weighted scans are hypointense on T_1-weighted images (the rest are isointense). Such hypointense lesions (sometimes called 'black holes') have long T_1 relaxation times. There is a strong correlation between T_1 relaxation time and MT ratio, and hypointense T_1 lesions have lower MT ratios than isointense lesions,[83] perhaps indicating greater tissue loss. One study has reported a

significant correlation between change in hypointense lesion load and change in EDSS over 2–3 years in secondary progressive MS.[84] While this looks a promising technique for treatment trials (being very easy to acquire), it is less quantitative than MT ratio measurement, it can be particularly difficult to decide when a 'grey hole' should be classed as hypointense or isointense, and modest variations in the MR parameters (TR, TE) may substantially influence lesion classification.

Atrophy Atrophy can be anticipated to result from axonal or myelin loss. Two difficulties have been:

- developing techniques which are sufficiently reproducible to allow the detection of subtle changes in volume over time
- the large range of volumes seen in normal individuals in the cerebral hemispheres, posterior fossa and spinal cord.

Fortunately, highly reproducible methods for measuring volumes in these structures have recently been developed using semiautomated segmentation algorithms[85,86] and, encouragingly, strong correlations have been found with EDSS and cord atrophy,[85] cerebellar atrophy,[87] and cerebral atrophy;[86] in the latter instance a serial study over 18 months showed a significant relationship between change in cerebral volume and change in EDSS.[86]

MR spectroscopy The proton MR spectrum of the normal brain shows a dominant peak due to *N*-acetyl aspartate (NAA). NAA is contained almost exclusively within neurones in the adult brain; thus a reduction suggests loss or dysfunction of neurones. A strong correlation exists between cerebellar white matter NAA concentration and disability.[87] In PP MS, a group which is notable for major disability but small lesion load on conventional MRI,[43] one small study has reported a reduction in NAA in normal appearing white matter, sug-

gesting that diffuse axonal loss or dysfunction is occurring.[88] Increased peaks at 0.9 and 1.3 ppm are also seen in acute enhancing plaques,[89] suggesting the presence of mobile lipid protons compatible with active breakdown of myelin. Thus, MR spectroscopy has the potential to monitor both demyelination and axonal loss separately; its main limitations are resolution (typically 1–4 cc because of the low concentrations of the metabolites), and difficulties in achieving reproducible, automated quantitation of metabolite concentrations.

Diffusion imaging Several MR methods can be used to measure the apparent diffusion coefficient (ADC) and its directional component in central nervous system (CNS) tissue. These methods probe the size, shape and orientation of water-containing spaces in tissues and also assess the permeability of membrane structures. White matter tracts show diffusion anisotropy (higher diffusion rates are seen parallel to the fibre tracts than perpendicular). An increase in ADC and a decrease in anistropy could therefore imply loss of fibre tracts and/or expansion of the extracellular space. MS lesions have an elevated ADC,[90,91] and studies are underway to see how diffusion abnormalities correlate with clinical state.

'Myelin' imaging: T_2 magnetization decay analysis A multi-echo train with a short interecho interval allows the determination of multiple tissue water compartments which have different T_2 relaxation times. A long T_2 (>200 ms) component probably indicates extracellular water and its increase may indicate tissue loss.[92] A moderate T_2 (80–100 ms) probably represents intracellular water and is the dominant feature of normal white matter. A very short T_2 (<10 ms) is probably due to bound water; in normal white matter this will be mainly myelin-associated water. MS plaques lose the short T_2 peak seen in normal

white matter.[93] This interesting method has yet to be studied in a large clinical cohort.

In summary, a number of the above techniques have shown promise in preliminary studies in correlating rather strongly with disability. Further studies of larger cohorts and with follow up are needed to consolidate the clinical correlates and experimental studies to correlate with pathology. The application of such techniques in clinical trials is crucial – not only might they provide an important treatment outcome measure, but also they will provide important natural history data in the placebo arm, something which will become difficult to obtain as disease-modifying therapies are increasingly introduced into routine clinical practice.

Normal Appearing White Matter (NAWM)

Microscopic pathology is found in macroscopically normal white matter in MS. Reported abnormalities include perivascular lymphocyte cuffs, small foci of myelin breakdown products and astrocyte hyperplasia.[94] Quantitative abnormalities of T_1, T_2, MT ratio and NAA have all been reported.[73,95,96] A consistent correlation with disability has not emerged. In a recent study, NAWM T_2 did not correlate with EDSS while T_2 lesion load did (r = 0.44).[97] Given the non-degenerative nature of microscopic NAWM pathology,[94] it is perhaps not surprising that it may impact less on function than macroscopic lesions. However, the reductions of NAA reported from NAWM raise the possibility of diffuse axonal dysfunc-

tion or loss, which could be functionally relevant.[97]

Cortical re-adaptation

Relapse and remissions are characteristic in the early years of the disease. The latter is probably due to multiple factors in the symptomatic lesion, i.e. resolution of inflammation and oedema, remyelination and insertion of sodium channels along the internodal membrane of demyelinated axons. Another potentially important mechanism is cortical readaptation, in which new cortical regions become activated in order to compensate for a deficit. Such a process could lead to functional improvement without any change in the pathology or MRI appearance of the symptomatic white matter plaque. The role of this mechanism can now be studied using functional MRI techniques.[41] These require rapid gradient echo or echoplanar imaging and rely on changes in the amount of deoxyhaemoglobin associated with regional increases in blood flow during cortical activation. A preliminary study in MS identified new regions of cortical activation during recovery from hemiparesis.[99]

Conclusion

MRI is clearly a valuable tool for monitoring new treatments in MS. It should not be the definitive outcome because its relationship to clinical outcome is still uncertain. But it is an indispensable tool, and it is quite possible that, with time, the objectivity, sensitivity and clinical predictive value will be sufficient to justify using MR as a fully fledged surrogate.

References

1. The IFNB Multiple Sclerosis Study Group. Interferon beta-1b is effective in relapsing–remitting multiple sclerosis. *Neurology* 1993; **43**: 655–661.

2. Jacobs LD, Cookfair DL, Rudick RA *et al.* Intramuscular interferon beta-1a for disease progression in relapsing multiple sclerosis. *Ann Neurol* 1996; **39**: 285–294.

3. Johnson KP, Brooks BR, Cohen JS *et al.* Copolymer-1 reduces relapse rate and improves disability in relapsing–remitting multiple sclerosis. Results from a phase III, multicentre, double-blind, placebo-controlled trial. *Neurology* 1995; **45**: 1268–1276.

4. Runmarker B, Anderson O. Prognostic factors in a multiple sclerosis incidence cohort with twenty-five years of follow up. *Brain* 1993; **116**: 117–134.

5. Harris JO, Frank JA, Patronas N *et al.* Serial gadolinium-enhanced magnetic resonance imaging scans in patients with early, relapsing–remitting multiple sclerosis: implications for clinical trials and natural history. *Ann Neurol* 1991; **29**: 548–555.

6. Thompson AJ, Miller D, Youl B *et al.* Serial gadolinium enhanced MRI in relapsing remitting multiple sclerosis of varying disease duration. *Neurology* 1992; **42**: 60–63.

7. Barkhof F, Scheltens P, Frequin STFM *et al.* Relapsing–remitting multiple sclerosis: sequential enhanced MR imaging vs clinical findings in determining disease activity. *Am J Radiol* 1992; **159**: 1041–1047.

8. Thompson AJ, Kermode AG, Wicks D *et al.* Major differences in the dynamics of primary and secondary progressive multiple sclerosis. *Ann Neurol* 1991; **29**: 53–62.

9. Kidd D, Thorpe JW, Kendall BE *et al.* MRI dynamics of brain and spinal cord in progressive multiple sclerosis. *J Neurol Neurosurg Psychiatry* 1996; **60**: 15–19.

10. Moreau T, Thorpe J, Miller D *et al.* Preliminary evidence from magnetic resonance imaging for reduction in disease activity after lymphocyte depletion in multiple sclerosis. *Lancet* 1994; **344**: 298–301.

11. McFarland HF, Frank JA, Albert PS *et al.* Using gadolinium-enhanced magnetic resonance imaging lesions to monitor disease activity in multiple sclerosis. *Ann Neurol* 1992; **32**: 758–766.

12. Nauta JJP, Thompson AJ, Barkhof F *et al.* Magnetic resonance imaging in monitoring the treatment of multiple sclerosis patients: statistical power of parallel-groups and cross-over designs. *J Neurol Sci* 1994; **122**: 6–14.

13. Paty DW, Li DKB. UBC MS/MRI Study Group *et al.* Interferon beta-1b is effective in relapsing–remitting multiple sclerosis. II. MRI analysis results of a multicenter, randomized, double-blind, placebo-controlled trial. *Neurology* 1993; **43**: 662–667.

14. Stone LA, Frank JA, Albert PS *et al.* The effect of beta interferon on blood brain barrier disruptions demonstrated by contrast enhanced MRI in relapsing remitting multiple sclerosis. *Ann Neurol* 1995; **37**: 611–619.

15. Pozzilli C, Bastianello S, Koudriavtseva T *et al.* Magnetic resonance imaging changes with recombinant human interferon-B-1a: a short term study in relapsing–remitting multiple sclerosis patients. *J Neurol Neurosurg Psychiatry* 1996; **61**: 251–258.

16. Edan G, Miller D, Clanet M *et al.* Therapeutic effect of mitoxantrone combined with methylprednisolone in multiple sclerosis: a randomised multi-centre study of active disease using MRI and clinical criteria. *J Neurol Neurosurg Psychiatry* 1997; **62**: 112–118.

17. Anderson O, Lycke J, Tollesson PO *et al.* Linomide reduces the rate of active lesions in relapsing–remitting multiple sclerosis. *Multiple Sclerosis* 1996; **1**: 348.

18. Karussis DM, Meiner Z, Lehmann D *et al.* Treatment of secondary progressive multiple sclerosis with the immunomodulator linomide: a double-blind, placebo-controlled pilot study with monthly magnetic resonance imaging

evaluation. *Neurology* 1996; **47**: 341–346.

19. Sorensen PS, Wanscher B, Schreiber K *et al*. A double-blind cross-over trial of intravenous immunoglobulin in multiple sclerosis: preliminary results. *Eur J Neurol* 1996; **3** (suppl 4): 34–35.

20. Durelli L, Bongianno MR, Cavallo R *et al*. Chronic, systemic high-dose recombinant interferon alpha-2a reduces exacerbation rate, MRI signs of disease activity, and lymphocyte interferon gamma production in relapsing–remitting multiple sclerosis. *Neurology* 1994; **44**: 406–413.

21. Mancardi GL, Sardanelli F, Parodi RC *et al*. The effect of copolymer-1 on serial gadolinium-enhanced magnetic resonance scans in relapsing–remitting multiple sclerosis. *Eur J Neurol* 1996; **3** (suppl 4): 33.

22. Tubridy N, Ader H, Bartchof F. Sample size calculations for MRI outcome pilot trials in multiple sclerosis: Relapsing-remitting versus secondary progressive subgroups. *Neurology* 1997; **48**: A175.

23. Kidd D, Thompson AJ, Kendall BE *et al*. Benign form of multiple sclerosis: MRI evidence for less frequent and less inflammatory disease activity. *J Neurol Neurosurg Psychiatry* 1994; **57**: 1070–1072.

24. Filippi M, Campi A, Martinelli V *et al*. Comparison of triple dose versus standard dose gadolinium-DTPA for detection of MRI enhancing lesions in patients with primary progressive multiple sclerosis. *J Neurol Neurosurg Psychiatry* 1995; **59**: 540–544.

25. Silver N, Good CD, Barker GJ *et al*. Sensitivity of contrast enhanced MRI in multiple sclerosis: effects of gadolinium dose, magnetisation transfer contrast and delayed imaging. *Brain* 1997 (in press).

26. Miller DH, Barkhof F, Nauta JJP. Gadolinium enhancement increases the sensitivity of MRI in detecting disease activity in multiple sclerosis. *Brain* 1993; **116**: 1077–1094.

27. Lai HM, Hodgson T, Gawne-Cain M *et al*. A preliminary study into the sensitivity of disease activity detection by weekly serial magnetic resonance imaging in multiple sclerosis. *J Neurol Neurosurg Psychiatry* 1996; **60**: 339–341.

28. Thorpe JW, Kidd D, Moseley IF *et al*. Serial gadolinium enhanced MRI of the brain and spinal cord in early relapsing–remitting multiple sclerosis. *Neurology* 1996; **46**: 373–378.

29. Filippi M, Yousry T, Campi A *et al*. Comparison of triple dose versus standard dose gadolinium-DTPA for detection of MRI enhancing lesions in patients with MS. *Neurology* 1996; **46**: 379–384.

30. Mehta RC, Pike BG, Enzmann DR. Improved detection of enhancing and non enhancing lesions of multiple sclerosis with magnetization transfer. *Am J Neuroradiol* 1995; **16**: 1771–1778.

31. Filippi M, Yousry T, Horsfield MA *et al*. A high-resolution three-dimensional T1-weighted gradient echo sequence improves the detection of disease activity in multiple sclerosis. *Ann Neurol* 1996; **40**: 201–207.

32. Filippi M, Horsfield MA, Campi A *et al*. Resolution dependent estimates of lesion volumes in magnetic resonance imaging studies of the brain in multiple sclerosis. *Ann Neurol* 1995; **38**: 749–754.

33. Filippi M, Yousry T, Baratti C *et al*. Quantitative assessment of MRI lesion load in multiple sclerosis. A comparison of conventional spin echo with fast fluid attenuated inversion recovery. *Brain* 1996; **119**: 1349–1355.

34. Gawne-Cain ML, O'Riordan JI, Thompson AJ *et al*. Multiple sclerosis lesion detection in the brain: a comparison of fast fluid attenuated inversion recovery and conventional T_2 weighted dual spin echo. *Neurology* 1997 (in press).

35. Stewart WA, Hall LD, Berry K *et al*. Magnetic resonance imaging (MRI) in multiple sclerosis (MS): pathological correlation in 8 cases. *Neurology* 1986; **36**: 320.

36. Ormerod IEC, Miller DH, McDonald WI *et al*. The role of NMR imaging in the assessment of multiple sclerosis and isolated neurological lesions. *Brain* 1987; **110**: 1579–1616.

37. Barkhof F, Filippi M, Miller DHG *et al*. Interobserver variation in reporting gadolinium-enhanced lesions in multiple sclerosis. *Proc Int Soc Magn Reson Med* 1996; **1**: 539.

38. Grimaud J, Lai M, Thorpe JW *et al*. Evaluation of a computer assisted quantification of MS lesions in cranial MRI. *Magn Res Imaging* 1996; **14**: 495–505.

39. Filippi M, Horsfield MA, Bressi S *et al*. Intra-

and inter-observer agreement of brain MRI lesion volume measurements in multiple sclerosis. A comparison of techniques. *Brain* 1995; **118:** 1593–1600.

40. Evans AC, Frank JA, Antel J *et al.* The role of MRI in clinical trials of multiple sclerosis: comparison of image processing techniques. *Ann Neurol* 1997; **41:** 125–132.

41. Kwong KK, Belliveau JHW, Chesper DA *et al.* Dynamic magnetic resonance imaging of human brain activity during primary sensory stimulation. *Proc Natl Acad Sci USA* 1992; **89:** 5675–5679.

42. Rudick RA, Antel J, Confavreux C *et al.* Clinical outcomes assessment in multiple sclerosis. *Ann Neurol* 1996; **40:** 469–479.

43. Thompson AJ, Kermode AG, MacManus DG *et al.* Patterns of disease activity in multiple sclerosis: clinical and magnetic resonance imaging study. *Br Med J* 1990; **300:** 631–634.

44. IFNB Study Group, University of British Columbia MS/MRI Analysis Group. Interferon beta-1b in the treatment of MS: final outcome of the randomized controlled trial. *Neurology* 1995; **45:** 1277–1285.

45. Ormerod IEC, McDonald WI, du Boulay EPGH *et al.* Disseminated lesions at presentation in patients with clinically isolated optic neuritis. *J Neurol Neurosurg Psychiatry* 1986; **49:** 124–127.

46. Jacobs L, Kinkel PR, Kinkel WR. Silent brain lesions in patients with isolated optic neuritis. A clinical and nuclear magnetic resonance imaging study. *Arch Neurol* 1986; **43:** 452–455.

47. Ormerod IEC, Bronstein A, Rudge P *et al.* Magnetic resonance imaging in clinically isolated lesions of the brain stem. *J Neurol Neurosurg Psychiatry* 1986; **49:** 737–743.

48. Miller DH, McDonald WI, Blumhardt LD *et al.* MRI of the brain and spinal cord in isolated noncompressive spinal cord syndromes. *Ann Neurol* 1987; **22:** 714–723.

49. Martinelli V, Comi G, Filippi M *et al.* Paraclinical tests in acute onset optic neuritis: basal data and results of a short follow up study. *Acta Neurol Scand* 1991; **84:** 231–236.

50. Frederiksen JL, Larsson HBW, Olesen J *et al.* Magnetic resonance imaging of the brain in patients with acute monosymptomatic optic neuritis. *Acta Neurol Scand* 1991; **83:** 343–350.

51. Ford B, Tampieri D, Francis G. Long term follow up of acute transverse partial myelopathy. *Neurology* 1992; **42:** 250–252.

52. Beck RW, Cleary PA, Trobe JD *et al.* The effect of corticosteroids for acute optic neuritis on the subsequent development of multiple sclerosis. *N Engl J Med* 1993; **329:** 1764–1769.

53. Morrissey SP, Miller DH, Kendall BE *et al.* The significance of brain magnetic resonance imaging abnormalities at presentation with clinically isolated syndromes suggestive of multiple sclerosis. *Brain* 1993; **116:** 135–146.

54. Soderstrom M, Lindqvist M, Hillert J *et al.* Optic neuritis: findings on MRI, CSF examination and HLA class II typing in 60 patients and results of short term follow up. *J Neurol* 1994; **241:** 391–397.

55. Campi A, Filippi M, Comi G *et al.* Acute transverse myelopathy: spinal and cranial MR study with clinical follow-up. *Am J Neuroradiol* 1995; **16:** 115–123.

56. Tas MW, Barkhof F, van Walderveen MAAA *et al.* The effect of gadolinium on the sensitivity and specificity of MR imaging in the initial diagnosis of multiple sclerosis. *Am J Neuroradiol* 1995 **16:** 259–264.

57. Miller DH, Albert PS, Barkhof F *et al.* Guidelines for the use of magnetic resonance techniques in monitoring the treatment of multiple sclerosis. *Ann Neurol* 1996; **39:** 6–16.

58. Rao SM, Leo GJ, Haughton VM *et al.* Correlation of magnetic resonance imaging with neuropsychological testing in multiple sclerosis. *Neurology* 1989; **39:** 161–166.

59. Ron MA, Callanan MM, Warrington EK. Cognitive abnormalities in multiple sclerosis: a psychometric and MRI study. *Psychol Med* 1991; **21:** 59–68.

60. Koopmans RA, Li DKB, Grochowski EW *et al.* Benign versus chronic progressive multiple sclerosis: magnetic resonance imaging features. *Ann Neurol* 1989; **25:** 74–81.

61. Filippi M, Campi A, Mammi S *et al.* Brain magnetic resonance imaging and multimodal evoked potentials in benign and secondary progressive multiple sclerosis. *J Neurol Neurosurg Psychiatry* 1995; **58:** 31–37.

62. Kidd D, Thorpe JW, Thompson AJ *et al.* Spinal cord MRI using multi-array coils and fast spin echo. II findings in multiple sclerosis. *Neurology* 1993; **43**: 2632–2637.

63. O'Riordan JI, Losseff N, Thompson AJ *et al.* High resolution brain and spinal cord MRI in clinically isolated syndromes. *Eur J Neurol* 1996; **3** (suppl 4): 6

64. Lycklama A, Niejeholt GJ, Barkhof F *et al.* Multiple sclerosis in the spinal cord: relevance of diffuse abnormality on magnetic resonance images. *Eur J Neurol* 1996; **3** (suppl 4): 4–5.

65. Hawkins CP, Munro PMG, Mackenzie F *et al.* Duration and selectivity of blood-brain barrier breakdown. *Brain* 1990; **113**: 365–378.

66. Katz D, Taubenberger JK, Cannella B *et al.* Correlation between magnetic resonance imaging findings and lesion development in multiple sclerosis. *Ann Neurol* 1993; **34**: 661–669.

67. Grossman RI, Gonzales-Scarano F, Atlas SE *et al.* Multiple sclerosis: gadolinium enhancement in MR imaging. *Radiology* 1986; **169**: 117–122.

68. Youl BD, Turano G, Miller DH *et al.* The pathophysiology of optic neuritis: an association of gadolinium leakage with clinical and electrophysiological deficits. *Brain* 1991; **114**: 2437–2450.

69. Smith ME, Stone LA, Albert PS *et al.* Clinical worsening in multiple sclerosis is associated with increased frequency and area of gadopentetate dimeglumine-enhancing magnetic resonance imaging lesions. *Ann Neurol* 1993; **33**: 480–489.

70. Khoury SJ, Guttmann CRG, Gray EJ *et al.* Longitudinal MRI in multiple sclerosis: correlation between disability and lesion burden. *Neurology* 1994; **44**: 2120–2124.

71. Losseff N, Kingsley DPE, McDonald WI *et al.* Clinical and magnetic resonance imaging predictors of disability in primary and secondary progressive multiple sclerosis. *Multiple Sclerosis* 1996; **1**: 218–222.

72. Moll C, Mourre C, Lazdunsky M *et al.* Increase of sodium channels in demyelinated lesions of multiple sclerosis. *Brain Res* 1991; **556**: 311–316.

73. Dousset V, Grossman R, Ramer KN *et al.* Experimental allergic encephalomyelitis and multiple sclerosis: lesion characterisation with magnetisation transfer imaging. *Radiology* 1992; **182**: 483–491.

74. Dousset V, Brochet B, Vital F *et al.* Imaging including diffusion and magnetisation transfer of chronic relapsing experimental encephalomyelitis – correlation with immunological and pathological data. *Proc Soc Magn Reson* 1994; **2**: 1401.

75. Dousset V, Brochet B, Vital A *et al.* Lysolecithin-induced demyelination in primates: preliminary in vivo study with MR and magnetization transfer. *Am J Neuroradiol* 1995; **16**: 225–231.

76. Dousset V, Armand JP, Degreze P *et al.* Progressive multifocal leucoencephalopathy studied by magnetisation transfer imaging. *Proc Soc Magn Reson* 1995; **1**: 284.

77. Silver NC, Barker GJ, MacManus DG *et al.* Decreased magnetisation transfer ratio due to demyelination: a case of central pontine myelinolysis. *J Neurol Neurosurg Psychiatry* 1996; **61**: 208–209.

78. Thorpe JW, Barker GJ, Jones SJ *et al.* Quantitative MRI in optic neuritis: correlation with clinical findings and electrophysiology. *J Neurol Neurosurg Psychiatry* 1995; **59**: 487–492.

79. Gass A, Barker GJ, Kidd D *et al.* Correlation of magnetization transfer ratio with clinical disability in multiple sclerosis. *Ann Neurol* 1994; **36**: 62–67.

80. Lai HM, Barker GJ, Gass A *et al.* Serial magnetisation transfer imaging in benign and secondary progressive multiple sclerosis. *Proc Int Soc Magn Reson Med* 1996; **1**: 537.

81. Lai HM, Davie CA, Gass A *et al.* Serial magnetisation transfer ratios in gadolinium enhancing lesions in multiple sclerosis. *J Neurol* 1997; **244**: 308–311.

82. Silver NC, Barker GJ, Losseff N *et al.* Magnetisation transfer ratio measurement in the cervical cord: a preliminary study in multiple sclerosis. *Neuroradiology* 1997 (in press).

83. Hiehle JF, Grossman RI, Ramer KN *et al.* Magnetization transfer effect in MR-detected multiple sclerosis lesions: comparison with gadolinium-enhanced spin-echo images and non-enhanced T1-weighted images. *Am J Neuroradiol* 1995; **16**: 69–77.

84. van Walderveen MAA, Barkhof F, Hommes OR *et al.* Correlating MR imaging and clinical

disease activity in multiple sclerosis: relevance of hypointense lesions on short TR/TE ("T1-weighted") spin-echo images. *Neurology* 1995; **45**: 1684–1690.

85. Losseff NA, Webb SL, O'Riordan JI *et al.* Spinal cord atrophy and disability in multiple sclerosis. A new reproducible and sensitive MRI method with potential to monitor disease progression. *Brain* 1996; **119**: 701–708.

86. Losseff NA, Wang L, Lai HM *et al.* Progressive cerebral atrophy in multiple sclerosis: a serial study. *Brain* 1996; **119**: 2009–2019.

87. Davie CA, Barker GJ, Webb S *et al.* Persistent functional deficit in multiple sclerosis and autosomal dominant cerebellar ataxia is associated with axonal loss. *Brain* 1995; **118**: 1583–1592.

88. Davie CA, Barker GJ, Webb S *et al.* ¹H MRS study of disability in multiple sclerosis. *Proc Int Soc Magn Reson Med* 1996; **2**: 942.

89. Davie CA, Hawkins CP, Barker GJ *et al.* Serial proton magnetic resonance spectroscopy in acute multiple sclerosis lesions. *Brain* 1994; **117**: 49–58.

90. Larsson HBW, Thomsen C, Frederiksen J *et al.* In vivo magnetic resonance diffusion measurement in the brain of patients with multiple sclerosis. *Magn Reson Imaging* 1992; **10**: 7–12.

91. Horsfield MA, Lai M, Webb SL *et al.* Apparent diffusion coefficients in benign and secondary progressive multiple sclerosis by nuclear magnetic resonance. *Magn Reson Med* 1996; **36**: 393–400.

92. Barnes D, Munro PMG, Youl BD *et al.* The longstanding lesion in multiple sclerosis. *Brain* 1991; **114**: 1271–1280.

93. MacKay A, Whittal K, Adler J *et al.* In vivo visualization of myelin water in brain by magnetic resonance. *Magn Reson Med* 1994; **31**: 673–677.

94. Allen IV, McKeown SR. A histological, histochemical, and biochemical study of the macroscopically normal white matter in multiple sclerosis. *J Neurol Sci* 1979; **41**: 81–91.

95. Miller DH, Johnson G, Tofts PS *et al.* Precise relaxation time measurements of normal appearing white matter in inflammatory central nervous system disease. *Magn Reson Med* 1989; **11**: 331–336.

96. Arnold DL, Matthews PM, Francis G *et al.* Proton magnetic resonance spectroscopic imaging for metabolic characterization of demyelinating plaques. *Ann Neurol* 1992; **31**: 235–241.

97. Gasperini C, Horsfield MA, Thorpe JW *et al.* Macroscopic and microscopic assessments of disease burden by MRI in multiple sclerosis: relationship to clinical parameters. *J Magn Reson Imaging* 1996; **6**: 580–584.

98. Norayanan S, Fu L, Pioro E *et al.* Imaging of axonal damage in multiple sclerosis: spatial distribution of magnetic resonance imaging lesions. *Ann Neurol* 1997; **41**: 385–391.

99. Clanet M, Berry I, Gracia-Meavilla I *et al.* Functional MRI assessment of motor deficit in multiple sclerosis. *Eur J Neurol* 1996; **3** (suppl 4): 2.

15

Measuring health outcomes in multiple sclerosis: why, which, and how?

Jeremy C Hobart

Introduction

This chapter concerns the measurement of health outcomes in multiple sclerosis (MS). The first section outlines what outcome measurement is, why it is important, why it has become central to the future of health care evaluation, and why it is now particularly relevant to MS.

The second section addresses which outcomes can be measured. A four-level classification is presented and clear definitions are given to help address confusion in the literature. The change in focus from physician to patient-based outcomes is explained. Disease-specific and generic health status measures in MS are discussed.

The third section addresses how outcomes can be measured and explains how abstract health concepts, such as disability and health-related quality of life, can be measured rigorously.

Measuring outcomes: why?

Outcomes are simply the results or effects of processes. Health outcomes refer specifically to results which can be attributed to health care interventions.[1] By measuring the outcomes associated with interventions health care professionals are able to answer two questions: does an intervention work? and what effect does it have? These questions are the basis of evidence-based clinical decision making.[2–6]

The central importance of outcomes measurement to health care evaluation immediately raises two fundamental questions. First, have health professionals not been interested in the results of their interventions until recently? Second, why has it taken until the 1980s to become a central theme of health care?

Interest in outcomes is not a new phenomenon; clinicians have always been interested in the results of their interventions.[5] The routine practice of asking 'how are you' and 'do you feel better' are almost certainly the oldest forms of health care evaluation, and formal collections of mortality rates have been undertaken for a century. Explicit concern with health outcomes first emerged at the beginning of this century through the work of the North American surgeon EA Codman, who recognized that multiple factors were probably at play in the determination of 'end results'.[7] This visionary surgeon asked physicians to systematically document the results of their interventions along with their clinical actions, the facilities of their centres, and the habits and pursuits of their patients. In this way he was able to identify factors producing undesirable end results and acquire a means of preventing future harm.[8] Unfortunately, Codman's approach failed to attract widespread support from medicine or society.[9]

The 1980s saw a resurgence of interest in outcomes measurement. This was precipitated by the extensive technological developments of the preceding decades which had expanded all aspects of disease management. These advances naturally resulted in two parallel developments: first, variations in clinical practice which raised concerns as to how conditions should be managed; and, second, escalating health care costs which were increasingly outstripping available resources. As a consequence there was a need for health care professionals to be accountable by demonstrating the benefit of their interventions and the relative benefits of different interventions. Only in this way could medical treatment be maximized, patients be accurately informed as to the benefits and limitation of the therapies available to them, and limited resources be allocated in an equitable manner. These problems could be tackled by systematic and rigorous measurement of health outcomes using reproducible techniques.

For the care of patients with MS the need for rigorous outcomes measurement has recently reached critical importance for a number of reasons. First, an increasing number of therapeutic pharmaceutical agents aimed at altering the disease course are being developed and introduced to the market and their effectiveness needs to be determined.[10] Second, the relative benefits of different interventions are likely to be marginal and so detailed analyses of comparative effectiveness are necessary.[11] Third, treatments are expensive and may well be required on a long-term basis; therefore, decisions about interventions based on short-term evaluation may have long-term economic implications. Fourth, within MS resources are required for other aspects of service provision, including rehabilitation and community support, and therefore resource allocation must be equitable. Finally, resources are increasingly limited and must be allocated appropriately.

Measuring outcomes: which?

The health outcomes to be measured are determined by multiple factors, especially the aims of the intervention(s) and the objectives of the study, and therefore are likely to vary considerably in individual situations. Consequently we will concern ourselves with a framework for classifying the different types of outcome, and then apply this to MS.

Classification of health outcomes

The World Health Organization's (WHO) classification of the consequences of disease as impairments, disabilities and handicaps[12] followed their re-definition of health[13] and is probably the most widely used framework for measuring health outcomes. The addition of pathology to this three-level system results in a logical continuum: underlying disease processes (pathology) result in symptoms and signs (impairment) which can lead to restriction in performing tasks (disability) and subsequently socio-economic limitations which are specific to an individual (handicap). Whilst this system is extremely useful we feel it is too limited and recommend a four-level framework which we have proposed before.[11,14] This is an extension of Gill's classification,[15] is by no means exhaustive but serves to illustrate a number of points.

Health outcomes can be considered from a physician-based assessment, by physiological parameters of disease (e.g. types of neuroimaging) and by clinical end-points (e.g. relapse and mortality rates, length of stay); or a patient-based assessment, by aspects of

Physician-based assessment
   (1) Physiological parameters of disease (e.g. types of neuro-imaging)
   (2) Clinical end-points (e.g. relapse and mortality rates, length of stay)

Patient-based assessment
   (3) Aspects of health status (e.g. disability)
   (4) Health related quality of life

Table 15.1 Health outcomes considered at the physician- and patient-based assessment levels.

health status (e.g. disability) and by health-related quality of life.

Physician-based assessment

Measurement at the first two levels (*Table 15.1*) can be termed physician-based assessments as they are defined and measured by clinicians to whom their results are of most interest despite their clear relevance to patients.[14] Traditionally, clinical medicine has been concerned with measuring outcomes at these two levels which provide cogent information on the presence, natural history, severity and activity of MS.

The most frequently studied physician-based outcomes in MS are magnetic resonance imaging (MRI) and relapse rate. The information derived from MRI and its limitations are discussed elsewhere in this book and will not be considered further. Although measuring relapse rate would at first appear straightforward it is complicated by the absence of a scientific way of defining a true relapse, an inability to quantify their severity, their unpredictability, the influence of age and duration of illness, and the concept of regression to the mean.[16] Furthermore, whilst the majority of

patients begin with a relapsing–remitting illness this is usually a feature of the early stages of the disease and in 60 per cent is superseded by a progressive stage. Consequently, pivotal studies have limited their inclusion criteria to a minority, and excluded the majority of the total MS population.[17,18]

Although physician-based outcomes have the patient's interests at heart they only address the pathological basis of MS and evaluate health in terms of quantity. They do not provide a complete picture of disease impact as they offer limited information about the diverse clinical consequences of MS and fail to incorporate subjective assessments of health.[19] As medical intervention is intended, for the most part, to maintain or improve functioning and well-being, measurement of the second and perhaps more important dimension of health, its quality, is necessary.[5] This requires a different set of indicators which can be termed patient-based assessments.[14,20]

Patient-based assessment

Patient-based assessments are results which are considered important to people with MS as they focus on the quality of their health. The resurgence of interest in outcomes in the 1980s was associated with a change of focus from physician-based to patient-based assessment. This was precipitated by developments in health care and changing social conditions which resulted in an increasing prevalence of chronic illnesses and led to a broader WHO definition of health as 'a complete state of physical, mental, and social well-being and not merely the absence of disease or infirmity'.[13] These changes, coupled with recent developments including diagnostic advances,[21] emergence of new treatments,[22] and the importance of incorporating the patient perspective,[9,23,24] highlighted the inadequacy of physician-based outcomes.

This change in outcomes focus is particularly relevant for MS where the disease has little effect on longevity and there is no recognized cure. Further support in the need to include patient-based outcomes is provided by clinical studies demonstrating that no clear relationship exists between MRI lesion load and disability,[25] and that a beneficial treatment effect in terms of MRI appearances and relapse rates fails to equate with a positive impact on disability.[17] In addition there is consistent evidence that patients, their clinicians, and their significant others (families and carers) each offered a unique and often conflicting perspective on health.[26–31]

Health status, or health-related quality of life, or both?

Confusion exists in the literature as to the terminology for patient-based outcomes. Some authors categorize all measures which define health beyond traditional indicators of biological function as quality of life measures.[32] Others use the terms functional status, health status, quality of life, and health-related quality of life interchangeably.[20,33] As no clear guidelines exist we use the terms aspects of health status and health-related quality of life for the following reasons:

(1) Quality of life is a multi-dimensional concept and health is just one of its dimensions.[33–35] In addition it is widely recognized to be subjectively determined. Health instruments cannot therefore measure quality of life.

(2) Health is also multi-dimensional, encompassing how well people function in everyday life and their personal aspects of well-being.[33–35] Whilst five generic dimensions of health have been defined,[20] different diseases will impact on diverse dimensions (e.g. MS and piles). Instruments designed to measure the five generic dimensions of health address general health status. Instruments designed to measure the generic dimension address general health status.[36] As health is not necessarily subjective, health status instruments include those which are both self- and observer-rated, generic- and disease-specific, and patient- and clinician-derived.

(3) Health-related quality of life defines the subjective assessment of health. As we have seen, health is multi-dimensional and disease specific. Therefore the term health-related quality of life instrument is strictly reserved for a specific type of health status measure, one that is self-report and whose health dimensions have been defined by people with the disease.[19,37]

As health-related quality of life is discussed in another chapter of this book we will concern ourselves only with health status measurement in MS.

Health-status measurement in MS

There are two basic approaches to health-status measurement:[38] the generic model uses measures designed to be broadly applicable across different types and severity of disease, medical interventions, and demographic and cultural groups, so as to permit comparisons across studies; the disease-specific model uses measures designed to reflect clinically relevant issues for a specific disease, rather than to establish global standards. Disease-specific instruments are more likely to be responsive to subtle change in outcome as they contain items of more relevance to patients and their clinicians.[33,38,39] It is important to note that disease-specificity does not always guarantee responsiveness.[40]

Disease-specific health-status measurement in MS

Whilst a number of instruments have been developed to assess the impact of MS, few have been widely adopted and none have been universally accepted for use in clinical trials.[41] The mainstay of health measurement in MS is the Kurtzke Expanded Disability Status Scale (EDSS),[42] which has superseded the earlier Disability Status Scale.[43] This is an observer (neurologist)-rated scale which grades 'disability' due to MS on a continuum of 0 (normal neurological examination) to 10 (death due to MS) in 20 steps. The instrument was developed on the basis of the extensive clinical experience of a neurologist specializing in MS. It addresses impairment (symptoms and signs) at the early levels (0–3.5), mobility in the middle range (4.0–7.5), and upper limb (8.0–8.5) and bulbar function (9.0–9.5) in the late stages.

Although the EDSS is the most widely used measure of outcome in clinical trials of MS[17,18,44] it has been repeatedly criticized for its poor reliability.[45,46] As reliability defines the confidence intervals around an individual's score poor reliability greatly reduces the scientific validity of interpreting individual change scores.[47] The responsiveness of the EDSS has also been criticized,[48] but this has only recently been evaluated and confirmed using accepted techniques.[49] The EDSS has not been subjected to comprehensive psychometric evaluation. A distinct advantage of the EDSS is its familiarity as a common language amongst neurologists. Unfortunately this does not guarantee rigorous outcome measurement and, given its scientific properties, this could be considered a lame excuse for the continued usage of the EDSS as the primary outcome measure in treatment trials in MS.

The Scripps Neurological Rating Scale (SNRS)[50] grades the extent of neurological abnormality from 0 (maximum) to 100 (normal examination). It is based on the standard neurological examination with additional categories for bladder, bowel and sexual dysfunction and is rated by a neurologist. The authors report high reliability[50] but validity and responsiveness have not been evaluated.[51,52] As with the EDSS the SNRS has not been comprehensively evaluated in terms of its measurement properties.

The Troiano functional scale was designed specifically for use in a study to determine the effectiveness of total lymphoid irradiation (TLI) in chronic progressive MS.[53] This instrument grades patients' 'practical' functional capabilities on three items: gait, activities of daily living and transfers. Item scores are summed to give an overall functional rating of 0–12. No details regarding development or scientific properties of the instrument are documented, but from its use the authors concluded that TLI appeared to be a promising new therapy for the treatment of chronic progressive MS.

The European Database for Multiple Sclerosis impairment scale[54] is a simplified version of the EDSS which is an observer (neurologist) rating scale. It grades 'disability' due to MS on a continuum of 0 (normal) to 10 (death due to MS) in 10 steps. It was developed as part of a European database for MS. Whilst its reliability is reported to be adequate[55] no further psychometric or clinical data exist.

The Cambridge Multiple Sclerosis Basic Score (CAMBS)[56] assesses clinical status in terms of disability and impairment, relapse, progression, and handicap. Each section has one item which is rated on a 5-point scale from 1 (best) to 5 (worst) by a trained interviewer. The CAMBS was not designed as an outcome measure in clinical trials, but as a shorthand record of clinical profile for routine practice. Preliminary reliability and validity are encouraging but responsiveness has not been assessed.

The Guy's Neurological Disability Scale (GNDS)[57] measures disability due to MS in 12 separate categories. Each category is rated from 0 (normal) to 7 (death due to MS) with individual items summated to give an overall score. The disability categories were determined by clinicians and ratings are undertaken by a trained interviewer. The scale is in its developmental stage although preliminary psychometric data are encouraging.

Three instruments have recently been developed: the Multiple Sclerosis Quality of Life-54 Instrument (MSQOL-54);[58] the Functional Assessment of Multiple Sclerosis quality of life instrument (FAMS);[37] and the Leeds Multiple Sclerosis Quality of Life Instrument.[59] As all three are self-report and developed in conjunction with MS patients they are by definition health-related quality of life measures; consequently they will not be discussed here.

In summary, none of the six health status measures described above provides the rigorous measurement required to evaluate currently available technologies in MS. All were developed using a 'common sense' approach based on the intuition and clinical experience of the author rather than in accordance with psychometric principles and item-measurement theory.[60] Patients were rarely directly involved in the construction of these instruments. All are clinician report (although the GNDS may become self-report) and have the associated problems of observer reliability (inter- and intra-rater), limited perspective,[28] and methodological limitations for study design.[11]

The three newer instruments show more promise, although the practice of adding a few disease-specific items to a generic core[37,58] is not truly disease-specific measurement as content validity is likely to be compromised. In addition, responsiveness is likely to be limited.[38] As the effects of new interventions in MS may well be marginal and the relative effects of different interventions even smaller, content validity and responsiveness are fundamental requirements of an instrument.

Generic health-status measurement in MS

Generic instruments are felt to be less appropriate than disease-specific measures in the evaluation of therapeutic effectiveness as they are likely to contain fewer relevant items and therefore be less responsive.[38] Although this is a logical and widely held belief supportive data is lacking. Indeed, there is evidence to the contrary[61] which probably reflects the lack of scientific rigour in the development of available instruments.

Whilst clinical medicine is littered with instruments which have not been designed and evaluated in accordance with psychometric principles there are many which satisfy these criteria. The reader is directed towards a series of texts which contain large numbers of instruments and provide extensive[62] or moderate[63–66] evaluation of their properties.

Although generic instruments have rarely been used in clinical trials of MS it is pertinent to discuss widely used measures here. The Barthel Index (BI) was developed in 1955 as a simple index of personal activities of daily living.[67,68] Scores for each of its 10 items are summed to give a total score which ranges from 0 (maximum disability) to 20 (minimum disability). The BI is well known to neurologists, has been recommended as a benchmark against which other instruments should be evaluated,[69] and has been advocated by the Royal College of Physicians of London as a standard assessment of activities of daily living (ADL) for elderly persons.[70] A number of studies have addressed its reliability[71–78] and validity,[67,79–82] and the available data are very encouraging. Although criticized for its simplicity and lack of responsiveness this is perhaps surprisingly not confirmed in studies.[61] The major limitation of the BI is that its content is only relevant to people with moderate and severe disability.

The Functional Independence Measure

(FIM) is an 18-item observer-rated instrument which measures disability in terms of burden of care.[83] Each item is rated on a seven-point ordinal scale, and item scores are summed to give six subscale, two domain or a total score. The FIM was specifically developed to fulfil the desperate need for a meaningful outcome measure in medical rehabilitation[84] and, as a consequence, is rapidly becoming the most widely used disability measure. Psychometric data is not extensive but supports it as a reliable, valid and responsive measure. The FIM has been used successfully in patients with MS[29,40] but studies of its head-to-head comparison with competing measures (e.g. the BI) have yet to be published. Such studies are important as there are financial (US$15,000 per annum) and practical (staff rater requirements) implications associated with its use. Consequently the incremental validity of the FIM above competitors must be demonstrated.

The Medical Outcomes Study Short Form 36 health survey (SF-36) is a 36 item instrument which assesses health status in eight health dimensions by self-report questionnaire.[36,85] Scores can be derived for each of the eight health dimensions[36] also two summary scores can be computed.[85] The reliability and validity of the SF-36 have been the subject of numerous studies which are summarized elsewhere.[36,85] The SF-36 is considered the gold-standard measure of health status and has been referred to as 'a Dow–Jones for health' and the 'optimum outcome measure'.[86] Despite these glowing references the SF-36 demonstrates pronounced floor effects and poor responsiveness in patients with advanced MS;[61,87] consequently it is likely to have a limited role in treatment trials of MS. This confirms the importance of demonstrating the appropriateness of measurement instruments to the patient populations under study.

Measuring outcomes: how?

Rigorous measurement is the *sine qua non* of science.[88] This applies equally to all four levels of our outcomes classification. Physiological parameters of disease and clinical end-points present few inherent measurement difficulties, as subjective judgement plays a minor role and issues of reproducibility and validity are usually amenable to technological solutions.[89] In contrast, aspects of health status and health-related quality of life are elusive, abstract and complex concepts. Ensuring their rigorous measurement is correspondingly complex and is the subject of this part of the chapter.

Many clinicians hold the view that because aspects of health status and health-related quality of life are abstract and subjective concepts they cannot be measured in a reliable and valid manner.[19] Some consider that the patient's perspective can only provide meaningful data after interpretation through the physician's objective filter.[24] Others feel that the psychosocial consequences of disease do not assume the same scientific importance as basic science concepts.[90] Despite these widely held beliefs there is irrefutable evidence that patients can provide reliable and valid judgements of health status and the benefits of treatment.[91,92] Indeed, patient-report has been described as the ultimate measure of health status.[86] In addition, self-report instrument administration affords considerable methodological advantages over other methods in terms of study design,[14] as large numbers of geographically disparate patients can be accessed by postal survey reducing selection bias, whilst minimizing patient discomfort and research staff involvement.

Rigorous measurement of abstract health concepts can be achieved by applying the principles of psychometrics.[89] Clinicians are often unfamiliar with the scientific techniques required to design and evaluate health measurement tools largely because the theoretical foundations and methodological concepts, which originated in the social sciences, have been slow to transfer to medicine.[47,93,94]

Psychometric theory proposes that when a concept cannot be measured directly (e.g. health status) it can be measured by asking a series of questions, known as items, each of which measures the same concept.[94] Analysis of a larger sample of potential items generated by clearly defined standard techniques allows one to reduce the number of items and to construct scales.[95] Instruments developed according to psychometric principles must then be formally evaluated to ensure that they measure the outcome of interest in a manner which is reliable (i.e. accurate, consistent, stable over time and reproducible), valid (i.e. measure what they purport or are intended to measure); and responsive (i.e. able to detect clinically important change over time).[89,95–103]

Psychometric theory: instrument development

Development of an outcomes measurement instrument in accordance with psychometric theory involves three stages: defining a conceptual model, generation of an item pool, and reduction of the item pool to form the final instrument. A conceptual model is the rationale for, and description of, the concept(s) which the measure is intended to assess.[47] The importance of a conceptual basis for measurement cannot be overemphasized,[104,105] but this is often absent or poorly defined for health measurement instruments.[62]

Potential items, based on the conceptual model, are generated from appropriate sources, including patients with the disorder under study, consensus opinion of experts in the field, literature review, and examination of other measures. From these sources items are

devised aiming to address the appropriate range and depth of concept(s) to be measured. These items are then pre-tested on a small sample to assess how easily they can be understood and completed. Appropriate alterations are made and this version is used in the preliminary field test.

The purpose of the preliminary field test phase is to reduce the number of items and to develop scales. The instrument is administered to a large sample of patients and the results are analysed using standard psychometric techniques for item analysis.[89,95] First, items with poor response rates and very high or low endorsement frequencies (proportion of people who give each response alternative to an item) are eliminated. The remaining items are analysed using exploratory factor analysis to determine the underlying dimensions (factors) of the instruments. Resulting factors are analysed for item redundancy, overlap, homogeneity and discrimination ability. Based on these results, items are retained or discarded and grouped into subscales to produce a final version of the instrument.

Psychometric theory: instrument evaluation

Despite seemingly rigorous development these instruments must now undergo comprehensive evaluation to determine whether they are both clinically useful and scientifically sound. If an instrument is to be clinically useful and acceptable such that it can be incorporated into daily practice, it must be appropriate to the patient group being studied, brief, user-friendly, practical to administer and cost effective. Unwieldy, time- and resource-consuming instruments have limited use in clinical practice. However, clinical utility does not guarantee scientific soundness in terms of rigorous measurement. The second, and perhaps more important, step in instrument evaluation is the assessment of three separate but intimately related scientific properties, reliability, validity and responsiveness, which ensure rigorous measurement of the health outcome of interest.

A reliable measure produces results which are accurate, consistent, stable over time and reproducible. The purpose of reliability testing is therefore to determine the extent to which random measurement error is present (high reliability = low error).[95] Random error refers to all chance factors that produce variations on repeated measurement. Reliability assessment, therefore, which evaluates the consistency of repeated measurements, determines the extent of random error associated with the measurement process. The potential sources of random error are protean, but can be attributed to errors in the measure itself, the person doing the measuring, or the person being measured.[102]

There are four types of reliability: internal consistency, test-retest, rater reliability (inter- and intra-rater), and parallel forms. Reliability is therefore a generic term, each type addressing different sources of random error and contributing to the overall evaluation of the reliability of measure. It is a common misconception that providing evidence for one type of reliability is sufficient; a comprehensive evaluation requires assessment of all relevant types.

Reliability coefficients are important as they determine the confidence intervals around a score and therefore poor reliability can have serious effects on all types of scientific inquiry by reducing the overall power of randomized studies,[106] attenuating the level of associations in observational studies,[99] and biasing conclusions in an unpredictable manner when confounding variables are present.[107–109] Finally, it sets limits to an instrument's validity.[96]

Measurement instruments which have been shown to be reliable have satisfied only one of the criteria for achieving scientific acceptance:

they must also be shown to be valid. Whilst reliability is necessary for an instrument to be valid, the latter is not guaranteed.[95]

Validity concerns the relationship between the concept being measured and the instrument used to assess that concept. It can be broadly defined as the extent to which the instrument measures the concept it purports, or is intended, to measure.[101,110–112] Validity of measurement cannot be proven, evidence in its support is gathered.[103] There are three types of validity evidence: content-related, criterion-related, and construct-related.[93] Whilst there is some conceptual overlap between the three types of validity, each takes a somewhat different approach to assessing the extent to which an instrument measures what it purports. Therefore, all three types of validity must be addressed for an overall evaluative judgement of the adequacy of inferences drawn from a test.[113]

Responsiveness is the ability of an instrument to measure clinically important change, and change over time.[114] Whilst reliability and validity are the major determinants of the scientific robustness of a measure, the ability of an instrument to detect clinically significant change is also essential when evaluating the relative benefits of different interventions.[39,115] This is particularly important when treatments are associated with small but significant differences (a feature of current day interventions in MS), which may be undetected by measures which are unresponsive. In such cases a clinically appropriate, reliable and valid but unresponsive instrument is of limited value.

Although several methods have been used to assess the responsiveness of an instrument,[114,116–119] there is no consensus as to which is the best.[119] Regardless of the method chosen, it is the comparative responsiveness of competing instruments which is important. This analysis is rarely undertaken.[120–122]

Conclusions

Prompted by variations in clinical practice and escalating health-care costs, outcome measurement has taken the centre stage in health-care evaluation. By answering the questions: does an intervention work? and what benefits does it have? outcomes measurement is the key to evidence-based clinical decision making and equitable resource allocation. Nowhere in medicine is this more pertinent than MS, a disorder with significant public health implications and an increasing number of potential therapeutic options.

Traditionally, outcomes measurement in MS has focused on physician-based assessments such as MRI and relapse frequency. Whilst these provide vital details about the pathological basis of disease and health in terms of its quantity, they afford limited information concerning health quality. It has become increasingly recognized that measures of health status and health-related quality of life are essential to provide a complete picture of the impact of MS.

Recognizing the inadequacy of physician-based assessment in a disorder which is chronic, progressive and has little effect on longevity, there has been a move towards patient-based outcomes measurement. Unfortunately the techniques required to ensure these instruments measure the abstract concepts of health in a reliable and valid manner have yet to fully transfer to clinical medicine from their foundations in the social sciences. None of the available patient-based instruments even approaches the scientific standards required for rigorous measurement. The inevitable price has been paid for using sub-optimal measures in a complex disorder as there is now controversy and confusion as to whether beta interferon delays the progression of disability in MS. The gradual introduction of psychometrics into neurology and the importance of patient perspective is witnessed by the recent development of three new health-related quality of life measures. They have yet to prove themselves as reliable, valid, and responsive.

As the pharmaceutical companies develop more preparations claiming to influence the natural history of MS their relative benefits are likely to be increasingly marginal. The gauntlet has been thrown down for MS clinicians to determine the relative effectiveness of these agents. This will require rigorous measurement of patient-based outcomes if evidence-based care for their patients is to be ensured.

References

1. UK Clearing House on Health Outcomes. Issues in Outcome Measurement. Outcomes Briefing 1993(1).
2. Hopkins A, Costain D, eds. *Measuring the Outcomes of Medical Care*, London: Royal College of Physicians of London 1990.
3. Frater A, Costain D. Any better? Outcome measures in medical audit. *Br Med J* 1992; **304:** 519–520.
4. Delmothe A, ed. *Outcomes into Clinical Practice*, 1st edn. London: BMJ Publications 1994.
5. Jenkinson C, ed. *Measuring Health and Medical Outcomes*, 1st edn. London: University College London Press 1994 [Bulmer M, ed. *Social Research Today*, Vol 3].
6. Rosenberg W, Donald A. Evidence based medicine: an approach to clinical problem-solving. *Br Med J* 1995; **310:** 1122–1126.
7. Codman EA. The product of a hospital. *Surg Gynec Obstet* 1914; **18:** 491–496.
8. Neuhauser D, Codman EA. End results of medical care. *Int J Tech Assess Health Care* 1990; **6:** 307–325.
9. Reiser SJ. The era of the patient. *J Am Med Ass* 1993; **269**(8): 1012–1017.
10. Thompson AJ, Noseworthy JH. New treatment for multiple sclerosis: a clinical perspective. *Curr Opin Neurol* 1996; **9**(3): 187–198.
11. Hobart JC, Thompson AJ. Clinical trials of multiple sclerosis. In: Reder AT, ed. *Interferon Therapy of Multiple Sclerosis*. New York: Marcel Dekker 1996; 499–508.
12. WHO. International Classification of Impairments, Disabilities and Handicaps (ICIDH): a manual of classification relating to the consequence of disease. Geneva: World Health Organization 1980.
13. WHO. The constitution of the World Health Organisation. *WHO Chron* 1947; **1:** 29.
14. Hobart JC, Freeman JA, Lamping DL. Physician and patient oriented outcomes in chronic and progressive neurological disease: which to measure? *Curr Opinion Neurol* 1996; **9**(6): 441–444.
15. Gill TM. Quality of life assessment. *J R Soc Med* 1995; **88:** 680–682.
16. Weinshenker BG. Natural history of multiple sclerosis. *Ann Neurol* 1994; **36:** S6–S11.
17. The IFNB Multiple Sclerosis Study Group. Interferon beta-1b is effective in relapsing–remitting multiple sclerosis. I Clinical results of a multi-center, randomised, double-blind, placebo-controlled trial. *Neurology* 1993; **43:** 655–661.
18. Jacobs LD, Cookfair DL, Rudick RA *et al.* Intramuscular interferon Beta-1a for disease progression in relapsing multiple sclerosis. *Ann Neurol* 1996; **39**(3): 285–294.
19. Peto V, Jenkinson C, Fitzpatrick R *et al.* The development and validation of a short measure of functioning and well-being for individuals with Parkinson's disease. *Qual Life Res* 1995; **4:** 241–248.
20. Ware JE. Standards for validating health measures: definition and content. *J Chron Dis* 1987; **40**(6): 473–480.
21. Thompson AJ, Miller DH. Magnetic resonance imaging in clinical practice. In: Kennard C, ed. *Recent Advances in Clinical Neurology* (Vol 7). London: Churchill Livingstone 1992; 199–219.
22. McDonald WI. New treatments for multiple sclerosis. *Br Med J* 1995; **310:** 345–346.
23. Hopkins A. Economic change and health service reform: likely impact on teaching, practice, and research in neurology. *J Neurol Neurosurg Psychiatry* 1994; **57:** 667–671.
24. Devinsky O. Outcomes research in neurology: incorporating health-related quality of life. *Ann Neurol* 1995; **37**(2): 141–142.
25. Fillipi M, Paty DW, Kappos L *et al.* Correlations between changes in disability and T2-weighted brain MRI activity in multiple sclerosis: a follow up study. *Neurology* 1995; **45:** 255–260.
26. Gothan A, Brown R, Marsden C. Depression in Parkinson's disease: a quantitative and qualitative analysis. *J Neurol Neurosurg Psychiatry* 1986; **49:** 381–389.

27. Brown R, MacCarthy B, Jahanshahi M *et al.* Accuracy of self-reported disability in patients with Parkinsonism. *Arch Neurol* 1989; **46**: 955–959.

28. Sprangers MAG, Aaronson NK. The role of health care providers and significant others in evaluating the quality of life of patients with chronic disease: a review. *J Clin Epidemiol* 1992; **45**(7): 743–760.

29. Brosseau L. The inter-rater reliability and construct validity of the Functional Independence Measure for multiple sclerosis subjects. *Clin Rehab* 1994; **8**: 107–115.

30. Hays RD, Vickrey BG, Hermann B *et al.* Agreement between proxy reports and self-reports of quality of life in epilepsy patients. *Quality of Life Res* 1995; **4**(2): 159–165.

31. Vickrey BG, Hays RD, Engel J *et al.* Outcome assessment for epilepsy surgery: the impact of measuring health-related quality of life. *Ann Neurol* 1995; **37**(2): 158–166.

32. Ware JE. The status of health assessment 1994. *Annu Rev Publ Hlth* 1995; **16**: 327–354.

33. Guyatt GH, Freeny DH, Patrick DL. Measuring health-related quality of life. *Ann Intern Med* 1993; **118**(8): 622–629.

34. Ware JE. Methodological considerations in the selection of health status assessment procedures. In: Wenger NK, Mattson ME, Furberg CD, eds. *Assessment of Quality of Life in Clinical Trials of Cardiovascular Therapies*, New York: Le Jacq Publishing Inc 1984; 87–111.

35. Bergner M. Quality of life, health status, and clinical research. *Med Care* 1989; **27** (suppl 3): S148–S156.

36. Ware JE. *SF-36 Health Survey Manual and Interpretation Guide*. Boston, MA: Nimrod Press 1993.

37. Cella DF, Dineen K, Arnason B *et al.* Validation of the functional assessment of multiple sclerosis quality of life instrument. *Neurology* 1996; **47**: 129–139.

38. Patrick D, Deyo R. Generic and disease specific measures in assessing health status and quality of life. *Med Care* 1989; **27** (suppl): 217–232.

39. Fitzpatrick R, Ziebland S, Jenkinson C *et al.* Importance of sensitivity to change as a criterion for selecting health status measures. *Qual Hlth Care* 1992; 89–93.

40. Hobart JC, Lamping DL, Freeman JA *et al.* Measuring disability in multiple sclerosis: reliability of the Functional Independence Measure. *J Neurol* 1996; **243** (6 suppl 2): S32.

41. Sharrack B, Hughes RAC. Clinical scales for multiple sclerosis. *J Neurol Sci* 1996; **135**: 1–9.

42. Kurtzke JF. Rating neurological impairment in multiple sclerosis: An expanded disability status scale (EDSS). *Neurology* 1983; **33**: 1444–1452.

43. Kurtzke JF. A new scale for evaluating disability in multiple sclerosis. *Neurology* 1955; **5**: 580–583.

44. Goodkin DE, Cookfair D, Wende K *et al.* Inter- and intra-rater scoring agreement using grades 1.0 to 3.5 of the Kurtzke Expanded Disability Status Scale (EDSS). *Neurology* 1992; **42**: 859–863.

45. Noseworthy JH, Vandervoort MK, Wong CJ *et al.* Interrater variability with the Expanded Disability Status Scale (EDSS) and Functional Systems (FS) in a multiple sclerosis clinical trial. *Neurology* 1990; **40**: 971–975.

46. Willoughby EW, Paty DW. Scales for rating impairment in multiple sclerosis: a critique. *Neurology* 1988; **38**: 1793–1798.

47. Scientific Advisory Committee of the Medical Outcomes Trust. Instrument Review Criteria. *Medical Outcomes Trust Bulletin* 1995; **3**(4): I-IV.

48. Whitaker JN, McFarland HF, Rudge P *et al.* Outcomes assessment in multiple sclerosis trials: a critical analysis. *Multiple Sclerosis* 1995; **1**: 37–47.

49. Hobart JC, Lamping DL, Freeman JA *et al.* Reliability, validity, and responsiveness of the Kurtzke Expanded Disability Status Scale (EDSS) in multiple sclerosis. *J Neurol Neurosurg Psychiatry* 1997; **62**(2): 212 (abstract).

50. Sipe JC, Knobler RL, Braheny SL *et al.* A neurological rating scale (NRS) for multiple sclerosis. *Neurology* 1984; **34**: 1368–1372.

51. Koziol JA, Frutos A, Sipe JC *et al.* A comparison of two neurologic scoring instruments for multiple sclerosis. *J Neurol* 1996; **243**: 209–213.

52. Hobart J, Thompson A. A comparison of two neurologic scoring instruments for multiple sclerosis: reply. *J Neurol* 1997; **244**(1): 60.

53. Cook S, Devereux C, Troiano R *et al.* Effect of total lymphoid irradiation in chronic progressive multiple sclerosis. *Lancet* 1986; **1**: 1405–1409.

54. Confavreux C, Compston DAS, Hommes OR *et al.* EDMUS, a European database for multiple sclerosis. *J Neurol Neurosurg Psychiatry* 1992; **55**: 671–676.

55. Amato MP, Hours M, Bartolozzi ML *et al.* European cross-national standardization in the use of the EDMUS database system for multiple sclerosis. *J Neurol* 1996; **243** (6 suppl 2): S82.

56. Mumford CJ, Compston A. Problems with rating scales for multiple sclerosis: a novel approach – the CAMBS score. *J Neurol* 1993; **240**: 209–215.

57. Sharrack B, Hughes RAC, Soudain S. Guy's Neurological Disability Scale. *J Neurol* 1996; **243** (6 suppl 2): S32.

58. Vickrey BG, Hays RD, Harooni R *et al.* A health-related quality of life measure for multiple sclerosis. *Qual Life Res* 1995; **4**: 187–206.

59. Ford HL, Tennant A, Johnson MH. The Leeds MSQoL scale: a disease specific measure of quality of life in multiple sclerosis. *J Neurol Neurosurg Psychiatry* 1997; **62**(2): 210 (abstract).

60. Lord FM. *Applications of Item Response Theory to Practical Testing Problems*, Hillside, New Jersey: Lawrence Erlbaum Associates 1980.

61. Hobart JC, Lamping DL, Freeman JA *et al.* The responsiveness of disability measures in multiple sclerosis. *J Neurol Neurosurg Psychiatry* 1997; **62**(2): 213–214 (abstract).

62. McDowell I, Newell C. *Measuring Health: A Guide to Rating Scales and Questionnaires*, 2nd edn. Oxford: Oxford University Press 1996.

63. Bowling A. *Measuring Health: A Review of Quality of Life Measurement Scales*, Buckingham: Oxford University Press 1991.

64. Bowling A. *Measuring Disease: A Review of Disease-specific Quality of Life Measurement Scales*, Buckingham: Open University Press 1995.

65. Wade DT. *Measurement in Neurological Rehabilitation*, Oxford: Oxford University Press 1992.

66. Wilkin D, Hallam L, Doggett M-A. *Measures of Need and Outcome for Primary Health Care*, Oxford: Oxford University Press 1992.

67. Wylie CM, White BK. A measure of disability. *Arch Environm Hlth* 1964; **8** (June): 834–839.

68. Mahoney FI, Barthel DW. Functional evaluation: the Barthel Index. *Maryland St Med J* 1965; **14**: 61–65.

69. Wade DT. Measurement in neurological rehabilitation. *Curr Opin Neurol* 1993; **6**(5): 778–784.

70. Royal College of Physicians. Standardised assessment scales for elderly people. Report of joint workshops of the Research Unit of the Royal College of Physicians and the British Geriatrics Society 1992.

71. Granger CV, Albrecht GL, Hamilton BB. Outcome of comprehensive medical rehabilitation: measurement by PULSES profile and Barthel Index. *Arch Phys Med Rehab* 1979; **60**(4): 145–154.

72. Shinar D, Gross CR, Bronstein KS *et al.* Reliability of the activities of daily living scale and its use in telephone interview. *Arch Phys Med Rehab* 1987; **68**(10): 723–728.

73. Roy CW, Togneri J, Hay E *et al.* An inter-rater reliability study of the Barthel Index. *Int J Rehab Res* 1988; **11**(1): 67–70 (Brief Research Report).

74. Shah S, Vanclay F, Cooper B. Improving the sensitivity of the Barthel Index for strike rehabilitation. *J Clin Epidemiol* 1989; **42**: 703–709.

75. Loewen SC, Anderson BA. Reliability of the Modified Motor Assessment Scale and the Barthel Index. *Phys Ther* 1988; **68**(7): 1077–1081.

76. Wolfe CDA, Taub NA, Woodrow EJ *et al.* Assessment of scales of disability and handicap for stroke patients. *Stroke* 1991; **22**(10): 1242–1244.

77. Gompertz P, Pound P, Ebrahim S. The reliability of stroke outcome measures. *Clin Rehab* 1993; **7**(4): 290–296.

78. Gompertz P, Pound P, Ebrahim S. A postal version of the Barthel Index. *Clin Rehab* 1994; **8**: 233–239.

79. Wade DT, Langton Hewer R. Functional abilities after stroke: measurement, natural history and prognosis. *J Neurol Neurosurg Psychiatry* 1987; **50**: 177–182.

80. Barer DH, Murphy JJ. Scaling the Barthel: a 10-point hierarchical version of the activities of daily living index for use with stroke patients. *Clin Rehab* 1993; **7**: 271–277.

81. McPherson K, Sloan RL, Hunter J *et al.* Validation studies of the OPCS scale – more useful than the Barthel Index. *Clin Rehab* 1993; **7**: 105–112.

82. Gompertz P, Pound P, Ebrahim S. Validity of the extended activities of daily living scale. *Clin Rehab* 1994; **8**: 275–280.

83. Hamilton BB, Granger CV, Sherwin FS *et al.* A Uniform National Data System for Medical Rehabilitation. In: Fuhrer MJ, ed. *Rehabilitation Outcomes: Analysis and Measurement*. Baltimore, MD: Paul H Brookes 1989; 137–147.

84. Granger CV, Hamilton BB, Keith RA *et al.* Advances in functional assessment for medical rehabilitation. In *Topics in Geriatric Rehabilitation*, Vol 1. Rockville: Aspen 1986; 59–79.

85. Ware JE, Kosinski MA, Keller SD. *SF-36 Physical and Mental Health Summary Scales: A User's Manual.* Boston: The Health Institute, New England Medical Centre 1994.

86. Ware JE. Measuring patients' views: the optimum outcome measure. *Br Med J* 1993; **306**(6890): 1429–1430.

87. Freeman J, Langdon D, Hobart J *et al.* The health-related quality of life of people with advanced multiple sclerosis. *J Neurol Rehab* 1996; **10**: 185–194.

88. Bohrnstedt GW. Measurement. In: Rossi PH, Wright JD, Anderson AB, eds. *Handbook of Survey Research*, New York: Academic Press 1983; 69–121.

89. Streiner DL, Norman GR. *Health Measurement Scales: A Practical Guide to Their Development and Use*, 2nd edn. Oxford: Oxford University Press 1995.

90. Deyo P, Patrick DL. Barriers to the use of health status measures in clinical investigation, patient care and policy research. *Med Care* 1989; **22** (suppl): S254–S268.

91. Stewart AL, Ware JEJ, eds. *Measuring Functioning and Well-being: the Medical Outcomes Study Approach*, Durham, NC: Duke University Press 1992.

92. Fitzpatrick R, Fletcher A, Gore S *et al.* Quality of life measures in health care. I: applications and uses in assessment. *Br Med J* 1992; **305**: 1074–1077.

93. Hobart JC, Lamping DL, Thompson AJ. Evaluating neurological outcome measures: the bare essentials. *J Neurol Neurosurg Psychiatry* 1996; **60**: 127–130.

94. Testa MA, Simonson DC. Assessment of quality-of-life outcomes. *New Engl J Med* 1996; **334**(13): 835–840.

95. Nunnally JC, Bernstein IH. *Psychometric Theory*, 3rd edn. New York: McGraw-Hill 1994.

96. Lord FM, Novick MR. *Statistical Theories of Mental Test Scores*, Reading, MA: Addison-Wesley 1968.

97. Brown FG. *Principles of Educational and Psychological Testing*, Hinsdale, IL: Dryden Press 1970.

98. Nunnally JC, Jr. *Introduction to Psychological Measurement.* New York: McGraw Hill 1970.

99. Allen MJ, Yen WM. *Introduction to Measurement Theory*, Monterey, CA: Brooks/Cole 1979.

100. Carmines EG, Zeller RA. *Reliability and Validity Assessment.* London: Sage Publications 1979.

101. American Educational Research Association, American Psychological Association and National Council of Measurement in Education. Standards for education and psychological testing. Washington DC: American Psychological Association 1985.

102. Anastasi A. *Psychological Testing*, 6th edn. New York: Macmillan 1988.

103. Kaplan RM, Saccuzzo DP. *Psychological Testing: Principles, Applications and Issues*, 3rd edn. Pacific Grove, CA: Brooks/Cole 1993.

104. DeVellis RF. *Scale Development: Theory and Applications.* London: Sage Publications 1991.

105. Kopec JA, Esdaile JM, Abrahamowicz M *et al*. The Quebec Back Pain Disability Scale: measurement properties. *Spine* 1995; **20**(3): 341–352.

106. Fleiss JL. *The Design and Analysis of Clinical Experiments*, New York: John Wiley 1986.

107. Lui K. Measurement error and its impact on partial correlation and multiple linear regression analysis. *Am J Epidemiol* 1988; **127**(4): 864–874.

108. Kupper LL. Effects of the use of unreliable surrogate variables on the validity of epidemiological research. *Am J Epidemiol* 1984; **120**(4): 643–648.

109. Greenland S. The effect of misclassification in the presence of covariates. *Am J Epidemiol* 1980; **112**(4): 564–569.

110. Cronbach LJ, Meehl PE. Construct validity in psychological tests. *Psychol Bull* 1955; **52**(4): 281–302.

111. Campbell DT, Fiske DW. Convergent and discriminant validation by the multitrait-multimethod matrix. *Psychol Bull* 1959; **56**(2): 81–105.

112. Campbell DT. Recommendations for APA test standards regarding construct, trait, or discriminant validity. *Am Psychol* 1960; **15**: 546–553.

113. Messick S. Test validity and the ethics of assessment. *Am Psychol* 1980; **35**(11): 1012–1027.

114. Guyatt G, Walter S, Norman G. Measuring change over time: assessing the usefulness of evaluative instruments. *J Chron Dis* 1987; **40**(2): 171–178.

115. Kirshner B, Guyatt G. A methodological framework for assessing health indices. *J Chron Dis* 1985; **38**(1): 27–36.

116. Deyo RA, Centor RM. Assessing the responsiveness of functional scales to clinical change: an analogy to diagnostic test performance. *J Chron Dis* 1986; **39**(11): 897–906.

117. Guyatt GH, Deyo RA, Charlson M *et al*. Responsiveness and validity in health status measurement: a clarification. *J Clin Epidemiol* 1989; **42**(5): 403–408.

118. Norman GR. Issues in the use of change scores in randomized trials. *J Clin Epidemiol* 1989; **42**(11): 1097–1105.

119. Deyo RA, Diehr P, Patrick DL. Reproducibility and responsiveness of health status measures: statistics and strategies for evaluation. *Controlled Clin Trials* 1991; **12**: 142s–158s.

120. Deyo RA, Inui TS. Toward clinical applications of health status measures: sensitivity of scales to clinically important change. *Hlth Serv Res* 1984; **19**(3): 275–289.

121. Liang MH, Larson MG, Cullen KE *et al*. Comparative measurement efficiency and sensitivity of five health status instruments for arthritis research. *Arthritis Rheum* 1985; **28**(5): 542–547.

122. Liang MH, Fossel AH, Larson MG. Comparisons of five health status instruments for orthopedic evaluation. *Med Care* 1990; **28**(7): 632–638.

16

Enhancing conduction in multiple sclerosis: is there a functional benefit?

Chris H Polman

Introduction

One of the cardinal pathological features of multiple sclerosis (MS) is the widespread demyelination in cerebrum, brain stem, cerebellum, spinal cord and optic nerves. It is well established that demyelination in the central nervous system (CNS) leads to block or slowing of nerve impulse conduction at the site of demyelination.[1] These conduction abnormalities are due to the resistive and capacitative leakage of current in the demyelinated region of the nerve fibre. Clinical symptoms and signs will develop if conduction block is present simultaneously in a significant proportion of the fibres within a given pathway. The inability of demyelinated fibres to transmit trains of impulses is due to an increase in depolarization threshold. Such an inability may contribute to the fading out of vision after looking at an object continuously for several seconds, and to the fatiguability of muscle strength experienced by patients with MS.

Conduction in demyelinated fibres can be restored by remyelination, although conduction might be slow and insecure until the remyelination is well established.[2,3] However, remyelination is not essential to restore nerve conduction: nerve conduction can be restored in fibres which are still demyelinated by interfering with neurophysiological mechanisms involved in nerve conduction.[4–6]

Mechanisms involved in the pathophysiology of conduction disturbances

Physiological consequences of demyelination include complete conduction block, failure to transmit high-frequency trains of impulses, slowing of conduction and temporal dispersion of impulses.[7]

In normal myelinated fibres, saltatory conduction is made possible by the following events: outward capacitative current driven by the preceding node of Ranvier (driving node) depolarizes the nodal membrane to threshold, and inward sodium current is initiated to drive the next node. The safety factor of transmission is defined as a ratio of the current available at a node to the threshold current of that node. The safety factor should be more than unity if conduction is to be successful. In demyelinative conduction block, current from the driving node is lost through the demyelinated segment of increased capacitance, falling short of the amount sufficient to depolarize the nodal membrane to threshold, resulting in a reduction of the safety factor below unity.

The available evidence indicates that mammalian myelinated fibres contain a repertoire of physiologically active membrane molecules, including a number of ion channels and an electrogenic Na/K-pump (for review see Black *et al.*[8]). Physiological properties of myelinated fibres reflect the distribution of these various

Channel type	Probable function	Primary location
Sodium (Na)	Depolarization phase of action potential	High density at node of of Ranvier, low density in internode
Potassium (K) (fast)	Rapid repolarization after action potential	Internode
Potassium (K) (slow)	Modulate repetitive firing; repolarization in response to prolonged depolarization	Node, internode
Inward rectifier (mixed Na/K conductance)	Modulate excitability; attenuate hyperpolarization	Node, internode

Table 16.1
Function and distribution of ion channels in myelinated axons.

types of channel and pump; their functions have been investigated by using specific blocking agents.[8]

The pathophysiology of demyelinated axons depends, in part, on their ion channel organization (*Table 16.1*). Sodium channels which are responsible for the depolarization phase of the action potential, are clustered in high density in the axon membrane at the node of Ranvier and are present at much lower densities in the internode. Fast potassium channels, present in the axon membrane under the myelin, are normally masked by myelin but are 'unmasked' by demyelination. After demyelination conduction will be impeded both by the low density of sodium channels in the internodal axon membrane and by unmasking of potassium channels. Slow potassium channels are activated during sustained depolarization and high-frequency discharge, and modulate repetitive firing patterns. A fourth type of ion channel, the 'inward rectifier' (electrogenic Na/K pump), which appears to be permeable to both sodium and potassium ions, probably plays a role in modulating the excitability of the axon or in controlling hyperpolarization of the axon membrane by reducing the resting membrane potential.

Very recently it was reported that cerebrospinal fluid (CSF) from MS patients reduces neuronal excitability by increasing sodium-current inactivation.[9] The nature of the factors in the CSF responsible for this effect was not identified. A number of studies have shown that antibody-mediated interference with axonal channel function might be an important disease mechanism in demyelinating disease of the peripheral nervous system.[10,11]

It can be derived from data presently

available that, theoretically, the safety factor for conduction can be increased by blocking sodium channel inactivation (which increases the duration of the action potential), by blocking fast potassium channels (which inhibits the rapid repolarization and thereby prolongs the depolarization of the action potential), or by blocking the electrogenic Na/K pump.

Treatment of conduction failure

In the search for effective treatment of conduction block, one approach has been to use agents which increase the current from the driving node.

4-Aminopyridine (4-AP), a blocker of fast potassium channel activation, prolongs the duration of nerve action potentials and thereby restores conduction in blocked demyelinated neurons.[12,13] In experimental studies using isolated animal nerve fibres the compound has been demonstrated to have a minimal effect on action potential waveform of normal mature myelinated fibres, whereas it significantly alters the action potential waveform and firing characteristics of demyelinated axons in which internodal potassium channels may be exposed and therefore are available to a potassium channel blocker.[14–16] This mechanism has been the putative basis for the clinical application of 4-AP in MS. However, 4-AP has other effects on axon excitability aside from action potential broadening. Multiple spike discharge, spontaneous impulse activity and alteration in refractory periods have also been reported and should be considered in the rationale for the clinical use of 4-AP.[16,17]

Other approaches, as indicated above, are suggested by observations that an additional increase in threshold is an important factor in rate-dependent block.[18] After high-frequency impulses, sodium concentration in axoplasm increases slightly. The electrogenic Na/K pump is immediately activated by this slight increase in sodium. The pump extrudes more sodium than potassium entry, causing membrane hyperpolarization, which in turn raises the threshold of the nodal membrane. As a consequence, conduction block follows high-frequency impulse activity. Cardiac glycosides are specific inhibitors of the Na/K pump and they therefore can be expected to improve rate-dependent block by reducing the threshold. It has indeed been demonstrated that administration of ouabain and digitalis can reverse conduction disturbances due to CNS demyelination by preventing hyperpolarization after high-frequency impulse activities and also by actively reducing the resting membrane potential.[19,20]

The venom of the scorpion Leiurus quinquestriatur, which acts principally by blocking sodium inactivation, has been shown to be able to prolong action potential duration quite impressively and irreversibly.[12] In contrast, drugs like lidocaine and other local anaesthetics, which reduce the rising phase of the action potential by blocking sodium channels, have been demonstrated to prevent impulse conduction in demyelinated segments of nerve fibres with low safety factors.[21]

Schauf and Davis,[22] using a theoretical model for predicting modifications in impulse conduction in MS, have shown not only that blocking of sodium channel inactivation and/or inhibition of potassium channel activation but also that a decrease in external calcium concentrations produces an increase in the nerve conduction safety factor. Influx of calcium into the intracellular compartment might also play an important role in the mechanism of myelin damage.

Can these approaches be clinically meaningful in MS?

It has been recognized for many decades that MS patients develop new symptoms or experience deterioration of existing symptoms following exercise or heat, a phenomenon later explained to be secondary to elevated body temperature.[23] Although challenged by some findings, the current hypothesis is that in MS hyperthermia induces a heat-linked neuroblockade of partially demyelinated axons.[24] Davis and colleagues[22] demonstrated that the temperature at which conduction block occurs is related to the degree of demyelination, and that even a small increase in temperature can block damaged axon function in an MS plaque. These findings strongly suggest that factors which interfere with the pathophysiology of nerve conduction have the potential to impose clinically meaningful effects in MS.

The effect of temperature decrease as a means of improving neurological function has been explored in many ways, varying from cold showers to sophisticated cooling suits, and has been found helpful by many patients.

For most of the pharmacological approaches indicated above only very small studies have been performed to answer the question of their clinical relevance in MS.

The cardiac glycoside digitalis has been given intravenously to seven patients with MS.[25] In three patients improvement of clinical deficits was observed concurrent with significant changes in evoked potential findings.

In two studies, involving only small numbers of patients, it has been demonstrated that experimentally-induced hypocalcaemia can be associated with transient improvement of visual function in MS patients with clinically stable optic nerve deficits.[26,27] Gilmore *et al.*[28] treated eight patients with stable MS intravenously with the calcium entry antagonist drug, verapamil, and found an improvement in evoked potential measurements, supporting the concept of acute facilitation of central nervous system electrical impulses by calcium-dependent processes.

Until now more extensive clinical experience in MS exists only for the aminopyridines.

Aminopyridines in MS

Based on the hypothesis that 4-AP acts to promote conduction by block of axonal potassium channels, a number of studies have been performed in MS to investigate the clinical usefulness of 4-AP. Initial clinical studies in MS, conducted by several groups, suggested that the drug caused improvement in temperature-sensitive neurological deficits, especially concerning motor and visual functions.[29–32] Definite conclusions, however, could not be drawn from these studies, since the drug was given to small groups of highly selected patients.

We enrolled 70 patients with clinically definite MS (Poser-criteria) in a two-phase, randomized, double-blind, placebo-controlled, cross-over trial.[33] The first phase was a placebo-controlled cross-over trial of short-term treatment with intravenously administered 4-AP. Improvements in visual contrast sensitivity, visual evoked response latencies and oculomotor function were seen. Sixty-nine patients subsequently entered phase two: a placebo-controlled cross-over trial of orally administered 4-AP (daily dose up to 0.5 mg/kg bodyweight in three divided dosages) with a treatment duration of three months for each period. Significant improvement in Kurtzke Extended Disability Status Scale (EDSS) was seen during the active treatment arm of the trial with ten patients improving and only three worsening, and no patients improving on placebo and eleven worsening ($p < 0.05$). A significant subjective improvement (defined as an improvement which significantly affected the activities of normal daily life) was indicated by 18 patients during 4-AP treatment and by 1 patient during placebo treatment ($p < 0.05$). Treatment-related improvements were also seen in quantitative tests of visual and oculomotor function. No serious side effects were encountered. However, subjective side effects such as paraesthesias, dizziness and light-headedness were frequently reported during 4-AP treatment. Analysis of subgroups revealed that especially patients with temperature-sensitive symptoms and patients characterized by a longer disease duration and a chronic progressive phase of the disease were likely to show clear clinical benefit. In this study the pharmacokinetics of 4-AP was extensively documented.[33] After both intravenous and oral administration there was a significant relationship between serum levels and 4-AP doses used. The amount of improvement in electrophysiological registration of eye movements was significantly related to 4-AP serum levels. The use of 4-AP in oral doses three times a day gives rise to a large variation and fluctuation in serum levels with high peaks related to subjective side effects. Perhaps a better control of 4-AP serum levels, for example by using a slow-release preparation, can have a favourable impact on the ratio between efficacy and side effects.

Follow-up in patients who continued open-label 4-AP has shown that efficacy of the drug tends to persist during continued usage.[34] Although, evaluating these data, a placebo effect cannot be excluded, the dynamics of the response in relation to the intake of the medication and the deterioration and subsequent improvement during and after a drug-free interval in a large majority of patients, are suggestive of a real and persistent effect induced by 4-AP. Improvements in fatigue and

in ambulation were particularly mentioned quite often by the patients as being responsible for the favourable overall effect. Major side effects, however, can be associated with the drug, two seizures and one possibly 4-AP related case of hepatitis being encountered during this follow-up.

In another small study we found that 4-AP does not induce significant effects on cognitive function in patients with MS, although a trend for improved performance during 4-AP could be detected for two of the neuropsychological tests used.[35] Bever *et al.*,[36] using a very elegant concentration-controlled study design, confirmed that 4-AP can induce clinically meaningful improvements in visual and lower extremity motor function in selected patients with MS. In this study it was shown that very high serum levels are associated with significant toxicity, a grand mal seizure and an acute confusional episode being reported.[36]

The fact that 3,4-diaminopyridine (DAP), although it crosses the blood–brain barrier less readily than 4-AP, is a more powerful potassium channel blocker than 4-AP has justified the investigation of the effects of DAP in MS. In two small studies a trend for efficacy has been demonstrated.[37,38] In a comparative study between 4-AP and DAP we demonstrated that, based on a reduced systemic tolerability (abdominal complaints) for DAP and on a clear preference for 4-AP, 4-AP is superior to DAP in the treatment of patients with MS.[39]

The future

More studies of 4-AP in MS are urgently needed. These studies should focus on the determination of the optimal dose regimen, taking into account aspects of both efficacy and toxicity. Patients with a moderate and stable disability can best be recruited for these studies and outcome measures should be selected which can provide objective and clinically meaningful measures of disability.

Up until now it was thought that the various approaches to enhance nerve conduction can only have functional effects in the absence of a structural substrate. There is evidence arising, however, which suggests that improvement of electrical activity can promote myelin formation in the CNS. In a recent study using a system of *in vitro* myelination it was shown that highly specific neurotoxins, which can either block or increase the firing of neurons by interfering with ion channel function, respectively inhibit and promote myelin production, thereby clearly linking neuronal electrical activity to myelinogenesis.[40] If these findings could be further substantiated, they would add a completely new dimension to future research in this field.

Conclusion

Present data suggest that 4-AP can induce a clinically meaningful benefit in a subgroup of MS patients. Potential side effects require careful medical supervision.

Although, in the studies performed, only small numbers of patients have been investigated, it can be concluded from these data that interference with the neurophysiological mechanisms involved in neural impulse transmission seems to have the potential to be clinically relevant for patients with MS.

References

1. McDonald WI, Sears TA. The effects of experimental demyelination on conduction in the central nervous system. *Brain* 1970 **93:** 583–598.
2. Smith KJ, Blakemore WF, McDonald WI. The restoration of conduction by central remyelination. *Brain* 1981; **104:** 383–404.
3. Honmou O, Falts PA, Waxman SG *et al.* Restoration of normal conduction properties in demyelinated spinal cord axons in the adult rat by transplantation of exogenous Schwann cells. *J Neurosci* 1996; **16:** 3199–3208.
4. Bostock H, Sears TA. The internodal axon membrane: electrical excitability and continuous conduction in segmental demyelination. *J Physiol* 1978; **280:** 273–301.
5. Smith KJ, Bostock H, Hall SM. Saltatory conduction precedes remyelination in axons demyelinated with lipophospatidyl choline. *J Neurol Sci* 1982; **54:** 13–31.
6. Waxman SG, Black JA, Kocsis JD *et al.* Low density of sodium channels supports action potential conduction in axons of neonatal rat optic nerve. *Proc Natl Acad Sci USA* 1989; **86:** 1406–1410.
7. Waxman SG, Conduction in myelinated, unmyelinated and demyelinated fibers. *Arch Neurol* (1977) **34:** 5585–5589.
8. Black JA, Kocsis JD, Waxman SG. Ion channel organization of the myelinated fiber. *TINS* 1990; **13:** 48–54.
9. Koeller H, Buchholz J, Siebler M. Cerebrospinal fluid from multiple sclerosis patients inactivates neuronal Na+ current. *Brain* 1996; **119:** 457–463.
10. Waxman SG. Sodium channel blockade by antibodies: a new mechanism of neurological disease? *Ann Neurol* 1995; **37:** 421–423.
11. Gutmann L, Gutmann L. Axonal channelopathies: an evolving concept in the pathogenesis of peripheral nerve disorders. *Neurology* 1996; **47:** 18–21.
12. Bostock H, Sherratt RM, Sears TA. Overcoming conduction failure in demyelinated nerve fibers by prolonging action potentials. *Nature* 1978; **274:** 385–387.
13. Targ EF, Kocsis JD. 4-Aminopyridine leads to restoration of conduction in demyelinated rat sciatic nerve. *Brain Res* 1985; **328:** 358–361.
14. Sherratt RM, Bostock H, Sears TA. Effects of 4-Aminopyridine on normal and demyelinated mammalian nerve fibers. *Nature* 1980; **283:** 570–572.
15. Bostock H, Sears TA, Sherratt RM. The effects of 4-Aminopyridine and Tetraethylammonium ions on normal and demyelinated mammalian nerve fibers. *J Physiol* 1981; **313:** 301–315.
16. Targ EF, Kocsis JD. Action potential characteristics of demyelinated rat sciatic nerve following application of 4-Aminopyridine. *Brain Res* 1986; **363:** 1–9.
17. Lees G. The effects of anticonvulsants on 4-aminopyridine-induced bursting: in vitro studies on rat peripheral nerve and dorsal roots. *Br J Pharmacol* 1996; **117:** 573–579.
18. Bostock H, Grafe P. Activity-dependent excitability changes in normal and demyelinated rat spinal root axons. *J Physiol* 1985; **365:** 239–257.
19. Kaji R, Sumner AJ. Effects of digitalis on CNS demyelinative conduction blocks in vivo. *Ann Neurol* 1989; **25:** 159–165.
20. Kaji R, Sumner AJ. Ouabain reverses conduction disturbances in single demyelinated nerve fibers. *Neurology* 1989; **39:** 1364–1368.
21. Sakurai M, Mannen T, Kanazawa I *et al.* Lidocaine unmasks silent demyelinative lesions in multiple sclerosis. *Neurology* 1992; **42:** 2088–2093.
22. Schauf CL, Davis FA. Impulse conduction in multiple sclerosis: a theoretical basis for modification by temperature and pharmacological agents. *J Neurol Neurosurg Psychiatry* 1974; **37:** 152–161.
23. Uhthoff W. Untersuchungen ueber die bei der multiplen Herdsklerose vorkommenden Augenstoerungen. *Arch Psychiat Nervenkr* 1890; **21:** 55–116 and 303–410.

24. Guthrie TC, Nelson DA. Influence of temperature changes on multiple sclerosis: critical review of mechanisms and research potential. *J Neurol Sci* 1995; **129**: 1–8.

25. Kaji R, Happel L, Sumner AJ. Effect of digitalis on clinical symptoms and conduction variables in patients with multiple sclerosis. *Ann Neurol* 1990; **28**: 582–584.

26. Davis FA, Becker FO, Michael JA *et al*. Effect of intravenous sodium bicarbonate, disodium edetate and hyperventilation on visual and oculomotor signs in multiple sclerosis. *J Neurol Neurosurg Psychiatry* 1970; **33**: 723–732.

27. Becker FO, Michael JA, Davis FA. Acute effects of oral phosphate on visual function in multiple sclerosis. *Neurology* 1974; **24**: 601–607.

28. Gilmore RL, Kasarskis EJ, McAllister RG. Verapamil-induced changes in central conduction in patients with multiple sclerosis. *J Neurol Neurosurg Psychiatry* 1985; **48**: 1140–1146.

29. Jones RE, Heron JR, Foster DH *et al*. Effects of 4-Aminopyridine in patients with multiple sclerosis. *J Neurol Sci* 1983; **60**: 353–362.

30. Stefoski D, Davis FA, Faut M *et al*. 4-Aminopyridine improves clinical signs in multiple sclerosis. *Ann Neurol* 1987; **21**: 71–77.

31. Davis FA, Stefoski D, Rush J. Orally administered 4-Aminopyridine improves clinical signs in multiple sclerosis. *Ann Neurol* 1990; **27**: 186–192.

32. Stefoski D, Davis FA, Fitzsimons WE *et al*. 4-Aminopyridine in multiple sclerosis: prolonged administration. *Neurology* 1991; **41**: 1344–1348.

33. van Diemen HAM, Polman CH, van Dongen MMMM *et al*. The effect of 4-Aminopyridine on the clinical signs in multiple sclerosis: a randomized, placebo-controlled, double-blind, cross-over study. *Ann Neurol* 1992; **32**: 123–130.

34. Polman CH, Bertelsmann FW, van Loenen AC *et al*. 4-Aminopyridine in the treatment of patients with multiple sclerosis: long-term efficacy and safety. *Arch Neurol* 1994; **51**: 292–296.

35. Smits RCF, Emmen HH, Bertelsmann FW *et al*. The effects of 4-aminopyridine on cognitive function in patients with multiple sclerosis: a pilot study. *Neurology* 1994; **44**: 1701–1705.

36. Bever CT, Young D, Anderson PA *et al*. The effects of 4-aminopyridine in multiple sclerosis patients. Results of a randomized, placebo-controlled, double-blind, concentration-controlled, crossover trial. *Neurology* 1994; **44**: 1054–1059.

37. Bever CT, Anderson PA, Leslie J *et al*. Treatment with oral 3,4 diaminopyridine improves leg strength in multiple sclerosis patients. *Neurology* 1996; **47**: 1457–1462.

38. Carter JL, Stevens JC, Smith B *et al*. A double-blind, placebo-controlled crossover trial of 3,4-diaminopyridine in the treatment of patients with multiple sclerosis. *Arch Neurol* 1994; **51**: 1136–1139.

39. Polman CH, Bertelsmann FW, de Waal R *et al*. 4-Aminopyridine is superior to 3,4-Diaminopyridine in the treatment of patients with multiple sclerosis. *Arch Neurol* 1994; **51**: 1136–1139.

40. Demerens C, Stankoff B, Logak M *et al*. Induction of myelination in the central nervous system by electrical activity. *Proc Natl Acad Sci USA* 1996; **93**: 9887–9892.

17

What is new in the symptomatic management of multiple sclerosis?

Michel G Clanet and Cécile Azais-Vuillemin

Introduction

Despite the proliferation of the new immunomodulatory regimens which may modify the natural history of the disease, many multiple sclerosis (MS) patients are severely affected by disabling symptoms. In neurological practice, the main therapeutic approaches consist of relieving these disabled patients from their daily difficulties rather than to rely on the putative beneficial effect of the newest marketed drug. Disabling symptoms usually vary according to the stage of the disease progression, its clinical form, relapsing–remitting or progressive, and the main functional systems affected by the lesions.

In the first stages of the relapsing–remitting period, the majority of patients do not suffer from major residual deficits after relapses. However, the diagnosis is revealed in this period, raising anxiety and sometimes depressive reactions in many patients. Sensory relapses are often followed by residual long-lasting painful paraesthesias, but bladder dysfunction is probably one of the most distressing symptoms because of its impact on the social life of these patients who remain completely active (see Goodwin and Fowler, Chapter 20). Sometimes residual visual disturbances are long-lasting, either loss of visual acuity or blurred vision, permanent diplopia or oscillopsia secondary to a lesion of the central oculomotor pathways. Uhthoff's phenomenon, a paroxysmal increase of functional deficit after a physical effort, is a frequent and specific effect of persistent central demyelination.

In the next stage irreversible deficit occurs, either after a severe relapse or at the beginning of the progressive phase. Walking becomes difficult owing to weakness, stiffness and proprioceptive loss of the lower limbs and locomotor ataxia. Many patients will reach the last stages with partial or total dependence secondary to major disturbances of neurological functions: spasticity and spasms, urinary incontinence and tract infections, action or truncal tremor, paralysis and pressure sores, nystagmus and abnormal eye movements which enhance visual difficulties, chronic pain and cognitive impairment.

Managing all these problems is often difficult and improving the quality of life requires a unique plan of action for every individual patient, with a combined drug treatment approach and rehabilitative procedures. This chapter will deal with some incapacitating symptoms such as spasticity, pain, tremor, visual disturbances secondary to abnormal visual movements and paroxysmal symptoms. The management of bladder dysfunction, fatigue and cognitive disturbances are covered in other chapters of this book.

Spasticity

Spasticity refers to muscular hypertonia expressing a hyperexcitability of the stretch reflex due to disinhibition of spinal cord reflexes.[1] Spasticity increases the resistance to passive movements in a velocity-dependent manner. Uncontrolled flexor responses and spasms reflect the spinal cord hyperreflexivity to exteroceptive stimuli, a condition often produced by intercurrent conditions such as urinary infection or pressure sores. Hypertonia is always accompanied by impaired voluntary motor function which is hidden behind spasticity and revealed by the excessive use of muscle relaxants.

In MS patients spasticity can have different effects: mild spasticity impairs the capacity to walk, increasing with effort and limiting the distance; severe and diffuse spasticity occurs in severely disabled patients who become paraplegic or quadriplegic, either in extension or in flexion; focal spasticity encountered in some patients requires specific therapeutic procedures; painful spasms increase the disabling aspects of hypertonia and produce fibrous contracture.

A wide range of treatments are available for managing spasticity which must be used according to the presentation and severity of each specific patient.[2]

Oral medications act at different levels of the pathophysiological mechanisms of spinal cord disinhibition. Major well established antispastic drugs are represented by baclofen, benzodiazepines, dantrolene and tizanidine. Threonine has been recently suggested as potentially effective.

Baclofen is a derivative of γ-aminobutyric acid (GABA), an inhibitory transmitter. It acts as an agonist of GABA β-receptor in the spinal cord which inhibits both mono- and poly-synaptic reflexes. The dose varies from 5 to 120 mg per day and reduces muscular stiffness and the frequency and intensity of the acute spasms. It is useful to increase the dose progressively to reach the maximal dose tolerated: side effects include sedation, nausea, mood depression, vertigo and confusion. Major complications are seizures and hallucinations which indicate the withdrawal of the drug. In patients with mild spasticity, or when used in sphincter hypertonia of the bladder, high doses are deleterious in creating excessive hypotonia which increases muscular weakness.

More recently, baclofen has been used intrathecally.[3] Suitability for treatment by this method is assessed using intrathecal injection of baclofen with increasing doses from 50 to 200 mg. An antispastic effect lasts for less than eight hours after the injection. When this antispastic effect improves the functional status of the MS patient continuous administration is obtained by an implantable drug delivery system. In MS the best indication for this procedure is fixed severe spasticity in the most disabled patient. Nursing is easier and painful spasms are abolished. This effect is long lasting. The frequency of refilling the drug reservoir varies according to every patient.

Technical problems are frequent, but usually easily resolved. Some patients suffer from central side effects of the drug including sedation or respiratory depression. Because of the difficulty in finding the accurate infusion rate, mildly spastic patients with spinal cord demyelinating lesions are not appropriate for the implantation procedure. However, it is possible to use it in some patients who are still ambulant with a careful titration of the dose. The major concern with this form of treatment is its high cost which limits the use to the most severe patients.

Benzodiazepines such as diazepam, tetrazepam or clonazepam, exert an antispastic effect by activating the GABA α-receptors, which increase presynaptic inhibition in the spinal cord and reduce the spontaneous firing of brainstem neurones, thus decreasing the descending spinal activity. Frequently used as muscle relaxants the benzodiazepines have major limiting side effects such as sedation, drowsiness and memory disturbances. They also induce drug tolerance and dependency.

Tizanidine has been introduced recently in some European countries as a new antispastic drug. It acts as an α2 adrenergic agonist by reducing excitability transmission in the spinal cord. It has a specific effect on paroxysmal spasms and a positive effect on muscle strength. Hypotension, drowsiness and sedation are its major reactions.

Dantrolene acts peripherally at the muscular level by a direct effect on the sarcoplasmic reticulum. It modifies the calcium release within the muscle fibre which impairs the excitation contraction mechanism. It reduces the hypertonic muscular tone and has a good efficacy in relieving acute contractures. It uncovers muscle weakness which is the limiting factor in clinical use. Moreover the higher doses (300 to 400 mg/day) can induce hepatotoxicity which must be carefully monitored.

The naturally occurring amino acid Threonine exerts its antispastic effect as a potential precursor for glycine synthesis in the spinal cord.[4] However, this compound has only been used in one limited trial and its beneficial action must be confirmed. As a GABA agonist, gabapentin warrants interest for alleviating spasticity, but trials have not yet started.

Focal disabling spasticity can be treated by peripheral nerve blocks or surgical procedures. Peripheral blocks consist of local injection of phenol or alcohol either into the nerve or directly in the muscle. A more recent procedure is the intramuscular injection of botulinum toxin which decreases temporarily the muscle contracture.[5] Its usefulness is not fully recognized and needs further assessment for defining its specific indications and its cost effectiveness.

Severe diffuse spasticity can be alleviated by intrathecal baclofen or surgical procedures. The latter includes either orthopaedic surgery with tenotomies or neurosurgery with irreversible procedures, such as selective functional microneurosurgery, peripheral neurotomy or lesioning of the dorsal root entry zone rather than radical neurosurgery (anterior or posterior rhizotomy).

Physical treatments are part of the rehabilitation programmes which are proposed to the spastic patients. They include cryotherapy and regular physiotherapy involving the Bobath method, self training for lengthening the muscles, and appropriate positioning of the lower limbs in daily care. Videos are available from some MS societies but these treatments are better initiated in rehabilitation centres.

Pain

Pain is a frequent symptom in MS patients.[6] It can be a direct manifestation of a demyelinating lesion affecting pain pathways or the consequence of other damage induced by the disease. Approximately 50 per cent of patients complain of chronic pain, and 30–65 per cent of patients experience pain at some time during the disease course. Less frequently, pain is a paroxysmal symptom like trigeminal neuralgia. Pain is more frequent in disabled and older patients. In the relapsing–remitting phase, it is associated with sensory relapses, and sometimes lasts several months after the acute phase, leading to depression and anxiety which enhance the symptom.

In MS patients pain can be classified into

three different categories: chronic, subacute and paroxysmal. Central neurogenic pain is caused by demyelination in the ascending or descending pathways which control the transmission and regulation of painful stimuli. It can be differentiated from other types of pain by some clinical characteristics: described as a grinding, gnawing or burning sensation, with topographical systematization as truncular or fascicular, it is associated with a decrease in sensation or hyperaesthesia, often mixing a chronic painful continuous sensation with acute exacerbations, spontaneous or provoked.

Trigeminal neuralgia is the most characteristic acute pain. It affects 1–2 per cent of patients, sometimes bilaterally, at any time during the course of the disease. It has been ascribed to plaques in the fifth nerve root entry zone. Ephaptic transmission is probably the major mechanism of painful stimulus.[7] Treatments for trigeminal neuralgia are aimed at:

- Reducing the abnormal neuronal excitability: carbamazepine is highly effective but, when the side effects are intolerable, other compounds can be used such as phenytoin, clonazepam, baclofen, amitriptyline, and opiate analgesics.
- Blocking the inflammation: trigeminal neuralgia is sometimes linked to a relapse which can be alleviated by a pulse steroid therapy. However, many patients complain of a chronic neuralgia with frequent exacerbations during the course of the disease. Misoprostol, a long-acting prostaglandin E_1 (PGE_1) analogue, has been found to be an effective and safe treatment either alone or in association with the other conventional drugs.[7] Its likely mechanism of action is directly associated with suppression of inflammation in the lesion.
- Surgical destruction of nociceptive path-

ways: in MS, thermorhizotomy of the nerve root is as efficient as in the idiopathic form. Glycerol instillation in the nerve vicinity would be a therapeutic procedure, but microsurgical decompression from pulsating arteries fails to relieve MS-associated trigeminal pain.

Other paroxysmal painful symptoms such as painful tonic seizures or Lhermitte's sign are generally relieved by carbamazepine, clonazepam or amitriptyline.

Subacute pain is usually symptomatic of an interfering event such as urinary retention, a pressure sore infection, or optic neuritis. In this last case, pain is provoked by the swollen optic nerve which stretches to the surrounding meninges. The treatment of the cause usually treats the pain.

Dysaesthesic extremity pain is the most common manifestation of chronic pain. Patients complain of a continuously burning sensation in the feet or legs, but sometimes also in arms and trunk. Pain is frequently worse at night or after exercise. Tricyclic antidepressants are the drugs of choice for this condition. Dorsal column electrostimulation and transcutaneous electrical nerve stimulation may be of some value in controlling this type of pain. The clinical effect is nevertheless modest. Chronic back and radicular pain are caused by the postural abnormalities induced by muscular weakness and spasticity, and are alleviated by physiotherapy with non-steroidal anti-inflammatory drugs if necessary. Painful leg spasms are part of spasticity management.

Tremor

Among the motor incapacitating symptoms, tremor is one of the most difficult to treat: it leads to the paradoxical situation in which a patient without any paralysis is unable to perform a voluntary movement owing to the action tremor intensity. Action tremor is the most common form of tremor in MS patients, followed by postural tremor. Rest tremor is one of the few symptoms rarely seen in MS.[8,9]

Action tremor is part of the Charcot and Vulpian clinical form, characteristic of long duration MS. It is also called intention tremor, goal directed tremor or hyperkinetic tremor. It means that the amplitude of the abnormal movement increases when reaching the target, often enhanced when the patient tries to be more accurate. In some cases the movement is completely incapacitating. These patients cannot drink, eat, write or generally perform any precise movement. This tremor is due to lesions of the cerebellum or the cerebellar outflow pathways. Its occurrence is independent of any relapse, expressing a secondary degenerative process in fine tuning control of the voluntary movement exerted by the dentato-rubro-thalamic pathway.

Postural tremor, occurring during sustained posture such as outstretching of the arms, is less common in MS. Orthostatic tremor leading to a postural tremor of the trunk or the head and neck is often associated with action tremor.

Symptomatic treatment is disappointing. Different drugs have been proposed with variable and generally inadequate results. Carbamazepine and isoniazid can be of some interest, but only anecdotally.[10,11] Low dose barbiturates, particularly primidone – at increasing doses of 20–50 mg or phenobarbitone – 50–100 mg per day – are sometimes useful to decrease the amplitude of tremor. Clonazepam can be tried when the former drug is not effective. Glutethimide, a piperidinedione derivative, and gabapentin, could be of some interest as has recently been reported.[12] Intravenous ondansetron, a serotonin HT3 antagonist, has recently shown some interesting results.[13] New generation anti-epileptic drugs and calcium channel blockers are under investigation.

Some orthostatic measures can be proposed, such as attaching small passive weights to the wrists. Computer-controlled mechanical damping is in a developmental phase.

Some patients can be referred for functional neurosurgery.[14,15] Thalamic surgery includes thalamotomy or thalamic electrostimulation. The target for stereotactic thalamotomy is the ventrolateral nuclei. The best patients for this treatment are those affected with unilateral action tremor without orthostatic tremor and cerebellar dyssynergia. A bilateral procedure is seldom performed because it induces speech disturbances. The procedure carries a high risk of complications such as worsened ataxia or hypotonic hemiplegia. Cerebral atrophy secondary to axonal loss, which is frequent in these patients, increases the risk of the stereotactic procedure. Thalamic electrostimulation uses mono- or multi-electrode devices implanted into the ventrolateral nuclei or into the adjacent areas. The suitable targets are determined by electrophysiological stimulations during surgery. Electrodes are connected to a stimulator which is implanted in the subclavicular region. This procedure compares favourably with thalamotomy in terms of complications and results, but is limited to the same category of patient, perhaps enlarged to those with bilateral involvement. In one third of patients, a tolerance occurs which decreases the efficacy of this chronic stimulation. The cost is high, which is a major limiting factor for the wide use of this procedure still under investigation in a small number of highly specialized centres.

Abnormal eye movements

Abnormal eye movements interfere with clear and stable vision because of an excessive drift of image on the retina or a displacement of the object of interest outside the fovea. Abnormal eye movements are a frequent clinical condition occurring in MS patients: all types of acquired nystagmus and saccadic intrusions can occur in MS.[16] With reduced visual acuity secondary to demyelination of the afferent pathways, oscillopsia contributes to the impairment of vision which is a frequent and disabling complaint of many severely involved patients.

The basic pathophysiological and neuropharmacological mechanisms of these abnormal movements are better understood, leading to the development of new therapeutic approaches, with either drugs or optical devices.[17]

Different drugs can act at the multiple pharmacological levels of oculomotor control pathways where disturbances are involved in abnormal eye movements. In some instances specific drugs are effective in treating symptoms due to well known mechanisms: periodic alternating nystagmus responds to the GABA β agonist baclofen. However, the therapeutic results are usually variable depending on the symptom and the patient. Downbeat and upbeat nystagmus can be influenced with clonazepam, baclofen, scopolamine or, as recently reported, with gabapentin.[18] Acquired pendular nystagmus, a frequent condition in MS patients, may respond to anticholinergics such as trihexyphenidyl, or barbiturates and isoniazid. Saccadic oscillations have been successfully treated with clonazepam, phenobarbitone, amphetamines or propanolol. In the majority of cases, results are moderate and increasing the dose only increases the side effects.

A number of optical devices have been proposed for the treatment of nystagmus, such as prisms or an optical system stabilizing the images on the retina. Botulinum toxin might be injected into selected extraocular muscles leading to a decrease in the amplitude of pendular acquired nystagmus. These therapeutic procedures are still under investigation and deserve more studies before clinical use.

Paroxysmal symptoms

The term paroxysmal symptoms refers to clinical conditions characterized by brief phenomena, sensitive or motor, often triggered by specific factors.[19] They are rather frequently encountered as 5–17 per cent of MS patients experience a wide range of paroxysmal symptoms, which share some common features: their brief duration, of less than a few minutes, their high frequency of occurrence, specific triggering conditions like hyperventilation, anxiety, or sustained posture of limbs. Their mechanism involves abnormal excitability of axons secondary to ephaptic transmission. The excitatory signal, reaching a demyelinated zone, may spread to the adjacent axons leading to its activation and clinical expression of symptoms which are sometimes unrelated.

The main clinical manifestations are tonic seizures or spasms, sensory disorders, dysarthria and ataxia, epilepsy and painful disorders.

Tonic seizures are highly characteristic and regarded as strong indicators of the disease. They are frequently triggered by acute emotional states, localized to the arm, the leg or the hemiface, occurring without any loss of consciousness or EEG abnormality. These hypertonic crises are very painful, but easily reproduced when patients are asked to perform short periods of hyperventilation. Carbamazepine is the drug of choice as the symptoms vanished shortly after its introduction. Other anticonvulsants are also active in the majority of the other paroxysmal symptoms.

Dysarthria and ataxia are less known although highly evocative of MS. Attacks are frequent, more than a few hundred per day, impairing speech with an increase in gait, ataxia and sometimes a limb dysynergia. Sensory symptoms can accompany dysarthria. Here, also, carbamazepine is a very efficient drug.

It is difficult to accept that epilepsy is an unusual symptom in MS. In fact it is a rare manifestation of the disease, occurring in fewer than 1 per cent of patients, suggesting an 'intercurring' event in a majority of cases. However, it has been suggested that a large subcortical plaque could be the cause in some patients. Seizures respond to the classical anticonvulsants.

Lhermitte's sign, commonly experienced by patients with demyelinative lesions in the cervical spinal cord, is an electric sensation passing down the spine after sudden flexion of the neck. It disappears spontaneously after a few months, or can be abolished with carbamazepine or benzodiazepines. Some patients report brief episodes of tonic seizures preceded by transient sensory disturbances in the involved limb.

In many instances, paroxysmal symptoms are consecutive to a disease attack and must be treated simultaneously with methylprednisolone.

Conclusion

The difficulty in managing the symptoms of MS is that current palliative treatments are seldom successful.[20] In the majority of cases, the limitation in the use of an efficient drug is the intensity of the side effects which are proportional to its activity. Unfortunately, no striking breakthrough has been made in this field in the last years, contrary to the immunomodulatory treatments recently available. As a final comment it should be mentioned that a recent report has provided some evidence for the efficacy of aerobic training on fitness and quality of life in MS,[21] suggesting once again the importance of all the rehabilitation procedures in the symptomatic management of MS (see Freeman and Thompson, Chapter 23).

References

1. Noth J. Trends in the pathophysiology and pharmacotherapy of spasticity. *J Neurol* 1991; **238**: 131–139.
2. Management of spasticity in MS. *The symptoms of MS and their management*. (Chairman: Clanet M). Proceedings of the MS Forum Modern management workshop, Paris 1994; 21–25.
3. Azouvi P, Mane M, Thiebaut JB *et al*. Intrathecal baclofen administration for control of severe spinal spasticity: Functional improvement and long term follow-up. *Arch Phys Med Rehabil* 1996; **77**: 35–39.
4. Hauser S, Doottle TH, Lopez-Bresnahan M *et al*. An antispastic effect of threonine in MS. *Arch Neurol* 1992; **49**: 923–926.
5. Snow BJ, Tsui JRC, Bhatt MH. Treatment of spasticity with botulinum toxin: a double blind study. *Ann Neurol* 1990; **28**: 512–515.
6. Clifford DB, Trotter JL. Pain in MS. *Arch Neurol* 1984; **41**: 1270–1270.
7. Reder AT, Arnason BGW. Trigeminal neuralgia in multiple sclerosis relieved by a prostaglandin E-analogue. *Neurology* 1995; **45**: 1097–1100.
8. Moulin DE, Foley KM, Ebers GC. Pain syndromes in MS. *Neurology* 1988; **38**: 1830–1834.
9. Management of tremor in MS. *The symptoms of MS and their management*, (Chairman: Clanet M). Proceedings of the MS Forum Modern Management Workshop, Paris 1994; 26–29.
10. Sechi GP, Zudas M, Predda M. Treatment of cerebellar tremor with carbamazepine: a controlled trial with long term follow-up. *Neurology* 1989; **39**: 1113–1115.
11. Hallet M, Lindsey JW, Adelstein BD. Controlled trial of isoniazid therapy for severe postural cerebellar tremor in MS. *Neurology* 1985; **35**: 1374–1377.
12. Aisen ML, Holzer M, Rosen M *et al*. Glutethimide treatment of disabling action tremor in patients with MS and traumatic brain injury. *Arch Neurol* 1991; **48**: 513–515.
13. Rice G, Dickey C, Lesaux J *et al*. Ondansetron for disabling cerebellar tremor. *Ann Neurol* 1995; **38**: 973.
14. Geny C, N'Guyen JP, Pollin B *et al*. Improvement of severe postural cerebellar tremor in multiple sclerosis by chronic thalamic stimulation. *Movement Disorders* 1996; **11**: 489–494.
15. Speelman JD, VanHaven J. Stereotactic thalamotomy for the relief of intention tremor in MS. *J Neurol Neurosurg Psychiatry* 1984; **47**: 596–599.
16. Frohman EM, Solomon D, Zee DS. Nuclear, supranuclear and internuclear eye movement abnormalities in MS. *Int MS J* 1996; **2**: 78–89.
17. Leigh RJ, Averbuch-Heler L, Tomsak RL *et al*. Treatment of abnormal eye movements that impair vision: Strategies based on current concept of physiology and pharmacology. *Ann Neurol* 1994; **36**: 129–141.
18. Averbuch-Heller L, Stahl JS, Rottach KG *et al*. Gabapentin as a treatment of nystagmus. *Ann Neurol* 1995; **38**: 972.
19. Management of paroxysmal symptoms in MS. *The symptoms of MS and their management* (Chairman: Clanet M), Proceedings of the MS Forum Modern Management Workshop, Paris 1994; 30–33.
20. Thompson AJ. Multiple sclerosis: symptomatic treatment. *J Neurol* 1996; **243**: 559–565.
21. Petajan JH, Gappmaier E, White AT *et al*. Impact of aerobic training on fitness and quality of life in MS. *Ann Neurol* 1996; **39**: 432–441.

18

Depression and suicide in multiple sclerosis

Ronald A Remick and A Dessa Sadovnick

Introduction

A relationship between mood disorders and multiple sclerosis (MS) has been acknowledged since the earliest clinical reports on this neurological disorder.[1-3] The historical explanation (or rationalization!) for depression in MS patients stated that this was an appropriate reaction to a very stressful illness, especially given its unpredictable episodic course and impact on personal, social and vocational functioning. An alternative explanation for depressive symptoms associated with MS was the progressive disability of the disorder.[2,4] More recent work,[5,6] however, has suggested that the increasing and specific central nervous system (CNS) involvement results in mood disorders associated with MS.

Mood disorders (depression, bipolar disorder or manic depressive illness) are among the most common medical disorders. Further, the vast majority of those afflicted can expect dramatic or complete recovery with appropriate treatment interventions.[7]

Our particular interest in the relationship between MS and depression was prompted by the alarming rate of suicide found in two Canadian MS clinics. In a study on causes of death among 3125 MS patients attending two MS clinics (Vancouver, British Columbia (BC); London, Ontario), the suicide rate among these patients was 7.5 times the rate for the age-matched general population.[8] This statistic, while high, was certainly consistent with

neurological clinical experience – all too often our colleagues have recounted the tragic and unexpected suicide of an MS patient.

In this chapter, we will review previous research on depression and MS, and then outline the current state of knowledge of mood disorders and MS. Finally, we will offer guidelines for the clinical assessment and treatment of mood disorders associated with MS.

Depressive symptoms and MS

Before reviewing the relationship between mood disorders and MS, it is important to emphasize the difference between depressive symptoms and a depressive syndrome or major depressive disorder. Major depression is a discrete operationally defined[9] medical syndrome with a constellation of mental and physical symptoms, only one of which may be a depressed mood. A depressed mood is not an unusual symptom in most serious medical disorders. Unfortunately, it is not clear in much of the early research on mood disorders and MS[2] whether the diagnosis is for a major depression and/or solely a depressed mood. In psychiatry, as is also true in other medical areas, the correct diagnosis is imperative if the goal is appropriate treatment intervention(s). We have already noted the efficacy of treatments for depression. Thus, this paper focuses only on previously published studies which clearly define the criteria used to diagnose a depressive syndrome.

Major depressive disorder and MS – a review

Whitlock and Siskind[3] compared 30 MS patients (excluding those with signs of dementia) with 30 patients diagnosed as having other chronic or progressive neurological syndromes (hereditary ataxias – 10; muscular dystrophy – 4; motor neuron disease – 3; dystrophia myotonia – 4; others – 13). All patients were interviewed by a research psychologist who diagnosed cases with endogenous depression (it is unclear how this diagnosis was defined) and completed the Beck Depression Inventory (BDI) – a valid psychometric rating scale for depression.[10] The diagnosis of endogenous depression was more frequent in the MS group (16 out of 30; 53 per cent) than the control group (5 out of 30; 17 per cent). The BDI was higher (i.e. more severe) in the MS group (mode 10–14) than in the control group (mode 0–4). Both of these results are statistically significant.

Rabins *et al.*[5] compared 87 MS patients who were not cognitively impaired with 16 stable spinal cord injury patients without known head injury. It was noted that 30 of the MS patients were receiving corticosteroid therapy which may have been a confounding factor and many of the MS patients were in the midst of an acute MS exacerbation (i.e. not stable). Patients in this study completed the General Health Questionnaire – Depression (GHQ-D) Scale[11] which, by current standards, is not the most sensitive psychometric for diagnosing depression. MS patient scores were higher (0.9 ± 1.4) than controls (0.5 ± 0.8) but not statistically significant.

Dalos *et al.*[12] also used the GHQ-D in a study of 64 MS patients and 23 spinal cord injury patients. Again, the GHQ-D scores were not statistically different between the MS (0.6 ± 0.9) and control (0.4 ± 0.8) groups. It

was noted, however, that the two groups differed significantly with respect to a number of important variables: age, duration of illness, age of onset of illness, and degree of disability.

Schiffer *et al.*[13] assessed 30 MS patients and 15 healthy volunteers. Depressive disorder was assessed using the Schedule for Affective Disorders and Schizophrenia–Lifetime Version (SADS-L),[14] which is an excellent diagnostic tool for the objective evaluation of major depression. Raters must be trained to use this instrument to ensure reliability. The methodology for this study did not describe raters and/or the reliability of their ratings. Nevertheless, 11 of the 30 (37 per cent) MS patients had a lifetime major depression diagnosis, compared with none of the healthy volunteers.

Minden *et al.*[15] used the SADS-L to assess 50 MS patients with moderate severity, but not on corticosteroids. There was no specific control group. A lifetime community prevalence rate for major depression of 20 per cent (current figures are similar at 17 per cent)[16] was used. MS patients were assessed by a psychiatrist. This study showed no difference in the prevalence of a major depression *before* the diagnosis of MS in MS patients (7 out of 50; 14 per cent) compared to the community rate (20 per cent). However, 27 of 50 (54 per cent) MS patients had a lifetime diagnosis of depression, significantly higher than the expected 20 per cent. The results of this study, which had several methodological improvements from earlier work, suggested a higher rate of major depression in MS patients compared with the community.

Joffe *et al.*[17] interviewed 100 MS patients seen in follow-up at an MS clinic. The SADS-L was completed by a psychiatrist who also made the diagnosis of a major depression using another excellent diagnostic instrument – Research Diagnostic Criteria (RDC).[18] Of these 100 MS patients, 42 (42 per cent) had a lifetime diagnosis of major depression.

The literature to date on depressive disorders in MS patients finds that the majority of studies have suggested that MS patients have a higher rate of depression compared to both neurological and normal controls. The rates, despite varying methodologies, have been relatively consistent with a lifetime prevalence between 37 and 54 per cent, i.e. two to three times the expected prevalence for the community[16] and groups with other neurological diseases.[19]

In summary, these earlier studies have been plagued by a number of methodological difficulties. First, with respect to psychiatric diagnosis, varying diagnostic criteria for major depression have been used but were seldom standardized. It was also often unclear who made the psychiatric diagnosis (psychiatrist, psychologist, research assistant, etc.) and what reliability measures were incorporated into the study. Further, many of the earlier studies used patients' subjective impressions of their mood state (Beck Depression Inventory) rather than objective impressions from the standardized instruments (e.g. SADS-L; RDC).

Another problem with the literature on depressive disorders in MS patients has been the difficulty of assessing a mood disorder without confounding factors from the actual disease influencing this assessment. For example, factors which may affect mood can include MS exacerbations, prescription drugs with psychoactive properties (e.g. corticosteroids) and 'self-help' techniques such as alcohol and drug abuse.

MS and depression – etiology

If a higher rate of mood disorders really exists in MS patients, one must question the etiology of the mood disorder. A number of studies[5,6,20] have suggested that the depressive *symptoms* in MS may correlate with increasing and specific CNS involvement. An important study by Honer *et al.*[21] compared magnetic resonance imaging (MRI) brain findings in eight MS patients with psychiatric impairment and eight control MS patients without psychiatric impairment. The two groups had similar lesion loads on MRI, but differed in lesion site distribution. Psychiatrically impaired patients had greater temporal lobe involvement. However, the small sample size of the Honer study and the failure to replicate these findings[22,23] have left understanding of any relationship between specific CNS involvement and depression unclear.

While the etiology of mood disorders remains unclear, genetic factors are recognized to play an important role in causation.[24] What is the genetic 'link', if any, between MS and depression? Only two previous studies[15,17] have examined this question with conflicting results. Joffe *et al.*[17] looked at the familial rate of depression in first-degree relatives of MS patients and found that it did not differ from the general population of individuals having a depression but not MS. They interpreted the data as evidence *against* a genetic link between MS and depression. In contrast, Minden *et al.*[15] found a high rate of depression in relatives of MS patients, suggesting a possible genetic link between MS and depression.

If data really do support a genetic link between MS and depression, a common etiology could be postulated. Conversely, if this is not suggested by the data, depressive syndromes occurring concurrently with MS could in fact have a different etiology (e.g. structural changes, immunological changes, etc.) from depressive syndromes in the absence of MS. It is important to determine which, if any, of the above are true as these findings could have potential implications for the treatment of the depression associated with MS.

Depression and MS: the Vancouver MS clinic experience

BC provided an excellent opportunity to study the relationship (if any) between MS and depression. A study was designed to examine the lifetime risk of major depression in a representative well defined MS group, avoiding as many as possible of the confounding variables noted in previous studies.[24]

Building on an ongoing collaboration between the Departments of Medical Genetics and Psychiatry, we compared the morbidity risks for depression among the first-degree relatives of MS patients with a current or lifetime diagnosis of depression with those first-degree relatives of MS patients not having a depression.

Over 80 per cent of MS patients in BC are seen at the Vancouver MS Clinic which, at the time of this study, was the only clinic in the Province. The study period was July 1, 1992 to June 30, 1993.

This study avoided problems with the diagnosis of MS. Each diagnosis was made by a neurologist experienced in the differential diagnosis of MS and in accordance with recognized criteria.[25] Only persons diagnosed with clinically definite MS were included in the study. To avoid other confounding factors, the study excluded: (1) MS patients with severe disability (Kurtzke Extended Disability Scale or EDSS >6.5),[26] (2) patients attending the Clinic because of an MS exacerbation, and (3) patients whose treatment protocol and/or lifestyle may confound psychiatric ratings (e.g. patients involved in clinical trials, patients with an active substance abuse problem as diagnosed after psychiatric evaluation).

The study group thus consisted of 221 MS patients, all of whom were assessed by trained interviewers who administered the structured clinical interview for DSMIIIR- non-patient (SCID-NP) edition.[27] The SCID-NP interview is specifically targeted to non-psychiatric patients such as outpatients who attended ambulatory medical clinics. The SCID-NP generated both current and lifetime psychiatric diagnoses and this study only reported on diagnoses of major depression. Throughout the study, inter- and intra-rater reliabilities were assessed.

Detailed genetic histories have been routinely obtained for all MS patients attending the Vancouver MS Clinic by a medical geneticist using multiple family informants.[24] A family history for depression was thus easily incorporated into the evaluation of the sample of 221 MS patients. In previous work we have developed an accurate and reliable methodology for assessing familial risks for depression in first-degree relatives using the patients (index case) and their relatives.[28] In our 221 MS patients, data were available on the psychiatric status (i.e. mood disorder diagnosis) of 1207 of their first-degree relatives. For more specific and detailed information on the methodology and data analysis for this study, see Sadovnick *et al.*[24]

In our sample of 221 MS patients, 76 patients (34.4 per cent) had a current or lifetime diagnosis of major depressive disorder by strict diagnostic criteria. The age-corrected risk[29] for a major depression among the 221 MS patients was 50.3 per cent by age 59 years (see *Fig. 18.1*).

Table 18.1 summarises the risk estimates[30] for a major depression in 1207 first-degree relatives of 221 MS patients. The overall risk estimate was 2.52 per cent. There were no statistical differences when the MS patients were separated into the following two groups: (1)

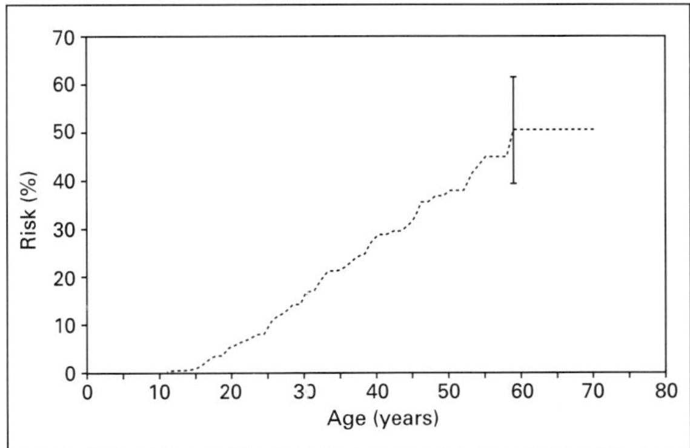

Fig. 18.1
Cumulative lifetime risk for a depression in 221 MS index cases.

76 MS patients with a mood disorder diagnosis and 397 of their first-degree relatives, and (2) 145 MS patients with no mood disorder diagnosis and 810 of their first-degree relatives. The risk estimates were 3.22 per cent

and 2.20 per cent, respectively. These estimates were compared with a 'control' group from our Mood Disorder Database[24] where 2840 first-degree relatives of 304 patients with major depression had a risk estimate for a mood disorder of 9.10 per cent.

In summary our data showed that the first-degree relatives of MS patients (with or without comorbid depression), showed a significantly lower risk for developing a depressive illness than did the first-degree relatives of a large well defined group of patients with 'non-neurological' major depression.

Summary

Our work and the work of others therefore suggests that there is a very high rate of major depression associated with MS. Our lifetime prevalence of 50.3 per cent is consistent with rates for earlier studies which have varied from 37 to 54 per cent. This extremely high

Group	No. of patients	Total no. of 1° relatives	Total no. affected 1° relatives (%)	Risk estimate (%)
MS (with depression)	76	397	8 (2.02)	3.22
MS (no depression)	145	810	12 (1.48)	2.20
Total MS group	221	1207	20 (1.66)	2.52
Depression control group	304	2840	182 (6.41)	9.10

Table 18.1
Lifetime risk estimates for depression in first-degree relatives of 'cases' and 'controls'.

prevalence appears to be specific to MS. Other chronic debilitating medical disorders, including other neurological disorders, such as Parkinson's disease, have rates which are one half to one third those for MS patients.[19,31]

The reason for the high rate of depression among MS patients remains unclear. Depression among MS patients does not appear to have a clear genetic basis, or at least the same genetic basis operating in families when depression occurs in the absence of MS. Whether there is a specific lesion, site of lesion, or load of MS lesions which results in depression is also unclear, although the research done in this area is very preliminary.

Treatment guidelines

Countless studies[16,32–34] have documented that the largest impediment to effective treatment of depression is the failure to recognize the syndrome. Perhaps up to 50 per cent of mood disorders go unrecognized and consequently untreated.

Clinicians treating MS patients should always be suspicious about the possibility of a mood disorder, given the known prevalence rates. Routine questioning concerning mood symptoms almost always elicits depressive symptoms if they are present.

The mnemonic prescription 'SIGE CAPS' outlines the eight key areas to question when assessing for depression:

S (Sleep):	'Is there a change in your sleep pattern (insomnia or hypersomnia)?'
I (Interest):	'Have you noticed you are less interested in things that typically give you pleasure?'
G (Guilt):	'Do you think you are more guilty or remorseful than usual about things you either have done or have not done?'
E (Energy):	'Has there been a change in your energy lately?' (This is often difficult to assess in MS patients and should not be pivotal in the decision about whether or not a mood disorder exists.)
C (Concentration):	'Do you find your memory or concentration less sharp than usual?'
A (Appetite):	'Has your appetite changed recently?' (i.e. too much or too little.)
P (Psychomotor):	Does the patient exhibit motor agitation or retardation?
S (Suicide):	'Have you felt life is not worth living? Have you contemplated suicide?'

Four of the above symptoms (excluding energy change or fatigue in MS patients) present for at least *two* weeks should result in a presumptive diagnosis of major depression. If a diagnosis of depression is confirmed, the mainstay of treatment for these individuals should be antidepressant chemotherapy.[35,36] There are approximately 20 effective antidepressants currently on the market in Canada – all of which result in symptomatic relief within two to four weeks in two thirds of patients. Mild forms of depression can be treated with psychotherapy. Severe or urgent cases may require electroconvulsive therapy (ECT).[35]

Depressive disorders have a significant mortality – predominantly from suicide. Indeed, 15 per cent of all patients with a mood disorder die by their own hands.[37,38] We have previously noted the high rate of suicide among MS patients.[8] Thus, the clinician must not only recognize a depressive disorder but evaluate the suicide risk. High risk patients need protection (family care, hospitalization), particularly if they suffer from a treatable illness such as depression.

Risk factors for suicide include males with a single marital status (especially divorced, widowed), unemployment, poor physical health, family history of suicide, past suicide attempts, alcohol/drug abuse, and a specific lethal suicide plan. Another mnemonic – the SADPERSONS Scale – can assist in identifying suicide risk. By scoring one point for:

S (Male Sex)
A (Above Age 40)
D (Depression)
P (Previous Attempt)
E (Ethanol/Drug Abuse)
R (Rational Thinking Loss)

S (Lack of Social Support)
O (Organized Suicide Plan)
N (No Spouse or Significant Other)
S (Sickness – i.e. Medical Disorder).

Using the above, patients with a total score of 0–2 can usually safely be sent home with family. A score of 3–4 requires arrangements for close follow-up (consider hospitalization). If the score is 5–6 strongly consider hospitalization. Patients with a score of 7–10 require immediate hospitalization/supervision.

Unfortunately, there are very few specific guidelines for treating depression in MS patients although all studies have indicated that treatment *per se* (whether psychotherapy or antidepressants) usually results in remission of depressive symptoms.[39,40]

Greater recognition of depression (and suicide risk) in MS patients will no doubt lead to more effective interventions, and will prevent the tragic loss of life from a treatable disorder.

References

1. Cottrell SS, Wilson SAK. The affective symptomatology of disseminated sclerosis. *J Neurol Psychopathol* 1926; **7**: 1–30.
2. Surridge D. An investigation into some psychiatric aspects of multiple sclerosis. *Br J Psychiat* 1969; **115**: 749–764.
3. Whitlock FA, Siskind M. Depression as a major symptom of multiple sclerosis. *J Neurol Neurosurg Psychiatry* 1980; **43**: 861–865.
4. McIvor GP, Riklan M, Reznikoff M. Depression in multiple sclerosis as a function of length and severity of illness, age, remission and perceived social support. *J Clin Psychol* 1984; **40**: 1028–1033.
5. Rabins V, Brooks BR, O'Donnell P *et al.* Structural brain correlates of emotional disorder in multiple sclerosis. *Brain* 1986; **109**: 585–597.
6. Campbell M, Fleming JA, Li D *et al.* Sleep disturbance, depression and lesion site in patients with multiple sclerosis. *Arch Neurol* 1992; **49**: 641–643.
7. Practice guidelines for major depressive disorder in adults. *Am J Psychiat* 1993; **150**: 4, April supplement.
8. Sadovnick AD, Eisen K, Paty DW *et al.* Cause of death in patients attending multiple sclerosis clinics. *Neurology* 1991; **41**: 1193–1196.
9. American Psychiatric Association: *Diagnostic and Statistical Manual of Mental Disorders*, 4th edn. Washington, DC: American Psychiatric Association 1994, 317–327.
10. Beck A, Ward C, Mendelson M *et al.* An inventory for measuring depression. *Arch Gen Psychiat* 1961; **4**: 561–571.
11. Goldberg D. *The Detection of Psychiatric Illness by Questionnaire*, London: Oxford University Press 1972.
12. Dalos WP, Rabins PV, Brooks BR *et al.* Disease activity and emotional state in multiple sclerosis. *Ann Neurol* 1983; **13**: 573–583.
13. Schiffer RB, Craine ED, Bamford KA *et al.* Depressive episodes in patients with multiple sclerosis. *Am J Psychiat* 1983; **140**: 1498–1500.
14. Endicott J, Spitzer RL. A diagnostic interview: the schedule for affective disorders and schizophrenia. *Arch Gen Psychiat* 1978; **35**: 837–844.
15. Minden S, Orav J, Reich P. Depression in multiple sclerosis. *Gen Hosp Psychiat* 1987; **9**: 426–434.
16. Blazer DG, Kessler RC, McGonagle KA *et al.* The prevalence and distribution of major depression in a national community sample: The National Comorbidity Survey. *Am J Psychiat* 1994; **151**: 979–986.
17. Joffe RT, Lippert GP, Gray TA. Depressions and multiple sclerosis. *Arch Neurol* 1987; **44**: 376–378.
18. Spitzer RL, Endicott J, Robins E. Research diagnostic criteria (RDC): rationale and reliability. *Arch Gen Psychiat* 1978; **35**: 773–782.
19. Tandberg E, Larsen JP, Aarsland D *et al.* The occurrence of depression in Parkinson's disease. *Arch Neurol* 1996; **53**: 175–179.
20. Ron MA, Feinstein A. Multiple sclerosis and the mind (editorial). *J Neurol Neurosurg Psychiatry* 1992; **55**: 1–3.
21. Honer WG, Hurwitz T, Li DK *et al.* Temporal lobe involvement in multiple sclerosis patients with psychiatric disorder. *Arch Neurol* 1987; **44**: 187–190.
22. Reischies FM, Baum K, Brau H *et al.* Cerebral magnetic resonance imaging findings in multiple sclerosis. Relation to disturbance of affect, drive, and cognition. *Arch Neurol* 1988; **45**: 1114–1116.
23. Feinstein A, Ron M, Thompson A. A serial study of psychometric and magnetic resonance imaging changes in multiple sclerosis. *Brain* 1993; **116**: 569–602.
24. Sadovnick AD, Remick RA, Allen J *et al.* Depression and multiple sclerosis. *Neurol* 1996; **46**: 628–632.
25. Poser CM, Paty DW, Scheinberg L *et al.* New diagnostic criteria for multiple sclerosis: guidelines for research protocols. *Ann Neurol* 1983; **13**: 227–231.
26. Kurtzke JF. Rating neurological impairment in multiple sclerosis: an expanded disability status

scale (EDSS). *Neurol* 1983; **33**: 1444–1452.

27. Spitzer RL, Williams J, Gibbon M *et al*. Structured clinical interview for DSMIIIR-nonpatient edition. Washington DC: American Psychiatry Press, 1990.

28. Sadovnick AD, Remick RA, Lam RW *et al*. Morbidity risks for depressions in 3,942 first-degree relatives of 671 index cases with single depression, recurrent depression, bipolar I or bipolar II. *Am J Hum Genet* 1994; **54**: 132–140.

29. Kaplan EL, Meier P. Non-parametric estimations from incomplete observations. *JASA* 1958; **53**: 457–581.

30. Risch N. Estimating morbidity risks with variable age of onset: review of methods and a maximum likelihood approach. *Biometrics* 1983; **39**: 929–939.

31. Wells KB, Golding JM, Burnam MA. Psychiatric disorders in a sample of the general population with and without chronic medical conditions. *Am J Psychiat* 1988; **145**: 976–981.

32. Keller MB, Klerman GL, Lavori PW *et al*. Treatment received by depressed patients. *J Am Med Ass* 1982; **248**: 1848–1855.

33. Bucholz KK, Robins LN. Who talks to a doctor about existing depressive illness? *J Affec Dis* 1987; **12**: 241–250.

34. Dew MA, Dunn LO, Bromet EJ *et al*. Factors affecting help-seeking during depression in a community sample. *J Affec Dis* 1988; **14**: 223–234.

35. Potter WZ, Rudorfer MV, Manji H. The pharmacologic treatment of depression. *New Eng J Med* 1991; **325**: 633–642.

36. Kaplan HI, Saddock BJ. *Pocket Handbook of Psychiatric Drug Treatment*, Baltimore: Williams and Wilkins 1990; 81–93.

37. Dyck RJ, Newman SC, Thompson AH. Suicide trends in Canada, 1956–1981. *Acta Psychiat Scand* 1988; **77**: 411–419.

38. Editorial: Depression and suicide: are they preventable? *Lancet* 1992; **340**: 700–701.

39. Larcombe NA, Wilson PH. An evaluation of cognitive-behavior therapy for depression in patients with multiple sclerosis. *Br J Psychiat* 1984; **145**: 366–371.

40. Schiffer RB, Windeman NM. Antidepressant pharmacotherapy of depression associated with multiple sclerosis. *Am J Psychiat* 1990; **147**: 1493–1497.

19

Cognitive dysfunction in multiple sclerosis. What are we measuring and why does it matter?

Dawn W Langdon

Introduction

A range of memory and other cognitive difficulties have been observed to occur in patients with multiple sclerosis (MS) since the first reports of the disease.[1] A review of several clinic-based studies found the prevalence of cognitive deterioration in MS patients to be between 54 and 65 per cent,[2] although the assessment method and sample recruitment both greatly influence the demonstrated prevalence. A community-based study found the prevalence to be 43 per cent.[3] A classical view of the cognitive impairment in MS is of a subcortical dementia;[4] however, cognitive dysfunction in MS follows a unique pattern and time course for each patient: some will encounter little or no cognitive difficulties, some will only experience difficulties in a few areas of cognition, whilst others may face severe and widespread dysfunction. In addition, cognitive deficits may occur and resolve in the same way as other impairments.[5]

It cannot be predicted precisely from any other aspect of the disease.[6] There is little or no significant relation between cognitive impairment and physical disability,[7–9] or disease duration,[7,10] or between the development of cognitive and neurological impairments,[11] for the individual patient. Indeed, significant cognitive impairment has been reported in the context of no sensorimotor dysfunction.[12,13] Some significant relations have been demonstrated between cognitive deficits and overall magnetic resonance imaging (MRI) lesion load.[14–18] In addition, some investigators have demonstrated a link between regional cerebral lesion load and poor performance on cognitive tests thought to rely on the integrity of the cerebral area with the greatest lesion load.[19,20]

Whilst cognitive assessment rarely contributes to diagnosis, it can provide an essential basis for the management and counselling of patients and their families throughout the disease. Indications for neuropsychological assessment have been described.[21] Patients should always be given an introduction to cognitive testing and a full explanation of its purpose and procedures. They may require some clarification about the difference between a psychologist and a psychiatrist and may also need to be reassured that the tests are not designed to address mental illness or instability. Full feedback should always be available to patients and their families if the patients wish. It should be presented in clear concrete terms, in a sensitive and constructive way, at a level of detail which is appropriate and helpful to the patient. The identification and description of their cognitive impairment is often a source of relief to patients and their families, who may have misinterpreted its effects as mental instability or the patient's lack of care for themselves or other family members.

What are we measuring?

The unpredictability of the pattern of cognitive dysfunction which a patient may experience makes cognitive assessment problematic and thorough cognitive assessment inevitably detailed and lengthy.[2] Short screening batteries designed for the bedside[7,22] and the mini mental state (MMS)[23] are only reliable when demonstrating severe cognitive impairment.[15] However, they are useful despite this limitation, because even severe cognitive impairment is not always accurately reported by patient or physician. In one large study, 14 per cent of patients were moderately to severely cognitively impaired on the MMS, compared with 9 per cent identified by self-report and 3 per cent by a neurologist from clinic interview.[24]

A Brief Repeatable Battery of Neuropsychological Tests (BRB-N)[25] has been developed to assess cognitive function in MS. It comprises five tests which were selected from a very extensive experimental battery as being the most sensitive to cognitive decline in MS. It tests verbal and spatial learning, symbol coding, auditory attention and word list generation. It can be administered in 20 or 30 minutes. It is sensitive to the degree of cognitive impairment and has a specificity of 94 per cent in discriminating cognitively impaired from cognitively intact MS patients.[3] The BRB-N is widely used in clinical trials and group studies.

Cognitive domains

Intelligence and reasoning

Perhaps the 'gold standard' test for intelligence, in terms of its international currency and established psychometric properties, the Wechsler Adult Intelligence Scale-Revised (WAIS-R)[26] comprises 11 subtests, six of them verbal tasks, five of them performance tasks. For English patient populations, the National Adult Reading Test[27] provides an estimate of pre-morbid IQ. The test consists of 50 single words, which are irregular, in that they do not obey the usual English letter-to-sound rules. There is evidence that the reading of irregular words is largely unaffected by disseminated neurological conditions,[28–30] although some reservations have been expressed.[31,32] An indication of pre-morbid optimum is very useful in detecting the first stages of cognitive impairment in the individual patient, because it can be compared with a measure of current function and the discrepancy, if any, between the two taken as the level of deterioration which has occurred in general intellectual function.

Abstract reasoning is often impaired in MS. The best-known test is the Wisconsin Card Sorting Test.[33] It consists of four key cards which are placed in a row before the patient (*Fig. 19.1*). A large pack of cards with abstract shapes, in various numbers and colours, is given to the patient. The patient places the top card from the pack below one

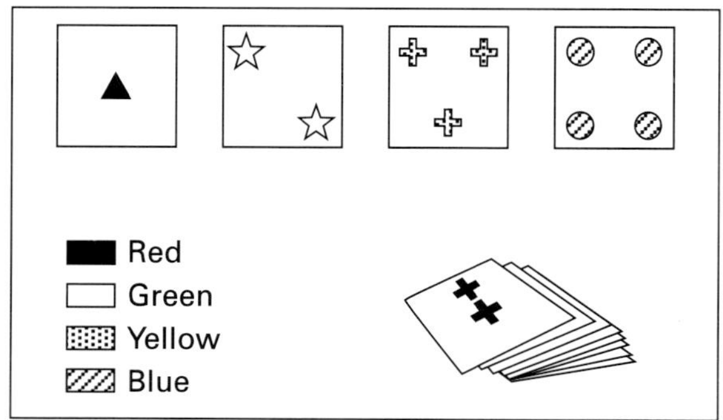

Fig. 19.1
The Wisconsin Card Sorting Test (reproduced from Milner 1963[33]).

of the four key cards, in an attempt to determine a sorting rule. The tester says whether the card is correctly or incorrectly placed after each sort. The patient must demonstrate consistency and flexibility, in line with the tester's feedback. Poor performance on the Wisconsin Card Sort and related tests have been reported in MS.[7,34] However, there is a general effect of any cerebral involvement on these tasks and it has proved hard to isolate a specific dysfunction in executive skills from the effects of a general intellectual deterioration, given the disseminated nature of the disease pathology.[35]

A new reasoning test has been developed for use with neurological patients,[36] designed to minimize the effects of physical and coincident cognitive deficits on test performance. The VESPAR comprises three sets of 25 verbal and 25 spatial items, matched for difficulty and format (*Fig. 19.2*). The VESPAR is designed to reduce the handicap of neurological impairment on reasoning test performance. The stimuli are large and clear to reduce demands on visual acuity. The multiple choice response format allows patients to respond by either speaking or pointing, allowing them to utilize their most efficient output mode. In addition, the test is untimed, which further reduces the penalties some other classical tests may impose, by timing the performance of MS patients with sensorimotor dysfunction. Concomitant cognitive deficits have also been considered. The stimuli are designed to be easily accessible. In addition, the problem and response alternatives are available for the patient's extensive inspection, to reduce both short-term memory load and also the requirement for sustained concentration.

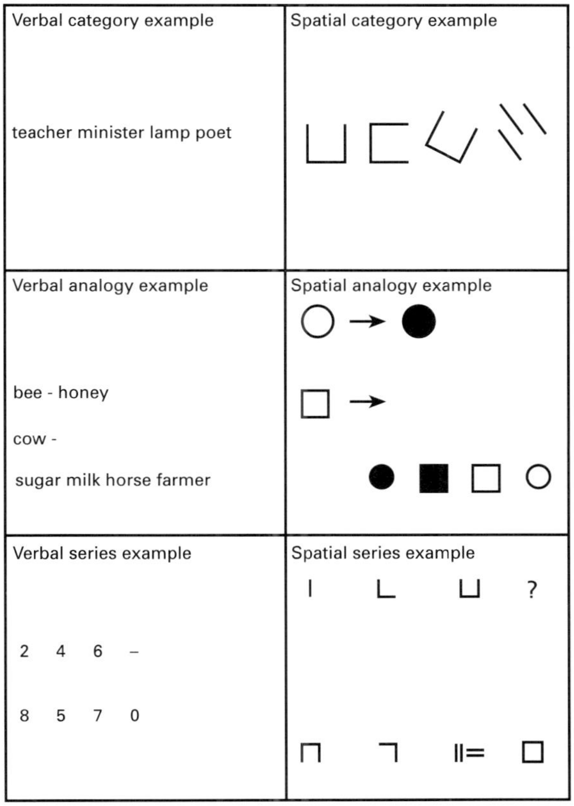

Memory

Memory deficits are a reliable finding in group studies of MS patients, especially when they are required to recall without cues or prompts.

Fig. 19.2
Sample items from each of the six sections of the VESPAR (reproduced with permission from LEA, Hove, Sussex).

For example, in one report, 36 per cent of patients performed at the same level of controls, 43 per cent had mild memory dysfunction and 21 per cent displayed moderate to severe impairment.[37] MS patients have tended to perform at a lower rate than controls[37,38] on the Wechsler Logical Memory test (WMS),[39] although the task demands include attention to, and comprehension of, spoken prose. As such, the WMS is not a pure test of memory function, but rather of a composite of cognitive skills, each of which is essential to task performance but which may be differentially affected by MS.[40] MS patients have also tended to be weaker than controls when learning which word is paired with another, termed paired associate learning.[41] Recognition tests, which provide a cue to remembering by offering stimuli which may or may not have been previously presented, and requiring the patient to distinguish between them, is generally less affected by MS.[37,42] This latter finding has led some to conclude that encoding is less compromised than retrieval in MS.

Little is known about how accurately scores on formal psychometric tests of memory function reflect the patients' own experience. A number of self-report measures are available to investigate the patients' viewpoint. The reports of memory function from MS patients and their relatives have been highly concordant, in terms of the most serious problems identified, the frequency with which failures in learning and memory were said to occur and overall functional level.[43] The patients' age was unrelated to their own and relatives' self-report of memory dysfunction. The reported prevalence of memory impairment in this sample from a national register was 9 per cent according to the patients themselves and 11 per cent according to their relatives.

Attention

Attention is the ability to sustain concentration effectively to complete a task. This may involve sharing or alternating attention between several points of information. Attention deficits, albeit subtle ones, have been reported even at very early stages of the disease, including patients with clinically isolated syndromes.[16] Simple tests of attention with low cognitive demands, such as repeating lists of digits (Digit Span) may not be sufficiently stringent to demonstrate the attention deficits which typically occur in MS.[44] Perhaps the test of attention which is most effective in MS is the Paced Auditory Serial Addition Task (PASAT).[45] This requires the patient to listen to an audio tape of random single digits, presented at one of a variety of constant rates, and to add together the last two numbers they have heard at any one time – a very exacting task.

Language

There have been few detailed studies of language function in MS. Naming and reading have been reported to be mildly affected, whilst spelling and comprehension was intact.[44] Chronic-progressive, but not relapsing–remitting, MS patients have performed below the level of controls on an aphasia test.[7] Linguistic disturbances developed in the course of a longitudinal study.[11] Aphasic syndromes have been associated with left cerebral hemisphere lesions.[46] Any aphasia battery is suitable, but for a quick indication a graded naming test is probably enough.[47]

Visual perception

The assessment of visual perceptual functions in MS is problematic, because of the many peripheral visual impairments which the patients may experience.[48] One perceptual battery which goes some way to minimize acuity and spatial demands, both of which might be affected by peripheral sensorimotor dysfunction, is the Visual Object and Space Perception Battery (VOSP).[49] It achieves this by using large, bold, mainly single stimuli, often in the form of black silhouettes.

Confounding factors

Neurological impairment

The disease process of MS confounds the measurement of cognitive function in several ways.[50] The methodological problems inherent in assessing cognitive function in this context are complex.[4,51] The pathology is diffuse in the cerebral hemispheres, which means that the assessment will be made in the context of physical impairments, which may compromise sensorimotor functions, on which many cognitive tests rely. For example, they can confound a patient's performance on a task which requires them to draw a complex pattern, such as the Rey–Osterreith Test, which was designed to examine visual memory function.[52] Some tests are timed and require manual dexterity to manipulate blocks or arrange small cards, such as the Block Design and Picture Arrangement subtests of the WAIS-R.[26] In addition some tests, such as the Picture Arrangement and Picture Completion subtest of the WAIS-R, require good visual function, which is often reduced by MS.

In addition, there are likely to be coincident cognitive deficits, which may affect the patient's performance on tests of related cognitive functions. For example, attention is often compromised by MS[53] and many cognitive tests rely on a restricted aural presentation of the task description and stimuli, for example the Arithmetic subtest of the WAIS-R. Difficulties in visual perceptual functions and visual spatial processing can alter performance on tests which rely on complex spatial stimuli, such as Raven's Progressive Matrices.[54] The patient is required to examine a complex abstract design from which a small piece is missing and then select the correct design to complete the pattern correctly, from a selection of alternatives.

A further complication in test interpretation is that the formats and content of cognitive tests are not typically matched across the verbal and spatial domains, thus the possibility of systematic bias resulting from test artefacts cannot be excluded. Artefacts which result from the formats of cognitive tests cannot be predicted precisely from any other aspect of the disease. Instead, it is also a source of error in comparisons of scores on several cognitive tests. Group studies of MS patients typically report greater verbal IQ scores than performance IQ scores. The discrepancy is usually ascribed to the reduced sensorimotor functions of the patients, handicapping them in the use of drawings and blocks, which the performance subtests require.[26] However, just as the performance subtests utilize a specific presentation mode, which happens to be visual perceptual and spatial, the verbal subtests have a specific presentation mode, which is the largely aural presentation of verbal material. Similarly, the response mode required by the performance subtests is generally manual, whereas the response mode required by the verbal subtests is speech. Because the formats of the two types of test differ, it is not possible to extricate the cognitive skill level from the effects of presentation and response mode.

The performance subtests of the WAIS-R present more novel problems (which require 'fluid' intelligence), than the verbal subtests, which rely on the application of learnt knowledge and routines (which has been termed 'crystallized' intelligence). MS patients' especial weakness on the performance scale might be the result of physical factors, or of a particular difficulty in fluid intelligence, or some combination of these two variables. This dilemma in interpretation is hard to resolve with conventional psychometric tests.

Fatigue

The role of fatigue in the cognitive function of

MS patients is not yet well understood, although it is an area of increasing interest. Most patients for whom fatigue is a significant problem report that when their fatigue becomes more apparent, they are simultaneously aware of compromised cognition, either as a non-specific decrement (such as 'concentration'), or a more specific problem (such as 'memory'). Self-rated fatigue has been significantly related to reading comprehension, phonemic fluency and anterograde memory in MS, perhaps because these tasks have high attentional demands, which may be specially susceptible to fatigue.[55] Pharmacological agents which treat fatigue have not been shown to improve cognitive function,[56] suggesting that the relationship may be complex. Some studies have compared MS patients with Chronic Fatigue Syndrome (CFS) patients, in an effort to control the effects of fatigue on cognition in MS, although fatigue in the two conditions may not be the same phenomenon. Matched groups of MS patients and CFS patients have performed significantly worse than control subjects on tests of attention, but may not differ significantly from each other.[57,58] However, when MS patients are matched to CFS patients for fatigue severity, the MS patients demonstrate more widespread cognitive deficits and a higher incidence of impairment than the CFS group (60 per cent versus 35 per cent).[59]

Emotion

Although MS patients have been demonstrated to be more depressed than 'matched' controls in group neuropsychological studies, there is generally no correlation between depression scores and memory test scores,[42,60] or reasoning ability,[22,61] or on more general cognitive batteries.[59,62] One study has related depression scores to frontal lobe dysfunction,[63] suggesting that the correlation arose because of the involvement of anatomically close structures. Patients' self-reports of everyday memory dysfunction have been shown to relate to their level of depression and not to their scores on objective memory tests.[64]

Why does it matter?

Although a consensus of clinical opinion acknowledges the impact of cognitive dysfunction, its effect on the everyday life of patients has proved more difficult to measure and investigate than the pure psychometric functions discussed in the first section. The extent of intellectual decline was an important independent predictor of handicap, second only to the Expanded Disability Status Scale (EDSS) score, in a longitudinal study which investigated the performance of everyday activities.[11] MS patients who were impaired on cognitive tests were less likely to be working[48] and also needed more personal assistance than those who were cognitively intact. An estimated 20 per cent of patients in this sample experienced cognitive deficits of sufficient severity to interfere with their employment and family duties.

There is no index or test result which will, by itself and as a rule, tell the clinician whether a patient with MS has a cognitive impairment which will interfere with their everyday function. The first step is to complete a full cognitive assessment, asking the patient and carers if they are aware of any difficulties, and then formally examining each of the cognitive domains outlined in the first section. An estimate of the patient's pre-morbid optimum intellectual level must then be considered, to form an impression of the degree of deterioration, if any, in each cognitive domain. Next, the patients' cognitive performance requirements should be considered in their home, social and employment activities. It is only by individually matching each patient's precise cognitive profile to their everyday functional needs that a clinically useful cognitive assessment can be produced.

Intelligence and reasoning

If a patient has experienced a decline in their intelligence or reasoning skills, they may appear to their relatives to be lethargic and less involved in family affairs. Sometimes this can be misinterpreted as wilful withdrawal from family responsibilities. If a patient is assumed to have deliberately adopted a passive role by a carer who is already feeling stretched by their own responsibilities, a great deal of distress and bitterness can occur. A family counselling session can sometimes be helpful in bringing these issues into the open and improving communication and understanding among family members. The provision of a timetable and the acknowledgement of the need for structure may be helpful in this situation. A deficit in abstract reasoning can lead a patient to have a very poor understanding of the implications of their decisions and actions relating to their future. A sensitive and detailed discussion of the options available, with full review and consideration of the outcomes likely to follow each option may help a patient with MS to become an active and involved member of their management programme.

Memory

Poor memory may not be understood or appreciated by the patient because, almost by definition, they must remember what they have forgotten. At interview, they may be unlikely to volunteer their most difficult or disabling symptom, without a systematic structured interview at the clinic, which addresses each possible area of difficulty in turn. Cues and prompts of a verbal, aural or pictorial nature may help initiate actions which would otherwise not be performed reliably. It is important that a health professional observe the patient actually remembering and performing important actions for their self care and health maintenance, if there is any doubt about the patient's memory function.

Attention

At first glance, good attention may seem a luxury and often the first signs of difficulty are not huge inconveniences, such as having to write down a telephone number as it is said, rather than hold it in the head whilst redialling. But a more severe attentional impairment can have very disabling aspects, for example as conversations can no longer be followed successfully. A woman with MS was found to have sustained a very small and circumscribed cognitive loss. Unfortunately, this impairment was in her attentional skills, which meant that she could no longer work confidently as a betting shop manageress, calculating the odds and payouts effortlessly in her head.

Language

Because language functions are often relatively unaffected in MS, it can be hard for the inexperienced or unwary clinician to become aware of, or address, a serious cognitive difficulty. This is why interviews on their own are not usually sufficient to alert a health care professional to the difficulties which a person with MS may be having.

Visual perception

Although visual perceptual deficits are hard to measure with accuracy and confidence in many MS patients, and they are probably rare, when they do occur they can seriously compromise many everyday activities. This is because locating and recognizing objects is a crucial part of negotiating the physical environment. Manual wheelchair users must compute trajectories to manoeuvre themselves in their chair along corridors, through doors and around corners and effect these trajectories by modulating the pressure and speed which they exert on the wheels. In an electric wheelchair, the trajectories must be effected by a variety of small movements of a joystick. The complexity of these calculations means that the perceptions of the walls and other obstacles must be almost exact, for collisions, reversing and realignment to be avoided. Similarly, any kitchen task requires a myriad of efficient object recognitions and spatial judgements, which a healthy person takes for granted.

Conclusions

Because each patient's experience of cognitive dysfunction in MS is unique and evolving, the clinician involved in this area is forced to adopt a problem-solving approach. A current neuropsychological assessment is often a crucial starting point for successful management of many aspects of some patients' disease. Many patients and their loved ones view cognitive function as fundamental to themselves and their relationships. Working with the patient to understand the dynamic relation of their cognitive status to their personal circumstances is a great challenge, but a worthwhile endeavour.

References

1. Charcot JM. *Lectures on the Disease of the Nervous System Delivered at La Salpetriere*, London: New Sydenham Society 1877.
2. Peyser JM, Rao Sm, LaRocca NG *et al.* Guidelines for neuropsychological research in multiple sclerosis. *Arch Neurol* 1990; **47**: 94–97.
3. Rao SM, Leo GJ, Bernardin L, Unversagt F. Cognitive dysfunction in multiple sclerosis. I. Frequency, patterns and predictions. *Neurol* 1991; **41**: 685–691.
4. Rao SM. Neuropsychology of multiple sclerosis: a critical review. *J Clin Exp Neuropsych* 1986; **8**: 503–542.
5. Rozewicz L, Langdon DW, Davie CA *et al.* Resolution of left hemisphere cognitive dysfunction in multiple sclerosis with magnetic resonance correlates: a case report. *Cog Neuropsychiat* 1996; **1**: 17–25.
6. Beatty WW, Goodkin DE, Hertsgaard D *et al.* Clinical and demographic predictors of cognitive performance in multiple sclerosis: do diagnostic type, disease duration and disability status matter? *Arch Neurol* 1990; **47**: 305–309.
7. Heaton RK, Nelson LM, Thompson DS *et al.* Neuropsychological findings in relapsing–remitting and chronic-progressive multiple sclerosis. *J Consult Clin Psychol* 1985; **53**: 103–110.
8. Rao SM, Glatt S, Hammeke TA *et al.* Chronic-progressive multiple sclerosis: relationship between cerebral ventricular size and neuropsychological impairment. *Arch Neurol* 1985; **42**: 678–682.
9. Rao SM, Hammeke TA, Speech TJ. Wisconsin card sorting test performance in relapsing–remitting and chronic-progressive multiple sclerosis. *J Clin Consult Psychol* 1987; **55**: 263–265.
10. Ivnik RJ. Neuropsychological test performance as a function of the duration of MS-related symptomatology. *J Clin Psychiat* 1978; **39**: 304–307.
11. Amato MP, Ponziani G, Pracucci G *et al.* Cognitive impairment in early-onset multiple sclerosis. Pattern, predictors and impact on everyday life in a 4-year follow up. *Arch Neurol* 1995; **52**: 168–172.
12. Franklin GM, Nelson LM, Filley CM *et al.* Cognitive loss in multiple sclerosis. *Arch Neurol* 1989; **46**: 162–167.
13. Hotopf MH, Pollock S, Lishman WA. An unusual presentation of multiple sclerosis. *Psychol Med* 1994; **24**: 525–528.
14. Medaer R, Nelissen E, Appel B *et al.* Magnetic resonance imaging and cognitive function in multiple sclerosis. *J Neurol* 1987; **235**: 86–89.
15. Franklin GM, Heaton RK, Nelson LM *et al.* Correlation of neuropsychological and MRI findings in chronic-progressive multiple sclerosis. *Neurology* 1988; **38**: 1826–1829.
16. Callanan MM, Logsdail SJ, Ron MA, Warrington EK. Cognitive impairment in patients with clinically isolated lesions of the type seen in multiple sclerosis: a psychometric MRI study. *Brain* 1989; **112**: 361–374.
17. Rao SM, Leo GJ, Haughton VM *et al.* Correlation of magnetic resonance imaging and cognitive functioning in multiple sclerosis. *Neurol* 1989; **39**: 161–166.
18. Anzola GP, Bevilacqua L, Cappa SF *et al.* Neuropsychological assessment in patients with relapsing–remitting multiple sclerosis and mild functional impairment: correlation with magnetic resonance imaging. *J Neurol Neurosurg Psychiatry* 1990; **53**: 142–145.
19. Swirsky-Sacchetti T, Mitchell DR, Seward J *et al.* Neuropsychological and structural brain lesions in multiple sclerosis: a regional analysis. *Neurol* 1992; **42**: 1291–1295.
20. Arnett PA, Rao SM, Bernardin L *et al.* Relationship between frontal lobe lesions and Wisconsin Card Sorting Test performance in patients with multiple sclerosis. *Neurol* 1994; **44**: 420–425.
21. Franklin GM, Nelson LM, Heaton RK *et al.* Clinical perspectives in the identification of cognitive impairment. In: Rao SM, ed. *Neurobehavioral Aspects of Multiple Sclerosis*, New York: Oxford University Press 1990; 161–174.

22. Peyser JM, Edwards KR, Poser CM. Psychological profiles in patients with multiple sclerosis: a preliminary investigation. *Arch Neurol* 1980; **37**: 577–579.

23. Folstein MF, Folstein SE, McHugh PR. Mini-Mental State: a practical method for grading the cognitive state of patients for the physician. *J Psychiat Res* 1975; **12**: 189–198.

24. Sanford ME, Petajan JH. Effects of multiple sclerosis on daily living. In: Rao SM, ed. *Neurobehavioral Aspects of Multiple Sclerosis*, New York: Oxford University Press 1990; 251–265.

25. Rao SM. *A Manual for the Brief Repeatable Battery of Neuropsychological Tests in Multiple Sclerosis*, New York: National Multiple Sclerosis Society 1990.

26. Wechsler D. *Wechsler Adult Intelligence Scale – Revised*, San Antonio, TX: Psychological Corporation 1981.

27. Nelson HE, Willison J. *Restandardisation of the NART Against the WAIS-R*, Windsor: National Federation for Educational Research 1992.

28. Nelson HE, O'Connell, A. Dementia: the estimation of pre-morbid intelligence levels using the new adult reading test. *Cortex* 1978; **14**: 259–267.

29. Paque L, Warrington EK. A longitudinal study of reading ability in patients suffering from dementia. *J Int Neuropsychol Soc* 1995; **1**: 517–524.

30. Maddrey AM, Cullum CM, Weiner MF *et al.* Premorbid intelligence estimation and level of dementia in Alzheimer's disease. *J Int Neuropsychol Soc* 1996; **2**: 551–555.

31. Patterson K, Hodges JR. Deterioration of word meaning: implications for reading. *Neuropsychologia* 1992; **30**: 1025–1040.

32. O'Carroll R. The assessment of pre-morbid ability: a critical review. *Neurocase* 1995; **1**: 83–89.

33. Milner B. Effects of different lesions on card sorting. *Arch Neurol* 1963; **9**: 90–100.

34. Rao SM, Hammeke TA, Speech TJ. Wisconsin card sorting performance in relapsing/remitting and chronic progressive multiple sclerosis. *J Consult Clin Psychol* 1987; **55**: 263–265.

35. Foong J, Rozewicz L, Quaghebeur G *et al.* Executive function in multiple sclerosis: the role of frontal lobe pathology. *Brain* (in press).

36. Langdon DW, Warrington EK. *VESPAR: a Verbal and Spatial Reasoning Test*, Hove, UK: Lawrence Erlbaum 1995.

37. Rao SM, Hammeke TA, McQuillen MP *et al.* Memory disturbance in chronic progressive multiple sclerosis. *Arch Neurol* 1984; **41**: 625–631.

38. Litvan I, Grafman J, Vendrell P *et al.* Multiple memory deficits in patients with multiple sclerosis. *Arch Neurol* 1988; **45**: 607–610.

39. Wechsler D. *Manual for the Wechsler Memory Scale – Revised*, New York: The Psychological Corporation 1987.

40. Rao SM, Grafman J, DiGuilio D *et al.* Memory dysfunction in multiple sclerosis: its relation to working memory, semantic encoding, and implicit learning. *Neuropsych* 1993; **7**: 364–374.

41. Grant I, McDonald WI, Trimble MR *et al.* Deficient learning and memory in the early and middle phases of multiple sclerosis. *J Neurol Neurosurg Psychiatry* 1984; **47**: 250–255.

42. Rao SM, Leo GJ, St Aubin-Faubert P. On the nature of memory disturbance in multiple sclerosis. *J Clin Exp Neuropsychol* 1989; **11**: 699–712.

43. Richardson JTE. Memory impairment in multiple sclerosis: reports of patients and relatives. *Br J Clin Psychol* 1996; **35**: 205–219.

44. Jambor KL. Cognitive functioning in multiple sclerosis. *Br J Psychiat* 1969; **115**: 765–775.

45. Gronwall DMA. Paced auditory serial addition task: a measure of recovery from concussion. *Percep Mot Skills* 1977; **44**: 367–373.

46. Achiron A, Ziv I, Djaldetti R *et al.* Aphasia in multiple sclerosis: clinical and radiologic correlations. *Neurol* 1992; **42**: 2195–2197.

47. McKenna P, Warrington EK. *The Graded Naming Test*, Windsor: NFER, Nelson 1983.

48. Rao SM, Leo GJ, Ellington L *et al.* Cognitive dysfunction in multiple sclerosis: II impact on employment and social functioning. *Neurol* 1991; **41**: 692–696.

49. Warrington EK, James M. *The Visual Object and Space Perception Battery*, Bury St Edmunds: Thames Valley Test Company 1991.

50. Mathews WB, Compston A, Allen IV *et al.* Course and prognosis. In: *MacAlpine's Multi-*

ple Sclerosis, 2nd edn. Edinburgh: Churchill Livingstone 1991, 139–163.

51. Fennell EB, Smith MC. Neuropsychological Assessment. In Rao SM (ed.), *Neurobehavioural Aspects of Multiple Sclerosis*, New York: Oxford University Press 1990, 63–81.

52. Osterreith P. Le test de copie d'une figure complexe. *Arch Psychol* 1944; **30**: 206–356.

53. Kujala P, Portin R, Revonsuo A *et al*. Automatic and controlled information processing in multiple sclerosis. *Brain* 1994; **117**: 1115–1126.

54. Raven JC. *Advanced Progressive Matrices*, London: Lewis 1962.

55. Grossman M, Armstrong C, Onishi K *et al*. Patterns of cognitive impairment in relapsing–remitting and chronic progressive multiple sclerosis. *Neuropsychiat Neuropsychol Behav Neurol* 1994; **7**: 194–210.

56. Krupp LB, Pollina DA. Mechanisms and management of fatigue in progressive neurological disorders. *Curr Op Neurol* 1996; **9**: 456–460.

57. DeLuca J, Johnson SK, Natelson BH. Information processing efficiency in chronic fatigue syndrome and multiple sclerosis. *Arch Neurol* 1993; **50**: 301–304.

58. DeLuca J, Johnson SK, Beldowicz D *et al*. Neuropsychological impairments in chronic fatigue syndrome, multiple sclerosis, and depression. *J Neurol Neurosurg Psychiatry* 1995; **58**: 38–43.

59. Krupp LB, Sliwinski M, Masur DM *et al*. Cognitive functioning and depression in patients with chronic fatigue syndrome and multiple sclerosis. *Arch Neurol* 1994; **51**: 705–710.

60. Grafman J, Rao S, Bernardin L *et al*. Automatic memory processes in patients with multiple sclerosis. *Arch Neurol* 1991; **48**: 1072–1075.

61. DePaulo JR, Folstein MF. Psychiatric disturbances in neurological patients: detection, recognition and hospital course. *Ann Neurol* 1978; **4**: 225–228.

62. Ron MA, Callanan MM, Warrington EK. Cognitive abnormalities in multiple sclerosis: a psychometric and MRI study. *Psychol Med* 1991; **21**: 59–68.

63. Filippi M, Alberoni M, Martinelli V *et al*. Influence of clinical variables on neuropsychological performance in multiple sclerosis. *Eur Neurol* 1994; **34**: 324–328.

64. Fischer JS. Objective memory testing in multiple sclerosis. In: Jensen K, Knudsen L, Stenager E *et al* eds. *Mental Disorders and Cognitive Deficits in Multiple Sclerosis*, London: Libbey 1989, 39–49.

20

Bladder, bowel and sexual dysfunction: recent advances

Robert J Goodwin and Clare J Fowler

Introduction

The complex innervation of the pelvic floor and pelvic viscera from both autonomic and somatic pathways mean that a degree of bladder, bowel and sexual dysfunction is almost universal in multiple sclerosis (MS) patients. The symptoms of detrusor hyper-reflexia – frequency, urgency and urge incontinence, and incomplete bladder emptying – are caused by spinal cord plaques disrupting the bulbospinal pathways from the pontine micturition centre.[1] The sacral origin of the nerve supply (caudal to the lumbosacral innervation of the legs) means that bladder involvement is likely in any patient with lower limb spasticity.[1]

Sexual function in both sexes also involves a complex interaction between different parts of the nervous system, the final pathway again involving the caudal part of the spinal cord. As well as the physical manifestations of erectile dysfunction, for example, psychological considerations must be taken into account when planning management. This is a complex interaction, as cerebral plaques may lead to psychological impairment, while the multiple physical manifestations of the disease will directly affect the psyche.

Effects of MS on bowel functioning will be discussed with reference to specific physical problems as well as the wider issues involved. The neurological pathways involved are less well understood than those controlling the bladder and sexual function. The associated symptoms can be equally, if not more, disabling. A multidisciplinary approach is as important in these problems as in other manifestations of MS.

The bladder

Introduction

Urinary symptoms affect 75–90 per cent of patients with MS. Difficulty with bladder control is as common a problem as is impaired mobility. Indeed, the two problems often go together because both disorders are due to spinal cord disease.[1] The parasympathetic and somatic nerve supply to the bladder and genitalia originate in the sacral cord, which is distal to the lumbosacral somatic supply to the legs so that, neurologically speaking, the bladder is below the legs (*Fig. 20.1*). This means that if there is a demyelinating disease in the spinal cord, for example in the cervical region (as shown by the stippling in the diagram), the nerves to both the legs and the bladder are likely to be affected. Clinically, therefore, as leg weakness and spasticity worsen, the patient's bladder control also deteriorates, making it increasingly difficult to respond to bladder urgency by hurrying to the toilet.

Spinal cord disease is the primary aetiology of detrusor hyper-reflexia.[1] A recent study has also correlated midbrain lesions on MRI scanning of the brain with the deterioration of bladder function in MS,[2] although this study

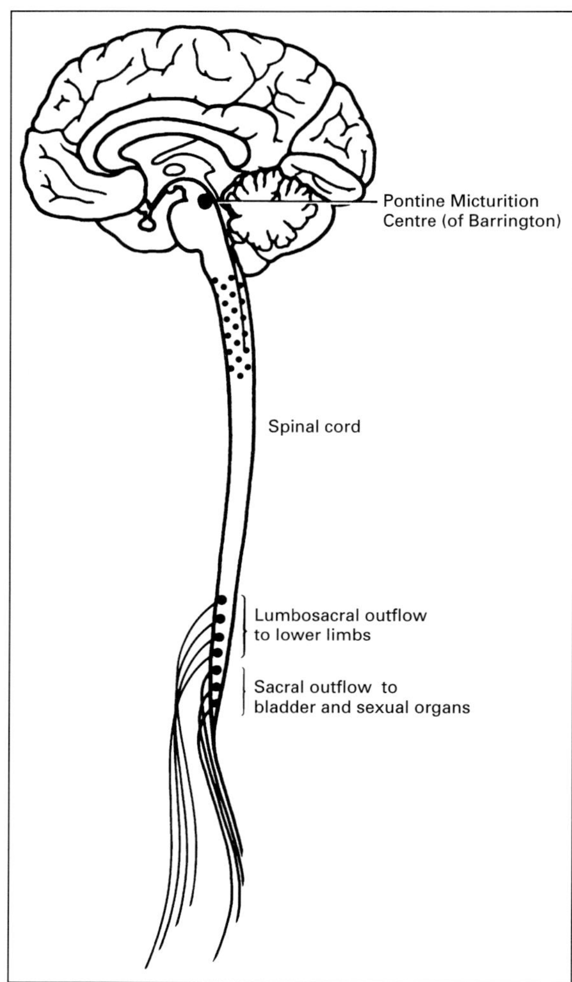

Fig. 20.1
The spinal cord in urogenital manifestations of MS.

did not address coexistent cord disease. Poor bladder control can be very disabling and many patients regard this as one of the worst aspects of their illness. Unpredictable urinary urgency with associated incontinence has an adverse effect on anyone, and many patients with this problem become housebound and unwilling to venture out where access to toilets is uncertain. Fortunately, recent years have seen important advances in the treatment of bladder dysfunction in MS.

Clinical features

History

Urinary urgency is the most common bladder symptom in MS, followed by frequency.[1] Urgency is often accompanied by urge incontinence, which can be very disabling. In addition, patients may have a sensation of incomplete emptying and it has been shown that if a patient feels that they have not emptied to completion, they are usually correct.

However, among those who feel that they have emptied completely, 50 per cent are wrong.[1] Incomplete bladder emptying is due to two problems, both related to spinal cord malfunction. Although the bladder becomes hyper-reflexic due to involvement of the spino-bulbospinal pathways connecting the pontine micturition centre (of Barrington) to the sacral cord, the detrusor contractions which occur are ineffective. In addition, the external (striated) sphincter may contract at the same time as the detrusor (detrusor–sphincter dyssynergia) and a combination of these two factors leads to incomplete bladder emptying.

Patients with MS may also admit on questioning to a poor stream and hesitancy of micturition, although these symptoms are volunteered less frequently than the complaints of frequency, urgency and urge incontinence.

Examination:

- General.
- Urological: pelvic examination should be performed especially if there is any gynaecological or urological history prior to the onset of neurological illness.
- Neurological: it is important to assess the lower limb reflexes, power, tone and

sensation as upper motor neurone signs in the legs may predict detrusor hyper-reflexia.

- Eye movements: internuclear ophthalmoplegia indicating pontine pathology may occur in patients with MS. Betts *et al.* have reported the combination of MS affecting the bladder and eye movements due to the involvement of the pontine micturition centre, without significant spinal cord demyelination.[1] However, it is unusual to have isolated problems with eye movements in the absence of upper motor neurone signs in the legs.

Investigations:

MSU

This investigation is used to exclude and treat urinary tract infections, which are commonly associated with incompletely emptying bladders.

Flow rate and ultrasound residual

This is the most important investigation in patients with MS presenting with urinary symptoms.[3] This investigation is known as an ultrasound cystodynogram (USCD) and involves the patient passing urine into a flow meter, followed by ultrasound scanning of the suprapubic region to measure the post-micturition residual volume. Generally speaking, a residual volume of more than 100 ml is significant and requires different management, as discussed later.

Ultrasound scanning of the bladder demonstrates common abnormalities associated with detrusor hyper-reflexia, including hypertrophy of the bladder wall and formation of diverticula.[4]

Renal ultrasound scanning

Renal ultrasound scanning is not routinely indicated, as it is rare to develop hydronephro-

sis in MS.[5,6] The incidence of upper tract involvement has been reported as 0–6 per cent.[1,7] The reason for this is unknown, because upper tract damage is a recognized hazard following spinal cord injury. It is possible that, despite detrusor hyper-reflexia, the bladder compliance in MS does not become poor enough to cause hydronephrosis. Ultrasound scanning of the kidneys is indicated in those patients with significant hesitancy and in severely disabled patients, especially those with long-term catheters and frequent urinary tract infections; upper tract dilatation in these patients may be as high as 20 per cent.[8]

Cystometry

This is not routinely indicated in patients with MS. Hyper-reflexia can be predicted by history alone, and this may be backed up by simple neurological assessment of the lower limbs. A history of urinary urgency, together with the diagnosis of MS and lower limb spasticity, is diagnostic and proving it by cystometry is unnecessary. It is rare to find detrusor areflexia in MS.[1,9] However, the controversy over this issue still persists, as areflexia has been reported in some series.[10] Taylor *et al.* in 1984 attributed acontractile bladders in MS to conus demyelination, although the claim has not been substantiated since then.[11]

Although cystometry does not form an important diagnostic tool in the routine management of bladder dysfunction, it is invaluable in certain situations; for example, before intravesical capsaicin treatment or before embarking upon any operative procedure such as augmentation cystoplasty.

Neurophysiological studies

These are not routinely indicated because if clinical examination shows evidence of spinal cord deficit, then tibial and pudendal evoked potentials will be abnormal.

Management of bladder dysfunction in MS

Management is directed towards treating detrusor hyper-reflexia and incomplete emptying (*Fig. 20.2*).

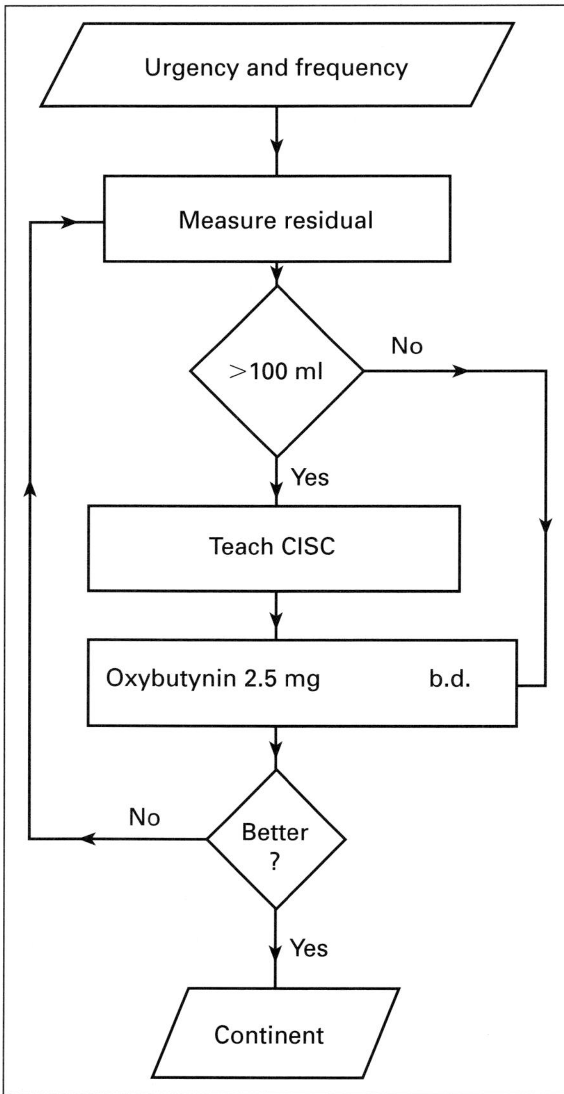

Fig. 20.2
Scheme showing management of bladder dysfunction.

Drugs

Anticholinergics The majority of patients with detrusor hyper-reflexia due to MS respond to oral anticholinergic drugs. The most commonly prescribed is oxybutynin which is commenced at a low dose of 2.5 mg twice daily. Oxybutynin is antimuscarinic and blocks the M3 subtype muscarinic receptor. Although the M3 subtype is not the most common muscarinic receptor, it is pharmacologically the most important in the bladder. Blockade of this receptor prevents the activity of acetylcholine and reduces the contractility of the hyper-reflexic bladder. Similar blockade occurs in other organs, including the salivary glands, and a dry mouth is the side effect most commonly reported. A patient not experiencing this is probably not taking a therapeutic dose. Constipation may be exacerbated and at higher doses blurring of vision may occur; the drug is contraindicated in closed angle glaucoma, which may be recognized clinically by reduced visual acuity, clouding of the cornea, an oval-shaped pupil and raised intraocular pressure. Patients are asked to adjust their medication carefully, adding an extra dose at intervals of some weeks so that their bladders are under control but their mouths are not too dry. The recommended maximum dose of oxybutynin is 5 mg t.d.s. Recent research is being directed towards drugs with higher M3 specificity.

Propantheline also has potent anticholinergic affects. In a controlled trial of oxybutynin versus propantheline, 67 per cent of patients with detrusor hyper-reflexia were shown to have a good response to oxybutynin, while only 36 per cent responded to propantheline. Oxybutynin has also been found to be more effective than propantheline in increasing the cystometric capacity.[12] If oxybutynin is found to be ineffective, the addition of a tricyclic antidepressant drug, such as imipramine, is occasionally found to be helpful.[13]

Desmopressin Desmopressin is an analogue of anti-diuretic hormone (ADH) and reduces urine formation by increased reabsorbtion of water at the collecting tubule of the kidney. It is particularly useful for treating troublesome nocturia in MS and is administered as a nasal spray. However, some authors recommend that serum sodium levels are monitored in these patients as there is a risk of hyponatraemia,[14] although other studies point to its safety;[15] it should be used with extreme caution in patients with significant renal or cardiovascular disease, and should generally not be used in the elderly.

Intrathecal Baclofen Although this is mainly used to treat spasticity, it has been found to be useful in some patients for improving bladder control.[16]

Alpha blockers These are primarily tried to improve bladder emptying[17] but their efficacy in MS has never been conclusively demonstrated.

Intravesical capsaicin Capsaicin is a neurotoxin derived from red chilli peppers and is particularly useful in patients who fail to tolerate the side effects of anticholinergics. Original experiments on rat bladder suggested that visceral pain could be induced by stimulation of C-afferent fibres via the vanilloid receptor.[18] In the human bladder, however, the vanilloid receptor has not been isolated and it is hypothesized that capsaicin modifies the density of C-fibres in the suburothelial layer directly.[19,20] Capsaicin proved efficaceous in treating painful bladders in humans at a dose of 0.1–10 μM. Following this, capsaicin at the same dose was tried in hyper-reflexia; the rationale for this came from de Groat's observations on spinal cats.[21] Following spinal injury, the afferent side of the micturition reflex appears to become mediated by C-fibres rather than the Aδ-fibres of intact animals. Furthermore, Aδ-fibres carrying the normal afferent supply are insensitive to capsaicin. Capsaicin, at the same dose as was effective in hypersensitive bladders, gives disappointing results in hyper-reflexia, and much higher doses are needed. To achieve this, the capsaicin must be used in solutions of 30–40 per cent alcohol, but controlled experiments indicate that the therapeutic benefit is not mediated by the alcohol.[22] Used at a dose of 1–2 mM it has been found to increase the bladder capacity and decrease hyper-reflexia, thus improving continence in patients with MS.[23,24] The effect of a single instillation of capsaicin lasts for an average of 3–4 months, after which it needs to be repeated. Side effects of burning and acute hyper-reflexic contractions during instillation may be ameliorated by prior instillation of lignocaine solution; initially, symptoms are worsened and many patients opt to use an indwelling catheter for the first ten days after instillation. Despite these drawbacks, the benefits mean that patients are willing to return for multiple instillations. The long-term safety and efficacy of capsaicin is still being evaluated. The use of intravesical capsaicin has generated worldwide interest as a useful treatment in intractable cases of detrusor hyper-reflexia.[25,26]

Alternative treatments A variety of other treatments have been reported; at best they are usually thought of as supplemental to mainstream treatments. For example, hyperbaric oxygen at 2 atmospheres is claimed by some authors to improve bladder symptoms in MS. The reports, however, are conflicting and it is therefore not established as a treatment modality. Improved bladder control has been reported by Zannini *et al.*[27] and Meneghetti *et al.*[28] but, equally, lack of beneficial effect has been reported by Barnes *et al.*,[29] Confavreux *et al.*[30] and Kindwall *et al.*[31]

Marijuana has a wide variety of pharmacological effects and has been claimed to have a beneficial effect on the bladder over and above the general feeling of well being it imparts.[32] However, no controlled therapeutic trial has been carried out. Active substances such as delta-9-tetrahydrocannabinol (9-THC) reduce spasticity and may improve the symptoms of hyper-reflexia, possibly by an anticholinergic mechanism.[33]

Clean Intermittent Self Catheterization (CISC)

Patients with significant post-micturition residual urine (>100 ml) need some means of emptying their bladder and CISC, in combination with anticholinergics, is an effective way of treating incomplete emptying. Anticholinergics are likely to lessen the ability of the bladder to contract and thereby worsen the already impaired ability to empty. The way around this is to deal with the problem of incomplete emptying first.

CISC was introduced by Lapides in 1972 and if a patient has the ability to write and feed himself then they are likely to have sufficient dexterity to perform CISC.[34] Leg spasms can make it particularly difficult to abduct the thighs and can prevent effective CISC. Visual impairment in either sex, however, does not seem to be a bar, provided that the patient is motivated and taught properly how to do it. A number of patients who are unable to catheterize themselves can have it performed by a carer. Most patients are recommended to catheterize 2–3 times daily, particularly last thing at night to minimize the symptom of nocturia.

Vibration

The use of a suprapubic vibrating stimulus to improve bladder emptying was first described by Nathan in 1977 at Queen Square, London.[35] A recent study of the technique has been conducted recently at the same hospital.

The stimulator, which is a hand-held, battery-operated, vibrating device, has been found to be effective in up to 80 per cent of patients with MS whose Kurtzke Pyramidal Function Scores are 3 or less and who are able to feel the vibrating stimulus in the suprapubic region. An improvement in flow and a reduction in residual volume are both seen, although complete emptying is rarely achieved.[36] There has been some debate about the mechanism of action, and whether this is a modification of 'tapping' used by patients with spinal injuries to provoke reflex voiding.[37] The technique appears to differ from tapping in that it does not appear to be a direct reflex: vibration does not work unless the patient perceives the stimulus, and blockade of local cutaneous afferent nerves abolishes its effect.[36] Vibration is a cheap, effective and non-invasive alternative to ISC for some patients with relatively mild neurological disability.

Long-term catheters and continence appliances

These usually become necessary in patients who have become severely disabled and who are unable to empty their bladders either by CISC or vibration. When long-term indwelling catheterization is planned, a suprapubic catheter is more comfortable than a urethral catheter and is easier to change. This should be done every 6–12 weeks, depending upon the patient's tendency to block their catheter. There are many problems associated with long-term indwelling catheters. Within a few days, a heavy bacterial growth will be associated with the catheter, even if meticulous aseptic conditions were used at the time of insertion. A commensal bacterial growth does not require antibiotics, but systemic symptoms such as fever and malaise, and local symptoms such as pain, may require a course of antibiotics and a change of catheter. Around 10 per cent of patients have a particular tendency to block and encrust their catheters, requiring more frequent changes; if the bladder is colonized by urease-producing organisms such as Proteus – which may occur after repeated courses of antibiotics – the urine will consequently be more alkaline and prone to stone formation. Long-term urethral catheterization may cause significant erosion of the distal urethra, which may be unsightly and painful and it may make it harder to change the catheter. The presence of a catheter in the urethra may cause it to dilate and the resultant patulous urethra may be unable to hold a catheter even with an extra large balloon. When this occurs the patient is invariably wet and surgical intervention (siting a suprapubic catheter and closure of the bladder neck) becomes necessary. For this reason, long-term indwelling catheterization is best via the suprapubic route from the outset in both sexes.

Patients can remain sexually active with long-term catheterization; a urethral catheter in a man can be doubled back and secured with a condom if necessary, or pulled upwards and out of the way in women. There are multiple factors affecting sexuality in the disabled; these will be discussed later.

Surgical operations and endourethral prostheses

Generally, operations for bladder management in MS are rarely indicated because most patients have progressive neurological disease, and bladder reconstruction, which often needs revision, is unsuitable for these patients. A clam ileocystoplasty may occasionally be indicated in a generally fit patient with a small capacity severely hyper-reflexic bladder which has failed to respond to primary medical treatment and CISC.[38] Before embarking upon this procedure it is important to make sure that the patient is able to perform CISC as 30–40 per

cent of patients will have incomplete bladder emptying after the operation. This is also one of the few indications for performing videocystometry in a patient with MS.

Persistent leakage around an indwelling catheter usually responds to simple measures, such as changing the catheter or adding anticholinergic medication, but very occasionally operative bladder neck closure with an indwelling suprapubic catheter may be indicated. Endourethral prostheses have been used for sphincter dyssynergia[39] but, again, their practical usefulness is limited to a very few patients in whom this isolated symptom is a primary problem.

Other treatments

Bladder training This has the advantage of avoiding urinary tract infections but requires a motivated patient since it involves timed voiding. Studies have reported that ultrasound-controlled bladder training can significantly reduce post-micturition volumes.[40] A more recent study has shown that bladder training in combination with CISC can be effective in the management of urinary symptoms in MS.[41] The authors' experience is that bladder training alone is seldom enough to significantly improve symptoms.

Aerobic training This has been reported by Petajan *et al.*[42] It is obvious that since leg spasticity is closely related to bladder dysfunction, improvement in mobility can indirectly be related to improvement in bladder control.

Electrical stimulation This was very fashionable in the 1970s and 1980s and various means of stimulation were reported. However, the efficacy of these can only be evaluated by controlled studies in centres equipped to treat patients with these modalities; such studies are lacking and electrical stimulation is not widely used, largely due to the lack of good evidence for its usefulness. Reported techniques include:

- intravaginal stimulation[43]
- PISCES (percutaneously inserted spinal cord electrical stimulation)[44]
- SES (spinal electrostimulation) 1988.[45–47] A 50–70 per cent effectiveness has been reported, but the response has not been found to be durable
- DSCS (Dorsal Spinal Cord Stimulation) – this is thought to work by alteration of neuropeptides and enkephalins. Several studies quote its usefulness.[48,49] Equally, however, there are studies reporting the opposite[50]
- ESES (Epidural Spinal Electrostimulation)[51,52]
- TENS (transcutaneous electrical nerve stimulation)[53]

Magnetic stimulation Single external application of low magnetic fields to the brain has been reported to be effective in bladder control in MS in up to 70 per cent of patients.[54] The mechanism of action remains unknown but it is possibly mediated by the pineal gland which releases melotonin and affects monoamine release.

Nerve blocks and neurectomies Responses to sacral blocks and neurectomies are variable and should only be carried out in a controlled setting.[55–57]

Summary

The importance of testing the reflexes and sensation in the lower limbs in a patient with MS presenting with urinary symptoms in order to establish the correct neurological basis, cannot be overemphasized. The most useful investigation is urinary flow rate followed by ultrasound estimation of post-micturition residual urine. In those patients with residuals >100 ml bladder emptying can be improved by the use of CISC or possibly suprapubic vibration. This can then be followed by oral anticholinergic medication to treat detrusor hyper-reflexia. If the post-void residual is less than 100 ml then oral anticholinergics alone are usually sufficient. The addition of Desmospray has been shown to be beneficial in patients with troublesome nocturia.[14]

It is now largely agreed that medical management should be instituted as first-line therapy to improve bladder symptoms in patients with MS[7,58] and the majority of patients respond to these simple measures. However, for some unfortunate patients these measures fail and something more is then needed. There are two categories of such patients: those who are generally very incapacitated, and those who, although not very severely disabled, have bladders which are so overactive that they have no storage capacity despite high doses of anticholinergic medication. In the former group of patients, an indwelling catheter becomes necessary and, in the latter, intravesical capsaicin is found to be useful. The debate over other treatment options such as hyperbaric oxygen, electrical and magnetic stimulation, sacral blocks and neurectomies and augmentation cystoplasty continues. Such treatment modalities are largely performed in a few specialized centres. Operative management is restricted to a few carefully selected patients who are not severely disabled.

Bowel problems in MS
Introduction

Bowel problems are very prevalent in MS, with 53 per cent of patients complaining of constipation,[59] while a larger study of 280 patients quoted that between 25 per cent (in the previous week) and 51 per cent (over three months) of patients had some faecal incontinence, 43 per cent had constipation and overall 68 per cent had some degree of bowel symptoms.[60,61] Chia reported that 52 per cent of patients with urinary symptoms in MS also had bowel symptoms.[62]

The neuroanatomical basis for bowel symptoms is less clear than that for the bladder. The central role of the spinal cord in bladder control is well known and in MS it is primarily spinal cord involvement which accounts for detrusor hyper-reflexia.[1] However, cord involvement does not seem to be the primary mechanism for bowel dysfunction since up to 32 per cent of patients with significant bladder symptoms and spinal cord disease reported no bowel symptoms at all.[62] A number of factors seem to contribute to bowel symptoms, including slow colonic transit times, pelvic floor spasticity, and poor perineal sensation. While bladder functioning is under continuous neural control (both for filling and voiding), the bowel smooth muscle is able to function when completely stripped of its central efferent nerve supply due to its intramural plexi; however, the somatic pathways for control of defaecation are commonly affected.

Clinical features

The principal symptoms are constipation and faecal incontinence. Slow colonic transit time has been demonstrated in MS patients[62–64] and contributory factors include poor mobility, anticholinergic drugs (used to treat bladder symptoms) and voluntary fluid restriction (again to minimize urinary incontinence). It has been hypothesized that vagal tone is deficient in these patients due to central MS involvement and that this contributes to constipation, but many patients without significant neurological features complain of severe constipation.[65] Another hypothesis is that this is a generalized phenomenon similar to that of fatiguability in MS, which also has no basis in terms of specific neuroanatomy.

Patients with more advanced disability often have difficulty commencing voluntary defaecation. Normally a complex series of neurologically mediated actions is initiated by rectal filling. When this occurs, and if it is judged appropriate to do so, defaecation is commenced by bearing down, causing pelvic floor descent. The internal anal sphincter pressure falls due to the rectoanal inhibitory reflex, and pubococcygeus and the external (striated) sphincter relax. The former relaxes the angle subtended by pubococcygeus, and the combination of events leads to the expulsion of faeces and rectal emptying. Significant pubococcygeal spasticity in advanced disease has been described by Gill *et al.* in a series of 11 patients, and some of these patients habitually required insertion of a digit (to pull the pubococcygeal impression on defaecating proctography) to allow sufficient effacement to occur for evacuation. Straining against a spastic pelvic floor may cause rectal intussusception, contribution to severe symptoms in 3 out of 11 patients.[66] Intussusception is a troublesome rectal mucosal prolapse leading to a continuous urge to defaecate and compounding the problem of prolonged straining.

Faecal incontinence is a function of three processes: failure of co-ordinated sphincter control characterized by weak sphincter squeeze pressures; concomitant constipation leading to rectal overloading and overflow; and diminished perineal and rectal sensation.[67] In addition, the presence of an underlying weakness (such as that caused by obstetric damage to the sphincters) may compound the problem.[68] In the presence of signifcant spinal cord disease, the rectoanal inhibitory reflex (a local intramural pathway) remains intact: thus, a patient whose rectum is full may have involuntary sphincter relaxation leading to incontinence, without the perception of fullness reaching the brain.[69] A chronically distended rectum will have a reduced compliance and be more subject to this reflex. Faecal incontinence is usually associated with constipation and patients who have incontinence without constipation should undergo more vigorous investigation of the lower bowel, for example with anal sphincter manometry.

Investigation

Detailed investigation of bowel symptoms is usually confined to specialist centres. Colonic transit times can be assessed by swallowing radiographic markers and a subsequent series of X-ray films.

Manometric studies of the sphincter and rectal contractions are used to investigate troublesome incontinence.

The most valuable investigation is defaecating proctography, which is performed by introducing radio-opaque barium paste into the rectum, and then observing defaecation by lateral X-ray screening. The pelvic floor and sphincter function can be assessed, with visualization of the effacement of pubococcygeus required for normal defaecation. This investigation will also identify intussusception.

Management

General measures have usually been taken before the patient sees a specialist. Stool softeners and bulking agents in combination with stimulant laxatives will improve symptoms caused by slow transit times. Increased fluid intake should be encouraged, and if necessary bladder symptoms treated to enable this. If these measures are inadequate, regular enemata may be required; this may help to reduce incontinence later in the day.

Specific problems such as intussusception may be surgically corrected although, again, patients with advanced disease and disability are poor candidates for major intervention. A recent series of patients using suprapubic vibration to treat incomplete bladder emptying in MS suggested that a significant number of them also noticed an improvement in symptoms of constipation;[36] further work on this and other treatments is required.

Conclusion

Bowel problems in MS – constipation, incontinence and difficulty in defaecating – are common. Such symptoms are not generally the primary interest of neurologists who may be somewhat dismissive of these problems, but an understanding of the common pathology is required. Beyond bulking agents, stimulant laxatives and enemata there is little specific treatment available to treat these problems. Vigorous investigation and surgical treatment should be reserved for patients whose bowel symptoms are disproportionate to the other clinical features of the progression of their MS or when a correctable cause, such as intussusception, may be identified and treated.

Sexual problems in MS
Introduction

Normal sexual function involves a complex series of neurologically controlled events, the final pathways involving the most caudal part of the spinal cord (as with the bladder). The multiplicity of dimensions of sexuality means that the majority of MS patients suffer from impaired sexual function: up to 75 per cent of men and 56 per cent of women.[70,71]

The physiological responses to sexual arousal are mediated by the limbic system and hypothalamus, with efferent and afferent activity in both the somatic and autonomic nervous system. The spinal cord carries this activity and thus sexual problems appear early in spinal cord disease.

Clinical features

Erectile dysfunction (impotence) is inadequate penile erection to achieve intercourse and is the most common complaint of male patients. The physiological sequelae of sexual arousal are similar in both sexes, but erectile dysfunction has a more profound effect than the equivalent in the female (increased vaginal engorement and lubrication), a failure of which can be overcome by a simple water-based lubricant such as KY Jelly™. Other problems presenting include reduced libido, impaired sensation or hypersensitivity (hyper-aesthesia), ejaculatory failure and infertility. Premature ejaculation is seen with the same incidence as in the normal population, and can be treated with clomipramine or (more recently) with fluoxetine.[72] Women may also suffer from vaginismus, and leg spasticity may lead to difficulty abducting the thighs. Incontinence even of small volumes of urine is upsetting and inhibits most people; rises in intra-abdominal pressure associated with intercourse may cause this. Ataxia and weakness make intercourse more difficult to achieve. The presence of an indwelling catheter may be physically and psychologically intrusive.

Plaque formation in the central nervous system (CNS) may affect libido directly. Antispasmodic, anticholinergic and antidepressant medication also influence this, and the inability to successfully arouse and achieve the plateau phase makes it virtually impossible to achieve orgasm. Psychological factors in chronic illness may contribute to a major extent to loss of libido.

Examination and investigation

There are few specific investigations required in assessing erectile dysfunction in MS. For the same reasons as with the bladder – the sacral parasympathetic and somatic outflow to the genitalia being neurologically below the legs – the cause of erectile dysfunction in MS is neurological and again correlates with leg spasticity due to spinal cord disease. Neurological assessment of the lower limbs should always therefore be performed. In patients with diminished libido, it is worth checking for endocrine failure, although this is more likely to be psychological and/or a manifestation of CNS involvement. Vasculogenic erectile dysfunction may be suspected in older patients especially if there is a history of vascular disease or evidence of reduced peripheral pulses on examination; this can be clinically evaluated by assessing the response to a small dose of an injected intracavernosal vasodilator. More complex vascular studies by cavernosography or duplex Doppler scanning are not generally useful: identifying a vascular deficit seldom leads to successful surgical intervention even in neurologically normal men.

Management of erectile dysfunction

For penile erection to occur, there must be adequate vascular inflow to the penile arteries. Arterioles in the corpora cavernosa undergo vasodilatation in response to parasympathetic activity mediated by cholinergic muscarinic receptors. In MS, the parasympathetic supply from the sacral cord via the pudendal nerves is interrupted by plaques within the cord, leading to loss of erectile ability. The most effective methods of treating this neurogenic erectile dysfunction are therefore locally acting vasodilators. While the sympathetic (adrenergic) innervation is not the primary mechanism of vasodilatation, sympathomimetic agents can be used to achieve tumescence by blockade of alpha-1 receptor activity.

Vacuum pumps

These devices are widely used and have the principal advantage that they are relatively non-invasive.[73] A vacuum chamber is placed around the penis, which engorges with mainly venous blood; this is maintained with a tourniquet at the base of the penis. However, the arterial fill of the sinusoids of the corpora cavernosa which occurs in normal erection does not occur, so the tumescence produced is more flaccid, cooler, and is confined to the distal part beyond the tourniquet. Petechiae and bruising often occur and the tourniquet should be removed within 30 minutes.

Drugs

Oral drugs There is unfortunately no single oral agent with specific activity to improve impotence. Yohimbine is a derivative of the bark of the yohimbine tree; although prescribable by specialists, it is not licensed for general usage in the UK. It is thought to improve erectile and ejaculatory ability by central pharmacological activity (adrenergic α-2 blockade); its principal peripheral effect is as a sympathetic α-1 agonist, which is paradoxically anti-erectile. Placebo-controlled trials have shown a slight benefit in men without an obvious physical cause for their erectile dysfunction.[74] However, the majority of impotent men with MS do have an obvious physical cause for it and therefore yohimbine has little benefit in MS in general, although it may be used on a 'nothing-to-lose' basis, for men unable to contemplate intracavernosal self injection, for early MS sufferers with primarily psychogenic aetiology, and for those patients with delayed ejaculation. Yohimbine may raise systemic blood pressure, and give side effects including dizziness and nausea. A dose of 10 mg is usually taken 1–2 hours before anticipated sex; the dose is titrated according to response and side effects, usually starting at 10 mg up to three times daily or as required.

Tradozone, a 5-HT antagonist, has recently been reported as being useful both alone and in combination with yohimbine.[75] *Clomipramine*, a tricyclic antidepressant, and more recently *fluoxetine*, may be used in ejaculatory dysfunction.[72,76]

Silfenadil, a phosphodiesterase inhibitor, has recently been reported as useful in general impotence.[77] Its use in MS has yet to be determined. Its pharmacological activity is directed towards blockade of type V phosphodiesterase, which breaks down intracellular second messengers cAMP and cGMP from the beta-adrenergic receptor-mediated G protein and nitric oxide pathways in corporeal arteriolar smooth muscle; this causes arteriolar smooth muscle relaxation and hence improved erection.

Topical drugs Topical *nitroglycerine* has been shown to improve erections but systemic absorption may lead to side effects including headache also affecting the partner, so that a condom is required to prevent this happening.[78] *Minoxidil* improves local blood flow, but has not been proved to have significant beneficial effects.[79] *Alprostadil* and *papaverine* – locally active vasodilatory drugs commonly used as injections – have been tried in topical and intraurethral formulations with limited success.[80,81]

Intracavernosal self injection The best way to achieve reliable and specific vasoactivity is to inject a drug directly into the corpus cavernosum. This will lead to the cascade of vascular events which result in successful erection – increased arteriolar inflow, closure of the emissary vein shunts and areteriolar fill of the sinusoids of the spongy erectile tissue. Adrenergic blocking agents such as *papaverine* and *phentolamine* have been used successfully for a number of years.[82] More recently, prostaglandin E2 derivatives (*alprostadil*) have been licensed and appear to be both safe and efficacious.[83] Drugs thought to act by nitric oxide donation such as *linsidomine* *chlorhydrate* have been used intracavernosally, but no benefit over PGE1 has been demonstrated in a controlled trial.[84]

The benefits of intracavernosal pharmacotherapy include a physiological erection which can be reliably induced, but there are several drawbacks. The injections are uncomfortable and may sting, and bruising at the injection site can occur. Some patients find it unacceptably invasive, and it requires reasonable manual dexterity, which may be a problem in men with MS. Acute priapism (hypersustained and painful erection) can develop, requiring hospital attention, aspiration of the corpora and pharmacological reversal to prevent irreversible corporal fibrosis. Patients should be warned in detail of this potential complication and exercise caution in dosage; for example, if an injection has not been effective, a second dose should not be given. Fibrous plaques of scar may develop in the corpora adjacent to the site of injection, and this complication seems more closely correlated to the injected dose than to the duration of injecting. Discontinuation of the injections usually leads to partial resolution of fibrosis. For these reasons injections should not be used more than twice weekly. Despite these disadvantages, intracavernosal injection therapy remains the treatment of choice for neurogenic erectile dysfunction. Injected pharmacotherapy has no significant effect on sensation or ejaculation, which are mediated by other pathways.

Operative implants

Malleable or deflatable prostheses may be implanted within the corpora to give a mechanically induced stiffness of the penis to allow intercourse. Adequately counselled patients in whom other methods have failed have a high rate of satisfaction with such operations. However, implants are rarely offered in neurogenic impotence because the numbness associated with MS leads to an unacceptably high rate of erosion and infection.

Management of other sexual problems

Anorgasmia is difficult to treat; yohimbine and clomipramine have been reported to have some use. Ejaculatory failure leading to infertility can be managed by a vibrating electro-stimulator, inducing reflex ejaculation, although the quality of sperm obtained in this way is often poor.[85,86]

Conclusion

Again, problem-orientated specialist treatment is required to treat the physical aspects of MS affecting sexual dysfunction. The coexistence of urinary symptoms and erectile dysfunction in many young men with MS makes the input of the uroneurologist central to the well-being of these patients. Unfortunately there is much less that can be done for sexual dysfunction in women. New methods of treatment require further appraisal and controlled trials within this group of patients.

References

1. Betts CD, D'Mellow MT, Fowler CJ. Urinary symptoms and the neurological features of bladder dysfunction in multiple sclerosis. *J Neurol Neurosurg Psychiatry* 1993; **56:** 245–250.
2. Grasso MG, Pozzilli C, Anzini A *et al.* Relationship between bladder dysfunction and brain MRI in multiple sclerosis. *Funct Neurol* 1991; **6:** 289–292.
3. Fowler CJ. Investigation of the neurogenic bladder. *J Neurol Neurosurg Psychiatry* 1996; **60:** 6–13.
4. Smith RB, Kettlewell MG. Rupture of a bladder diverticulum in multiple sclerosis. *Br J Urol* 1976; **48:** 382.
5. Kasabian NG, Krause I, Brown WE *et al.* Fate of the upper urinary tract in multiple sclerosis. *Neurourol Urodyn* 1995; **14:** 81–85.
6. Koldewijn EL, Hommes OR, Lemmens WA *et al.* Relationship between lower urinary tract abnormalities and disease-related parameters in multiple sclerosis. *J Urol* 1995; **154:** 169–173.
7. Sirls LT, Zimmern PE, Leach GE. Role of limited evaluation and aggressive medical management in multiple sclerosis: a review of 113 patients. *J Urol* 1994; **151:** 946–950.
8. Sliwa JA, Bell HK, Mason KD *et al.* Upper urinary tract abnormalities in multiple sclerosis patients with urinary symptoms. *Arch Phys Med Rehabil* 1996; **77:** 247–251.
9. Philp T, Read DJ, Higson RH. The urodynamic characteristics of multiple sclerosis. *Br J Urol* 1981; **53:** 672–675.
10. Blaivas JG, Bhimani G, Labib KB. Vesicourethral dysfunction in multiple sclerosis. *J Urol* 1979; **122:** 342–347.
11. Taylor MC, Bradley WE, Bhatia N *et al.* The conus demyelination syndrome in multiple sclerosis. *Acta Neurol Scand* 1984; **69:** 80–89.
12. Gajewski JB, Awad SA. Oxybutynin versus propantheline in patients with multiple sclerosis and detrusor hyperreflexia. *J Urol* 1986; **135:** 966–968.
13. Rabey JM, Moriel EZ, Farkas A *et al.* Detrusor hyperreflexia in multiple sclerosis. Alleviation by a combination of imipramine and propantheline, a clinico-laboratory study. *Eur Neurol* 1979; **18:** 33–37.
14. Eckford SD, Carter PG, Jackson SR *et al.* An open, in-patient incremental safety and efficacy study of desmopressin in women with multiple sclerosis and nocturia. *Br J Urol* 1995; **76:** 459–463.
15. Kinn AC, Larsson PO. Desmopressin: a new principle for symptomatic treatment of urgency and incontinence in patients with multiple sclerosis. *Scand J Urol Nephrol* 1990; **24:** 109–112.
16. Broseta J, Morales F, Garcia March G *et al.* Use of intrathecal baclofen administered by programmable infusion pumps in resistent spasticity. *Acta Neurochir (Suppl Wien)* 1989; **46:** 39–45.
17. Nordling J. Alpha-blockers and urethral pressure in neurological patients. *Urol Int* 1978; **33:** 304–309.
18. Maggi CA, Abelli L, Giuliani S *et al.* The contribution of sensory nerves to xylene-induced cystitis in rats. *Neuroscience* 1988; **26:** 709–723.
19. Dixon JS, Gilpin CJ. Presumptive sensory axons of the human urinary bladder: a fine structural study. *J Anat* 1987; **151:** 199–207.
20. Dasgupta P, Chandiramani VA, Fowler CJ. Intravesical capsaicin: its effect on nerve densities in the human bladder. *Neurourol Urodyn* 1996; **15:** 373–374.
21. Guimares M, Silva C, Cruz F *et al.* Intravesical capsaicin facilitates storage of urine in hyperactive and hypersensitive bladders. *Eur Urol* 1996; **30** (suppl 2): 237.
22. Chandiramani VA, Peterson T, Duthie GS *et al.* Urodynamic changes during therapeutic intravesical instillations of capsaicin. *Br J Urol* 1996; **77:** 792–797.
23. Fowler CJ, van Kerrebroeck PE, Nordenbo A *et al.* Treatment of lower urinary tract dysfunc-

tion in patients with multiple sclerosis. Committee of the European Study Group of SUDIMS (Sexual and Urological Disorders in Multiple Sclerosis). *J Neurol Neurosurg Psychiatry* 1992; **55**: 986–989.

24. Fowler CJ, Beck RO, Gerrard S *et al*. Intravesical capsaicin for the treatment of detrusor hyperreflexia. *J Neurol Neurosurg Psychiatry* 1994; **57**: 169–173.

25. De Ridder D, Van Poppel H, Baert L. Intravesical capsaicin as a treatment for detrusor hyperreflexia in multiple sclerosis: results in 41 patients. *Neurourol Urodyn* 1996; **15**: 376–377.

26. de Groat WC, Kawatani M, Hisamitsu T *et al*. Mechanisms underlying the recovery of urinary bladder function following spinal cord injury. *J Auton Nerv Syst* 1990; **30** (suppl): S71–S78.

27. Zannini D, Formai C, Bogetti B *et al*. [40 cases of multiple sclerosis treated with hyperbaric oxygen therapy.] Osservazioni su 40 casi di sclerosi multipla trattati con ossigenoterapia iperbarica. *Minerva Med* 1982; **73**: 2939–2945.

28. Meneghetti G, Sparta S, Rusca F *et al*. Hyperbaric oxygen therapy in the treatment of multiple sclerosis. A clinical and electrophysiological study in a 2 year follow-up. *Riv Neurol* 1990; **60**: 67–71.

29. Barnes MP, Bates D, Cartlidge NE *et al*. Hyperbaric oxygen and multiple sclerosis: final results of a placebo-controlled, double-blind trial. *J Neurol Neurosurg Psychiatry* 1987; **50**: 1402–1406.

30. Confavreux C, Mathieu C, Chacornac R *et al*. [Ineffectiveness of hyperbaric oxygen therapy in multiple sclerosis. A randomized placebo-controlled double-blind study.] Inefficacite de l'oxygenotherapie hyperbare dans la sclerose en plaques. Essai randomise controle par placebo en double aveugle. *Presse Med* 1986; **15**: 1319–1322.

31. Kindwall EP, McQuillen MP, Khatri BO *et al*. Treatment of multiple sclerosis with hyperbaric oxygen. Results of a national registry. *Arch Neurol* 1991; **48**: 195–199.

32. Greenberg HS, Werness SA, Pugh JE *et al*. Short-term effects of smoking marijuana on balance in patients with multiple sclerosis and normal volunteers. *Clin Pharmacol Ther* 1994; **55**: 324–328.

33. Ungerleider JT, Andyrsiak T, Fairbanks L *et al*. Delta-9-THC in the treatment of spasticity associated with multiple sclerosis. *Adv Alcohol Subst Abuse* 1987; **7**: 39–50.

34. Lapides J, Diokno AC, Silber SJ *et al*. Clean, intermittent self-catheterization in the treatment of urinary tract disease. *J Urol* 1972; **107**: 458–461.

35. Nathan P. Emptying the paralysed bladder [letter]. *Lancet* 1977; **1**(8007): 377.

36. Dasgupta P, Haslam C, Goodwin RJ *et al*. The "Queen Square bladder stimulator": a device for assisting emptying of the neurogenic bladder. *Br J Urol* 1997 (in press).

37. Dimitrijevic MR, Spencer WA, Trontelj JV *et al*. Reflex effects of vibration in patients with spinal cord lesions. *Neurology* 1977; **27**: 1078–1086.

38. Shah J, Dasgupta P, Selim A. A twelve year experience with "clam" ileocystoplasty: a safe and successful procedure. [Abstract]. *Eur Urol* 1996; **30** (suppl 2): 769.

39. Joseph AC, Juma S, Niku SD. Endourethral prosthesis for treatment of detrusor sphincter dyssynergia: impact on quality of life for persons with spinal cord injury. *SCI Nurs* 1994; **11**: 95–99.

40. Christ KF, Kornhuber HH. Treatment of neurogenic bladder dysfunction in multiple sclerosis by ultrasound-controlled bladder training. *Arch Psychiatr Nervenkr* 1980; **228**: 191–195.

41. Kornhuber HH, Schutz A. Efficient treatment of neurogenic bladder disorders in multiple sclerosis with initial intermittent catheterization and ultrasound-controlled training. *Eur Neurol* 1990; **30**: 260–267.

42. Petajan JH, Gappmaier E, White AT *et al*. Impact of aerobic training on fitness and quality of life in multiple sclerosis. *Ann Neurol* 1996; **39**: 432–441.

43. Primus G. Maximal electrical stimulation in neurogenic detrusor hyperactivity: experiences in multiple sclerosis. *Eur J Med* 1992; **1**: 80–82.

44. Tani S, Shimizu H, Ishijima B *et al*. [Our experiences of PISCES (percutaneously inserted spinal cord electrical stimulation) in SMON

and other neurologic disorders]. *No To Shinkei* 1984; **36**: 383–388.

45. Ronzoni G, De Vecchis M, Rizzotto A *et al.* [Long-term results of spinal cord electrostimulation in the treatment of micturition disorders associated with neurogenic bladder] Resultats a long terme de l'electro-stimulation de la moelle dans le traitement des troubles mictionnels des neurovessies. *Ann Urol Paris* 1988; **22**: 31–34.

46. Abbate AD, Cook AW, Atallah M. Effect of electrical stimulation of the thoracic spinal cord on the function of the bladder in multiple sclerosis. *J Urol* 1977; **117**: 285–288.

47. Dooley DM, Sharkey J. Electrostimulation of the nervous system for patients with demyelinating and degenerative diseases of the nervous system and vascular diseases of the extremities. *Appl Neurophysiol* 1977; **40**: 208–217.

48. Berg V, Bergmann S, Hovdal H *et al.* The value of dorsal column stimulation in multiple sclerosis. *Scand J Rehabil Med* 1982; **14**: 183–191.

49. Hawkes CH, Myke M, Desmond A *et al.* Stimulation of dorsal column in multiple sclerosis. *Br Med J* 1980; **280**(6218): 889–891.

50. Young RF, Goodman SJ. Dorsal spinal cord stimulation in the treatment of multiple sclerosis. *Neurosurgery* 1979; **5**: 225–230.

51. Illis LS, Read DJ, Sedgwick EM *et al.* Spinal cord stimulation in the United Kingdom. *J Neurol Neurosurg Psychiatry* 1983; **46**: 299–304.

52. Klingler D, Kepplinger B, Gerstenbrand F *et al.* [Epidural spinal electrostimulation (ESES) in patients with chronic pain and central motor disturbances (author's transl)] Die epidurale spinale Elektrostimulation (ESES) bei chronischen Schmerzzustanden und zentralen motorischen Storungen. *Wien Klin Wochenschr* 1981; **93**: 688–695.

53. Flanigan RC, August HM, Jr, Young B *et al.* Cutaneous stimulation of the bladder in multiple sclerosis: a case report. *J Urol* 1983; **129**: 1047–1048.

54. Sandyk R, Iacono RP. Improvement by picoTesla range magnetic fields of perceptual-motor performance and visual memory in a patient with chronic progressive multiple sclerosis. *Int J Neurosci* 1994; **78**: 53–66.

55. Susset JG, Zinner N, Archimbaud JP. Proceed-ings: Differential sacral blocks and selective neurotomies in the treatment of incomplete upper motor neuron lesion. *Urol Int* 1974; **29**: 236–248.

56. Rockswold GL, Bradley WE, Chou SN. Effect of sacral nerve blocks on the function of the urinary bladder in humans. *J Neurosurg* 1974; **40**: 83–89.

57. Markland C, Merrill D, Chou S *et al.* Sacral nerve root stimulation: a clinical test of detrusor innervation. *J Urol* 1972; **107**: 772–776.

58. Nordenbo A, Van Kerrebroeck P, Van Poppel H *et al.* Treatment of lower urinary tract dysfunction in patients with multiple sclerosis. European Group on SUDIMS [letter; comment]. *J Neurol Neurosurg Psychiatry* 1993; **56**: 1137.

59. Sullivan SN, Ebers GC. Gastrointestinal dysfunction in multiple sclerosis [letter]. *Gastroenterology* 1983; **84**: 1640.

60. Hinds JP, Eidelman BH, Wald A. Prevalence of bowel dysfunction in multiple sclerosis. A population survey. *Gastroenterology* 1990; **98**: 1538–1542.

61. Hinds JP, Wald A. Colonic and anorectal dysfunction associated with multiple sclerosis. *Am J Gastroenterol* 1989; **84**: 587–595.

62. Chia YW, Fowler CJ, Kamm MA *et al.* Prevalence of bowel dysfunction in patients with multiple sclerosis and bladder dysfunction. *J Neurol* 1995; **242**: 105–108.

63. Glick ME, Meshkinpour H, Haldeman S *et al.* Colonic dysfunction in multiple sclerosis. *Gastroenterology* 1982; **83**: 1002–1007.

64. Weber J, Grise P, Roquebert M *et al.* Radiopaque markers transit and anorectal manometry in 16 patients with multiple sclerosis and urinary bladder dysfunction. *Dis Colon Rectum* 1987; **30**: 95–100.

65. Chia YW, Gill KP, Jameson JS *et al.* Paradoxical puborectalis contraction is a feature of constipation in patients with multiple sclerosis. *J Neurol Neurosurg Psychiatry* 1996; **60**: 31–35.

66. Gill KP, Chia YW, Henry MM *et al.* Defecography in multiple sclerosis patients with severe constipation. *Radiology* 1994; **191**: 553–556.

67. Nordenbo A, Anderson JT, Anderson J. Disturbances of anorectal function in multiple sclerosis. *J Neurol* 1996; **243**: 445–451.

68. Swash M, Snooks SJ, Chalmers DH. Parity as a

factor in incontinence in multiple sclerosis. *Arch Neurol* 1987; **44**: 504–508.

69. Lubowski D, Nicholls R, Swash M *et al.* Neural control of internal sphincter function. *Brit J Surg* 1987; **74**: 668–670.

70. Hulter BM, Lundberg PO. Sexual function in women with advanced multiple sclerosis. *J Neurol Neurosurg Psychiatry* 1995; **59**: 83–86.

71. Mattson D, Petrie M, Srivastava DK *et al.* Multiple sclerosis. Sexual dysfunction and its response to medications. *Arch Neurol* 1995; **52**: 862–868.

72. Kaplan PM. The use of serotonergic uptake inhibitors in the treatment of premature ejaculation. *J Sex Marital Ther* 1994; **20**: 321–324.

73. Heller L, Keren O, Aloni R *et al.* An open trial of vacuum penile tumescence: constriction therapy for neurological impotence. *Paraplegia* 1992; **30**: 550–553.

74. Susset JG, Tessier CD, Wincze J *et al.* Effect of yohimbine hydrochloride on erectile impotence: a double-blind study. *J Urol* 1989; **141**: 1360–1363.

75. Montorsi F, Strambi LF, Guazzoni G *et al.* Effect of yohimbine-trazodone on psychogenic impotence: a randomized, double-blind, placebo-controlled study. *Urology* 1994; **44**: 732–736.

76. Althof SE, Levine SB, Corty EW *et al.* A double-blind crossover trial of clomipramine for rapid ejaculation in 15 couples. *J Clin Psychiat* 1995; **56**: 402–407.

77. Eardley I, Morgan R, Dinsmore W *et al.* Oral administration of Sildenafil improves penile erections in patients with male erectile dysfunction (MED). A double-blind, placebo con-trolled study with patient and partner outpatient diary as efficacy end points. [Abstract] *Eur Urol* 1997; **30** (suppl 2): 573.

78. Heaton JP, Morales A, Owen J *et al.* Topical glyceryltrinitrate causes measurable penile arterial dilation in impotent men. *J Urol* 1990; **143**: 729–731.

79. Cavallini G. Minoxidil versus nitroglycerine: a prospective, double-blind, controlled trial in transcutaneous therapy for organic impotence. *Int J Impot Res* 1994; **6**: 205–212.

80. John H, Lehmann K, Hauri D. Intraurethral prostaglandin improves quality of vacuum erection therapy. *Eur Urol* 1996; **29**: 224–226.

81. Kim ED, el Rashidy R, McVary KT. Papaverine topical gel for treatment of erectile dysfunction. *J Urol* 1995; **153**: 361–365.

82. Kirkeby HJ, Poulsen EU, Petersen T *et al.* Erectile dysfunction in multiple sclerosis. *Neurology* 1988; **38**: 1366–1371.

83. Porst H. The rationale for prostaglandin E1 in erectile failure: a survey of worldwide experience. *J Urol* 1996; **155**: 802–815.

84. Truss MC, Becker AJ, Djamilian MH *et al.* Role of the nitric oxide donor linsidomine chlorhydrate (SIN-1) in the diagnosis and treatment of erectile dysfunction. *Urology* 1994; **44**: 553–556.

85. Belker AM, Sherins RJ, Bustillo M *et al.* Pregnancy with microsurgical vas sperm aspiration from a patient with neurologic ejaculatory dysfunction. *J Androl* 1994; **15** (suppl): 6S–9S.

86. Denil J, Ohl DA, McGuire EJ *et al.* Treatment of anejaculation with electroejaculation. *Acta Urol Belg* 1992; **60**: 15–25.

21

Mechanisms, measurement, and management of fatigue in multiple sclerosis

Lauren B Krupp

Introduction

Fatigue in multiple sclerosis (MS) is frequent and often debilitating.[1,2] Patients rate their fatigue as more disabling compared to healthy or hypertensive controls and MS fatigue greatly detracts from quality of life.[2–7] While there has been progress in understanding MS fatigue, we are still refining its definition and testing pathogenic mechanisms, and identifying major covariates. These efforts should lead to more effective drug therapies.

Fatigue is defined as an overwhelming sense of tiredness, lack of energy, or feeling of exhaustion. It is distinguished from symptoms of depression, which include lack of self-esteem, despair, or feelings of hopelessness. Fatigue is also distinct from limb weakness. It is most easily conceptualized as a feeling of exhaustion which, in healthy individuals, often accompanies mild 'flu-like illness. For patients with MS, fatigue can be chronic and severe.

MS fatigue: frequency, characteristics and relationships

Between 76 and 92 per cent of MS patients experience fatigue.[9,10] For some, fatigue is the most severe MS symptom.[3,4,8] Vercoulen and co-workers found that over 85 per cent of MS patients experience fatigue daily.[11] Between 55 and 75 per cent of patients consider it one of their three most disabling symptoms.[2,3] The majority (more than 90 per cent) of MS patients report that heat dramatically worsens fatigue, while cool temperatures relieve fatigue.[2] This sensitivity to heat, while typical of other MS symptoms, is not a feature shared by fatigued patients with systemic lupus erythematosus (SLE), Lyme disease, or by healthy controls.[2,6]

New onset of fatigue in the MS patient may be an important harbinger of other problems. Fatigue can be the first sign of an impending relapse. In other medical disorders associated with severe fatigue, such as SLE, fatigue may also signal other impending systemic involvement.

MS patients have an associated feeling of tiredness with activities such as using a wheelchair, moving about, or working. Feelings of tiredness have also been associated with aching, feeling stiff, or new responsibilities such as child-rearing.[7] In a study of the psychosocial correlates of fatigue among 139 MS patients, fatigue was found to limit social, work and overall role performance.[12] A low sense of control of the environment was closely associated with both global fatigue and fatigue-related stress.[12] These findings underscore the interrelationship of fatigue, physical activity, pain, and social engagement.

While MS fatigue is closely associated with perceived general and mental health,[3] it does not correlate highly with patient age or level of neurologic impairment (as measured by the Expanded Disability Status Score (EDSS)) or by Ambulation Index.[1–3,5,6,8–10,13] On questionnaires MS patients' responses on subscales of thinking and fatigue are not closely associated with measures of motility.[14] Two reports describe fatigue as more severe in chronic-progressive versus relapsing–remitting MS patients,[3,13] but others do not find this difference.[14] Fatigue is clearly a problem which spans all levels of neurologic disability and subcategories of MS.

Fatigue and motor function

Despite the minimal relationship between fatigue and EDSS[2,3,8–10] physical activity is probably related to some aspects of fatigue. For example, some MS patients associate their fatigue with impaired physical activity rather than mental activity.[7] In one study more than 90 per cent of patients picked activities such as walking, housework, going out, or grooming as most affected by fatigue rather than concentration or attention.[10]

Fatigue in MS has been associated with impaired motor function as defined with measures of maximal force decay as generated during exercise.[15] Using an isometric strain gauge to measure the force generated by muscle contraction and dividing the integral of the force–time curve by the maximal force generated by a patient, a fatigue index is created. This fatigue index was found to be significantly elevated in MS compared to healthy controls and another medical comparison group, chronic fatigue syndrome (CFS) patients.[15] MS patients with pyramidal tract signs had a greater index and the index worsened during MS relapses, in which there was increased pyramidal tract dysfunction.[15] Other motor deficits demonstrated in MS include decreased motor unit firing rates, inadequate motor unit recruitment,[16,17] and impaired mus-

cular activation and metabolism during isometric exercise. Impaired drive to the motor cortex without frequency-dependent conduction block has also been proposed as a mechanism for fatigue.[18] These deficits limit the MS patients' ability to produce voluntary muscle force and may contribute to motor fatigue.[19]

Relationship between fatigue, sleep, and mood

A variety of studies show that fatigue and mood disturbance overlap but have low correlations, and should be considered distinct symptoms. In two multi-center fatigue treatment studies depression and fatigue were not significantly correlated.[9,10] In one of the studies change in depression showed a modest correlation with vitality, the inverse of fatigue, but was not significantly correlated with change on an MS-specific fatigue measure. While it is clear that fatigue and depression may show only a modest association,[2,5,6,8,9] patients who report being more depressed may report more severe fatigue.[12] These findings reaffirm that fatigue and depression may in some patients be linked, and in others represent clearly distinct phenomena.

Sleep disturbance is common in MS[20–22] and may be missed as a cause for fatigue. However, sleep problems do not fully explain fatigue. Patients' reports of sleep disturbance have not been significantly associated with fatigue or vitality.[20] In an investigation using tests of daily activity (actinography) and sleep pathology (multiple sleep latency test), no evidence of a disturbance in generalized circadian rhythm in MS patients was observed, nor were specific sleep disorders causing fatigue identified.[21] Abnormalities of sleep such as nocturnal myoclonus, sleep apnea, periodic leg movement disorder, and poor sleep efficiency occur in MS,[22] and should be ruled out as contributing factors. However, many MS patients with fatigue lack these sleep disorders. At present the relationship between sleep quality and efficiency to MS fatigue needs further study.

Fatigue and cognitive loss in MS

Some of the cognitive effects of fatigue in MS have been delineated. MS patients when fatigued have prolonged reaction times compared to when they are less fatigued.[23] Fatigue can also affect tests of complex attention[13,24–26] and sustained cognitive effort.[27] On successive trials of a test of sustained attention MS patients' performance worsened over time, in contrast to controls.[27] This decrement in performance was attributed to fatigue. Thus, fatigue may be an important aspect of cognition. Grossman and co-workers[13] found that when fatigue and depression were included with neuropsychological measures in a stepwise discriminant analysis, they predicted 62 percent of the memory dysfunction in MS and increased both the sensitivity and specificity for the classification of neurobehavioral diagnosis in MS.[13]

Despite these findings, most standard neuropsychological tests of memory and visual–spatial function are not significantly associated with fatigue in MS.[12,25] Geisler and colleagues did not find a significant correlation between measures of memory, visuospatial ability, and cognitive flexibility and fatigue.[25] A study of 139 MS patients evaluated with a multidimensional fatigue scale and neuropsychological tests showed that cognitive performance was not associated with fatigue.[12] This result was similar to an earlier pilot study of Leo and co-workers which also found little association between fatigue and cognition.[28] Identifying the effects of mental fatigue on cognitive functioning may require experimental neuropsychological testing procedures which examine sustained attention and mental processing speed rather than the more standard cognitive

measures used in most MS neurobehavioral studies.

Treatment of fatigue has little effect on most cognitive deficits associated with MS. Although one study showed that amantadine treatment improved performance on several neuropsychological measures, compared to placebo,[29] these findings were not confirmed in a subsequent investigation.[27]

Fatigue: mechanisms

There is no one proven universal etiology for fatigue. The mechanism for fatigue differs among diverse neurologic and medical disorders. In MS, pathogenic mechanisms proposed for fatigue have included immune dysfunction with release of pro-inflammatory cytokines. One reason to emphasize the importance of immune mechanisms is the overlap between MS fatigue and fatigue associated with other autoimmune disorders such as SLE. Another proposed explanation for MS fatigue relies on the motor deficits and the observed impairments in nerve conduction, muscular oxidative capacity, and motor drive, which in turn contribute to physical deconditioning. Disturbed sleep and psychological factors are also important problems which relate to fatigue.

A patient's premorbid psychological vulnerability may be closely linked to their tendency to develop fatigue with illness. Several studies have found that individuals with prior histories of increased psychological stress, poor coping, or greater psychological vulnerability have prolonged recoveries complicated by persistent fatigue following influenza or experimental viral inoculation.[30–33] These findings demonstrate the importance of healthy coping skills in dealing with fatigue.

Immune mechanisms for fatigue have been suggested from the response of patients treated with cytokines. Interferon (INF)-γ and INF-α may cause severe fatigue in MS patients as well as in patients receiving these treatments for other conditions.[34,35] Pro-inflammatory cytokines such as tumor necrosis factor (TNF) and interleukin (IL)-1 also cause fatigue and provoke slow wave sleep.[36,37] Immunologic factors, including elevated cytokines, are frequently considered in the pathogenesis of MS fatigue[38] and have been studied in animal models of fatigue.[39] However, immune system abnormalities in relationship to fatigue in MS are inconsistent.

The contribution of muscular defects in fatigue differs across MS patients. Defects in phosphocreatine resynthesis have been noted during exercise. These findings have been interpreted as a defect in oxidative capacity of skeletal muscle which could partially explain muscular fatigue and deconditioning in MS.[40]

Fatigue measurement

A variety of instruments have been developed to assess fatigue in MS. Several are listed in *Table 21.1*. Despite efforts to identify objective correlates of fatigue, most investigators have not found that laboratory measures are reliable predictors of fatigue severity. Furthermore, since fatigue is inherently a subjective experience analogous to pain, the most appropriate measure of the symptom is a self-report instrument which can quantify what the patient experiences.

Some studies of fatigue use a visual analogue scale to measure fatigue.[2] In this instance, a patient is asked to indicate on a line their degree of fatigue with 'none' being indicated along the left margin of the line and 'most severe' along the right margin. The dis-

Scale	Advantages	Disadvantages
Rand index of vitality[41]	Easy to score and administer	Covers limited aspects of fatigue
Fatigue impact scale[3]	Assesses physical, emotional, and social dimensions	Long and established for MS only
Chalder fatigue scale[48]	Examines physical and mental aspects	Forces patients into dichotomous thinking
Fatigue severity scale[4]	Brief, easy to administer, proven reliability	May be less sensitive than other scales
Multidimensional fatigue assessment[46]	Covers severity, intensity, psychosocial dimensions, good validity	Some items overlap or may be misinterpreted

Table 21.1
Fatigue scales.

tance where the patient bisects the line is calculated and a number signifying intensity of fatigue is generated. Although quick to administer, this measure is vulnerable to impulsive answers and does not assess qualitative aspects of fatigue. It is also possible that older subjects or those with visual impairment will have greater difficulty with this method. The process of measuring the distance on each line is also cumbersome unless special computer software is available.

Other fatigue instruments involve structured self-report questionnaires. Many developed for general medical disorders can also be applied to MS. One example is the subset of items which cover energy and fatigue as part of the Medical Outcome Survey (MOS).[41,42] The MOS measures mental and psychologic states and general health, and was developed as a result of a health survey conducted by the Rand Health Organization. It includes a four-item questionnaire used to assess energy levels in the general population which has been referred to as the Rand Index of Vitality. It is short, simple to score, and is inversely related to fatigue. Disadvantages are that it does not assess fatigue's impact on daily living, or provide information regarding conditions which worsen or improve fatigue.

The Fatigue Impact Scale was developed by Fiske to examine fatigue in MS.[3] It was a strong predictor of mental and general health in a population of 85 MS patients. It demonstrates significant differences between fatigue in MS versus hypertensive patients. It contains 40 items and is completed by the patient using a rating scale of 1–4. Whether it will be sensitive to treatment effects is likely to be addressed in a current ongoing clinical trial.

The Fatigue Severity Scale[4] is a nine-item scale which assesses the effect of fatigue on activities of daily living. It has been used to examine fatigue in MS,[4] Parkinson's disease,[43] SLE,[4] Lyme disease,[44] and CFS.[6,26] It is derived from a 29-item questionnaire which includes items assessing which conditions enhance and ameliorate fatigue. It provides some data on differential diagnostic features of fatigue. It is brief, easy to administer, and demonstrates reliability and internal consistency. This scale is useful in the classification of patients but may not be sensitive to changes associated with treatment.[9,45]

Another useful scale is the Multidimensional Assessment of Fatigue (MAF) scale developed by Belza and colleagues[46] for the study of medical populations, and more recently studied in MS.[12] This 16-item likert scale measures four dimensions of self-reported fatigue: severity, distress, timing, and interference. These fatigue dimensions cover subjective aspects, frequency and variability, and 14 activities of daily living.

Only a limited number of MS fatigue studies have been applied in treatment studies. An MS-specific fatigue scale which contains only six items detected changes in a medication treatment study of fatigue in MS.[9] However, for optimum efficacy it is best administered by a health provider to the patients. Another measure which was sensitive to an exercise program designed to alleviate fatigue was the 'tiredness/vigor' subscale of the Profile of Mood States.[47] This self-report measure has been used to assess several different psychological states in a variety of clinical populations and has established reliability and sensitivity.

Other fatigue scales used in neurologic and medical populations have distinguished medical and physical components of fatigue[48] or emphasized activities affected by fatigue.[49]

Evaluation

The evaluation of fatigue is outlined in *Table 21.2*. An important question in evaluating the fatigued patient with MS is whether there are signs of an impending relapse. New neurologic symptoms or signs accompanying fatigue could indicate increased disease activity. The possibility of new infection or heat exposure causing a pseudo exacerbation should be considered. Medication history is important to review when fatigue has changed. Medications such as those used for spasticity, beta blockers, tricyclic antidepressants, benzodiazepines, and anticonvulsants, can worsen fatigue.

It is critical to evaluate other symptoms which may contribute to fatigue. Potential problems include pain, poor sleep, psychological stress, and deconditioning. Approximately 40 per cent of MS patients experience severe pain. This may disrupt sleep, adding stress and making fatigue, which was previously mild, unmanageable. For example, among patients with cancer and rheumatoid arthritis, pain is the most important correlate of fatigue.[46,50] A review of systems approach which focuses on headache, muscle pain, and radicular or back pain, may reveal that these are contributing to a patient's lack of energy. Sleep disorder may be experienced as fatigue.[51] Rarely comorbid conditions in MS such as sleep apnea, nocturnal myoclonus, or narcolepsy cause fatigue.[20–22] Careful assessment of a patient's sleep habits are helpful. Observations by the patient's spouse or partner on quality of sleep, number of nocturnal awakenings, and apneic episodes may help identify previously undiagnosed sleep disorders.

Assessment of mood is very valuable. Most patients with MS have elevated depressive symptoms although they may not meet criteria for major depression. A simple quick office approach is to use self-report questionnaires. Inclusion of a brief history for family psychiatric illness, examining the nature of the family unit and support systems, and evaluating current level of self-esteem or anxiety are also important.

Self-report instruments with demonstrated reliability and validity for depression which have been widely used are the Beck depression inventory[52] and the Center for Epidemiologic Studies Depression Scale (CES-D).[53] Both scales provide cut off scores which can identify a patient at risk for clinical major depression.

At least at some point in their course patients should be evaluated with a laboratory screen to exclude other fatigue-producing conditions. Testing should include thyroid function tests (TFTs), complete blood cell count, electrolytes, glucose, tests of liver function, ANA, ESR, and urinalysis and culture.

For patients in whom overwhelming fatigue is associated with severe depression, or in patients who are refractory to all forms of fatigue therapy, psychiatric referral may be of value. Psychiatric evaluation may disclose previously unrecognized psychosocial or psychiatric problems, help in the management of major depression, or may simply rule out the possibility of psychological factors, so that more aggressive medical treatment is pursued. Before considering treatment for fatigue with amphetamine-type medication, we often have patients assessed by a psychologist or psychiatrist.

Fatigue management

Fatigue management requires a multi-disciplinary approach which should encompass the various factors which may contribute to fatigue severity, such as mood, level of physical activity, pain, medication, and sleep. Among the non-pharmacologic treatments, education and support are very important. Patients directly benefit when their symptom is recognized as genuine. Education and reassurance are effective therapy.

Exercise is a powerful means to combat deconditioning and enhance self-esteem. The advantages of exercise on fatigue were demonstrated in a study of 54 patients randomly assigned to either 15 weeks of aerobic training or a non-exercise condition.[45] Patients in the exercise condition experienced a significant reduction in fatigue as measured by the Profile of Mood States at week 10, and had improvement in quality of life as measured by the Sickness Impact Scale.[44] However, improvement was not sustained at week 15. Self-reported physical state, social interaction, emotional behavior and home management also improved.

While a graded exercise program is useful, over-exertion can be detrimental. For some patients selected reductions in some activities is something they must learn to accept. Rest periods during the work day and avoidance of environmental factors which worsen fatigue (such as heat) are also beneficial, i.e. fatigue management programmes.

Behavioral modification therapy when applied to CFS can reduce associated symptoms of depression, and fatigue components caused by mood disorder.[54,55] Behavioral therapies may be effective on an individual or group basis and should also be considered for MS patients experiencing coping difficulties. They are structured in a format analogous to chronic pain treatment groups, and have been shown for some patients to provide a major benefit.

Often non-pharmacologic measures must be supplemented with drug therapy. Current treatments shown to be effective for MS fatigue in randomized double-blind placebo-controlled trials are magnesium pemoline (pemoline), a central nervous system (CNS) stimulant and amantadine hydrochloride (amantadine), an antiviral agent which also has anti-parkinson effects.[8–10,56]

In a Canadian multi-center MS fatigue treatment trial, using a cross-over design, amantadine significantly improved fatigue relative to placebo.[10] In a multi-center study comparing pemoline and placebo, no significant differences emerged but there was a trend in favor of pemoline.[56] Forty-six per cent of treated patients had excellent or good relief with pemoline compared to only 19.5 per cent with placebo. Poorly tolerated side effects occurred in 25 per cent of the pemoline group.[56] A randomized study comparing pemoline, amantadine, and placebo in the treatment of MS fatigue using a parallel group design, showed a benefit with amantadine but not pemoline when compared to placebo.[9] Side effects with either medication in this study were infrequent.

Based on the relative benefit with amantadine, and its low side effect profile, we believe this is the first-line medication to use for MS fatigue. If no benefit is seen then a second option is pemoline, since pemoline, particularly at doses higher than 56.25 mg, may help some patients. The possibility of a placebo response from either agent is high.

The mechanism for amantadine's fatigue treatment effect is not known. In one fatigue treatment study using amantadine, higher levels of β-endorphin-β-lipotropin and lower levels of lactate were present in responders compared to non-responders.[57] These changes may have been due to direct effects of the drug or concomitant metabolic changes associated with lowered fatigue.

Other medications used on an anecdotal basis for fatigue include CNS stimulants such as methylphenidate (ritalin) or dextroamphetamine. CNS stimulants should be used with caution but in selected cases have value. They are contraindicated in patients with abuse potential. In a study examining long-term efficacy and safety of 4-aminopyridine treatment in MS, fatigue was a symptom frequently reported as improved with therapy[58] (see

History

- Assess for increased disease activity
- Review medications
  (antispasticity agents, antidepressants, anticonvulsants)
- Assess related symptoms
  (pain, sleep, memory, depression)
- Determine onset of fatigue

Neurologic/medical exam

- Check for new deficits
- Mental status
- Administer fatigue and depression measures

Laboratory screen

- Complete blood cell count, glucose, electrolytes, tests of liver function, ANA, ESR, TSH, U/A, urine culture

Special studies

- Polysomnography
- MRI

Psychiatric referral

- For depression or if treatment with amphetamine is planned

Table 21.2
Evaluation of fatigue.

Polman, Chapter 16). A pilot study in MS with 3,4-diaminopyridine reported subjective fatigue improvement in six of eight treated subjects but no change in physiological fatigue measures.[59] Future studies of 4-aminopyridine in the treatment of MS fatigue are under consideration.

Another pharmacologic strategy for fatigue consists of antidepressant medication. This is clearly the treatment of choice for patients with coexisting major depression, which is common in MS.[60] However, even patients who deny depressive symptoms may have definite responses to antidepressant medication. Agents with the least sedating properties are preferable such as fluoxetine (Prozac), sertraline (Zoloft), nefazodone hydrochloride (serzone), and desipramine (Norpramin).

In patients in whom fatigue is associated with sleep disorder, improved sleep hygiene is important. Exercise six hours before sleep can help, and patients should be cautioned not to look at the time every few minutes. Medications for insomnia may also lower fatigue in selected cases. Occasionally fatigue is associated with anxiety. Alleviating anxiety or panic attacks with appropriate therapies may have a beneficial effect on fatigue in such cases.

More direct treatments for MS fatigue are under current investigation. At the time of this writing a multi-center clinical trial using INF-β-1b for the treatment of secondary progressive MS is in progress which incorporates a measure of fatigue (similar to the Fiske scale and the MOS) as a secondary outcome. This study hopefully will help determine whether immune therapies may lessen fatigue.

Summary

Fatigue is a multi-faceted problem. It is common in neurologic disorders and is very frequent in MS. For many patients it is the primary complaint. Interest in fatigue has grown in recent years and has led to improvement in our methods of evaluation and treatment.

References

1. Freal JE, Kraft GH, Coryell JK. Symptomatic fatigue in multiple sclerosis. *Arch Phys Med Rehabil* 1984; **65**: 135–138.
2. Krupp LB, Alvarez La, LaRocca NG *et al*. Clinical characteristics of fatigue in multiple sclerosis. *Arch Neurol* 1988; **45**: 435–437.
3. Fisk JD, Pontefract A, Ritvo PG *et al*. The impact of fatigue on patients with multiple sclerosis. *Can J Neurol Sci* 1994; **21**: 9–14.
4. Krupp LB, LaRocca NC, Muir-Nash J *et al*. The fatigue severity scale applied to patients with multiple sclerosis and systemic lupus erythematosus. *Arch Neurol* 1989; **46**: 1121–1123.
5. Pepper C, Krupp LB, Friedberg F *et al*. Comparison of psychiatric characteristics in chronic fatigue syndrome, multiple sclerosis, and depression. *J Neuropsychiat Clin Neurosci* 1993; **5**: 1–7.
6. Schwartz J, Jandorf L, Krupp LB. The measurement of fatigue: A new scale. *J Psychosom Res* 1993; **37**: 753–762.
7. Monks J. Experiencing symptoms in chronic illness: fatigue in multiple sclerosis. *Int Disability Stud* 1989; **11**: 78.
8. Murray TJ. Amantadine therapy for fatigue in multiple sclerosis. *Can J Neurol Sci* 1985; **12**: 251–254.
9. Krupp LB, Coyle PK, Doscher C *et al*. Fatigue therapy in multiple sclerosis: results of a double-blind randomized parallel trial of amantadine, pemoline, and placebo. *Neurology* 1995; **45**: 1956–1961.
10. Canadian MS Research Group. A randomized controlled trial of amantadine in fatigue associated with multiple sclerosis. *Can J Neurol Sci* 1987; **14**: 273–278.
11. Vercoulen J, Hommes OR, Swanink C *et al*. The measurement of fatigue in patients with multiple sclerosis: A multidimensional comparison with patients with chronic fatigue syndrome and healthy subjects. *Arch Neurol* 1996; **53**: 642–649.
12. Schwartz CE, Coulthard-Morris L, Zeng Q. Psychosocial correlates of fatigue in multiple sclerosis. *Arch Phys Med Rehabil* 1996; **77**: 165–170.
13. Grossman M, Armstrong C, Onishi K *et al*. Patterns of cognitive impairment in relapsing–remitting and chronic progressive multiple sclerosis. *Neuropsychiat Neuropsychol Behav Neurol* 1994; **7**: 194–210.
14. Cella DF, Dineen K, Arnason B *et al*. Validation of the functional assessment of multiple sclerosis (FAMS); quality of life instrument. *Neurology* 1996; **47**: 129–139.
15. Djaldetti R, Ziv I, Achiron A *et al*. Fatigue in multiple sclerosis compared with chronic fatigue syndrome: A quantitative assessment. *Neurology* 1996; **46**: 632–635.
16. Rice CL, Vollmer TL, Bigland-Riticheie B. Neuromuscular responses of patients with multiple sclerosis. *Muscle Nerve* 1992; **15**: 1123–1132.
17. Sharma KR, Kent-Braun J, Mynhier MA *et al*. Evidence of an abnormal intramuscular component of fatigue in multiple sclerosis. *Muscle Nerve* 1995; **18**: 1403–1411.
18. Sheean GL, Murray MF, Rothwell JC *et al*. An electrophysiological study of the mechanism of fatigue in multiple sclerosis. *Brain* 1997; **120**: 299–316.
19. Kent-Braun JF, Sharma KR, Weiner MW *et al*. Effects of exercise on muscle activation and metabolism in multiple sclerosis. *Muscle Nerve* 1994; **17**: 1162–1169.
20. Caruso LS, LaRocca NC, Tyron W *et al*. Activity monitoring of fatigued and non-fatigued persons with MS. *Sleep Res* 1991; **20**: 368.
21. Taphoorn MJ, van Someren E, Snoek FJ *et al*. Fatigue, sleep disturbances, and circadian rhythm in multiple sclerosis. *J Neurol* 1993; **240**: 446–448.
22. Giancarlo T, Kapen S, Saad J *et al*. Analysis of sleepiness and fatigue in multiple sclerosis. *Ann Neurol* 1987; **22**: 187.
23. Sandroni P, Walker C, Starr A. "Fatigue" in patients with MS. *Arch Neurol* 1992; **49**: 517–524.

24. DeLuca J, Johnson SK, Beldowicz D *et al.* Neuropsychological impairments in chronic fatigue syndrome, multiple sclerosis, and depression. *J Neurol Neurosurg Psychiatry* 1995; **58**: 38–63.

25. Geisler MW, Sliwinski M, Coyle PK *et al.* The effects of amantadine and pemoline on cognitive functioning in multiple sclerosis. *Arch Neurol* 1996; **53**: 185–188.

26. Krupp LB, Sliwinski M, Masur D *et al.* Cognitive functioning and depression in patients with chronic fatigue syndrome and multiple sclerosis. *Arch Neurol* 1994; **51**: 705–710.

27. Kujala P, Portin R, Revonsuo A *et al.* Attention related performance in two cognitively different subgroups of patients with multiple sclerosis. *J Neurol Neurosurg Psychiatry* 1995; **59**: 77–82.

28. Leo GJ, Rao SM, St. Aubin-Faubert P *et al.* Correlates of fatigue in multiple sclerosis. *Ann Neurol* 1987; **22**: 152.

29. Cohen RA, Fisher M. Amantadine treatment of fatigue associated with Multiple Sclerosis. *Arch Neurol* 1989; **46**: 676–680.

30. Canter A, Cluff LE, Imboden JB. Hypersensitive reactions to immunization innoculations and antecedent psychological vulnerability. *J Psychosom Res* 1972; **16**: 99–101.

31. Cope H, David A, Pelosi A *et al.* Predictors of chronic "postviral" fatigue. *Lancet* 1994; **344**: 864–868.

32. Cohen S, Tyrrell AJ, Smith AP. Psychological stress and susceptibility to the common cold. *N Eng J Med* 1991; **325**: 606–612.

33. Imboden JB, Canter A, Cluff LE. Convalescence from influenza. A study of the pscyhological and clinical determinants. *Arch Intern Med* 1961; **108**: 393–399.

34. Panitch HS, Hirsch RL, Schindler J *et al.* Treatment of multiple sclerosis with gamma interferon: Exacerbations associated with activation of the immune system. *Neurology* 1987; **37**(2): 1097–1102.

35. Adams F, Quesada JR, Gutterman JU. Neuropsychiatric manifestations of human leukocyte interferon therapy in patients with cancer. *J Am Med Ass* 1984; **252**: 938–941.

36. Moldofsky H, Lue FA, Eisen J *et al.* The relationship of interleukin-1 and immune functions to sleep in humans. *Psychosom Med* 1986; **48**: 309–318.

37. Krueger JM, Walter J, Dinarello CA *et al.* Sleep-promoting effects of endogenous pyrogen (interleukin-1). *Am J Physiol* 1984; **246**: R994–R999.

38. Bertolone K, Coyle PK, Krupp LB *et al.* Cytokine correlates of fatigue in MS. *Neurology* 1993; **43**: 769S.

39. Chao CC, DeLa Hunt M, Hu S *et al.* Immunologically mediated fatigue: a murine model. *Clin Immunopath* 1992; **64**: 161–165.

40. Kent-Braun JA, Sharma KR, Miller RG *et al.* Postexercise phosphocreatine resynthesis is slowed in multiple sclerosis. *Muscle Nerve* 1994; **17**: 835–841.

41. Brook RH, Ware JE, Davies A *et al.* Overview of adult health status measures fielded in the Rand's Health Insurance Study. *Med Care* (supplement) 1979; **17**: 1–55.

42. Stewart AL, Hays RD, Ware JE. The MOS Short Form General Health Survey – Reliability and validity in a patient population. *Ed Care* 1988; **26**: 724–735.

43. Friedman J, Friedman H. Fatigue in Parkinson's disease. *Neurology* 1993; **43**: 2016–2018.

44. Krupp LB, Schwartz JE, Jandorf L. Fatigue in Lyme disease. In: Coyle PK, ed. *Lyme Disease*, St. Louis: Mosby Year Book 1993.

45. Petajan JH, Gappmaier E, White AT *et al.* Impact of aerobic training on fitness and quality of life in multiple sclerosis. *Ann Neurol* 1996; **39**: 432–441.

46. Belza BL, Henke CJ, Yelin EH *et al.* Correlates of fatigue in older patients with rheumatoid arthritis. *Nurs Res* 1993; **42**: 93–99.

47. McNair DM, Lorr M, Droppleman LF. *Profile of Mood States (POMS)*, San Diego: Educational and Industrial Testing Service 1992.

48. Chalder T, Berelowitz G, Pawlikowska T *et al.* Development of a robust fatigue scale. *J Psychosom Res* 1993; **37**: 147–153.

49. Piper BF, Lindsey AM, Dodd MJ *et al.* The development of an instrument to measure the subjective dimension of fatigue. In: Funk SG, Tornquist EM, Champagne MT *et al.*, eds. *Key Aspects of Comfort; Management of Pain, Fatigue, and Nausea*, New York: Springer Publishing Co. 1989.

50. Pickard-Holley S. Fatigue in cancer patients: a descriptive study. *Cancer Nurs* 1991; **14**: 13–19.

51. Krupp LB, Jandorf L, Coyle PK *et al*. Sleep in chronic fatigue syndrome. *J Psychosom Res* 1993; **37**: 325–331.

52. Beck AT, Ward CH, Mendelson M. An inventory for measuring depression. *Arch Gen Psych* 1961; **4**: 561–571.

53. Radloff LS. CES-D scale: A self-report depression scale for research in the general population. *Appl Psychol Meas* 1977; **1**: 385–401.

54. Friedberg F, Krupp LB. A comparison of cognitive behavioral treatment of chronic fatigue syndrome and primary depression. *Clin Infect Dis* 1994; **18**(S1): 105–110.

55. Butler S, Chalder T, Ron M *et al*. Cognitive behaviour therapy in CFS. *J Neurol Neurosurg Psychiatry* 1991; **54**: 153–158.

56. Weinshenker BG, Penman M, Bass B. A double-blind, randomized, crossover trial of pemoline in fatigue associated with multiple sclerosis. *Neurology* 1992; **42**: 1468–1471.

57. Rosenberg GA, Appenzeller O. Amantadine, fatigue, and multiple sclerosis. *Arch Neurol* 1988; **45**: 1104–1106.

58. Polman CH, Bertelsmann FW, van Loenen AC *et al*. 4-Aminopyridine in the treatment of patients with multiple sclerosis: long-term efficacy and safety. *Arch Neurol* 1994; **51**: 292–296.

59. Sheean G, Murray N, Rothwell J *et al*. An open labelled clinical and electrophysiological study of 3,4 Diaminopyridine in the treatment of fatigue in multiple sclerosis. *J Neurol* 1996; **6** (suppl 2): 243.

60. Minden SL, Schiffer R. Affective disorders in multiple sclerosis. *Arch Neurol* 1990; **47**: 98–104.

22

Assessing the quality of life of patients with multiple sclerosis

Lilian EMA Pfennings, Leo Cohen and Henk M Van der Ploeg

Introduction

'Susan is 31 years old and is living with John, who is 30 years old. She was recently told that she had MS. Suddenly Susan's (and John's) future was very unsure. They alternately felt confused, angry and sad. Many questions crossed their minds. Could they ever start a family? Would it be possible to stay at work? Would she be in a wheelchair or, even worse, be bed-bound within a few years?

Susan decided to stay at work as long as possible. She had a price to pay, however. When she came home she was very fatigued, so time and energy to meet friends, family and colleagues were limited. An attendant problem is that her friends did not know how to react. They were used to old people with a chronic disease, but not to a chronically ill person of their own age.'

This chapter provides information necessary for the judgment of publications on quality of life (QoL) in multiple sclerosis (MS) and for carrying out studies in this field. Since understanding the concept of QoL is essential in measuring QoL in MS patients, the first part of the chapter consists of general information on the concept of QoL and its measurement. In the second part information specific to MS is provided. The literature on QoL in MS is reviewed and practical guidelines in the measurement of QoL in persons with MS are described. The problems which may arise from the measurement are then outlined. The last part of the chapter deals with the issue how QoL in MS can be improved.

The concept of QoL

Most researchers acknowledge that QoL has three characteristics: (1) multi-factoriality; (2) self-administration; and (3) subjectivity. The first characteristic refers to the idea that QoL consists of several dimensions. Unfortunately, no consensus exists as to the dimensions and the number of dimensions which have to be measured. In the eight articles concerning QoL in MS, which are described in detail on pp. 301–306 the number of QoL domains varies from three to five, which corresponds with the number of dimensions mentioned by most researchers. Vickrey *et al.*[1] mention that 'health-related quality of life is a multidimensional construct that includes physical, mental and social health'. Lankhorst *et al.*[2] add functional health to Vickrey's definition of QoL. Rudick *et al.*[3] give no definition of QoL, but in their standardized interview they use questions grouped in four clusters: functional and economic, social and recreational, affect and life in general, and medical problems. Aronson[4] views QoL as consisting of five components: health, job or major activity, housing, finances, and family and friendships. Some researchers add a dimension involving economic status and economic factors, which is inappropriate in assessing QoL in clinical trials but might be useful in studies concerning cost-effectiveness.[5]

The second (self-administered) and the third characteristic (subjective) of the QoL paradigm are closely linked. The use of methods of self-administration fits in with the idea that QoL is a personal (subjective) perception which can be measured only by determining the opinions of the patient. The perception of a situation is strongly influenced by a person's values and norms. Through these the same circumstance can be perceived totally differently by different persons.

In this chapter we will use the following definition of QoL: *the status of a person as judged by himself/herself in three important domains of life: physical, psychological and social functioning*. In this definition physical functioning refers to impairments and disabilities as perceived by a patient. Frequently posed questions related to physical functioning concern strength, energy, and the ability to carry on expected normal activities. These questions approximate most nearly to the outcome measures traditionally used by physicians. The psychological parameters most often measured are anxiety, depression and fear.[5] Sometimes questions are posed concerning the underlying pattern of emotions at the time of diagnosis, at the approaching of reassessment or in moments of diagnostic and therapeutic uncertainty.[5] When assessing the psychological status of a patient it is very important to ask the patient himself/herself, because doctors involved in traditional medical care appeared to be poor estimators of a patient's psychological state.[5] The moderate correlations with reports from patients themselves on their psychological functioning might be attributed to the less observable nature of the psychological functioning compared to physical functioning, or to the shortage of attention doctors pay to the psychological status of their patients. Social functioning not only relates to social support and contacts with other people, but also to role fulfilment. Within social interaction social contacts are often seen as a hierarchy:[5] family, close friends, work, vocational associates, and general community. Role fulfilment refers to the extent to which a person fulfils his/her role as a father, mother, husband, wife, neighbour, etc.

Measurement of QoL

QoL assessment is suitable for both patient care and clinical trial purposes, although one gets the impression from the literature that it is used more in clinical trials. In patient care QoL can be used to monitor the effectiveness of treatment of individuals. This is useful since there is often a discrepancy between the QoL as assessed by the patient and by the treating physician.[6–8] It appears that physicians often underestimate the difficulties which patients have with the activities of daily living and basic social routines.[6] Measuring QoL can provide them with a better insight into the lives of their patients and can thereby lead to improved patient care. Besides, the use of QoL assessment fits in with the development in medicine to give more attention to the patient as a whole, instead of just taking care of physical problems. In clinical trials QoL is – next to physiological and other parameters – used to evaluate the effectiveness of treatment among groups. By using QoL as an outcome the subjective perception of the drug by a patient can be taken into account. This might be important for drugs with few side effects. A patient may judge side effects on psychological functioning to be more important than better physical functioning.

Methods of measurement

Direct observations, face-to-face interviews, telephone interviews, and self-administered questionnaires, as well as interviewer-supervised questionnaires, are used to assess QoL.[9] Many researchers prefer the use of questionnaires, probably because they are less time consuming. QoL questionnaires are divided into two groups: general and specific instruments.[10] General QoL instruments are designed for use across a wide range of populations. They have the advantage that results gathered with them can be compared across (patient) populations. A drawback is that they are not always adequately focused on the specific problems of a particular (patient) population.[11] Specific scales are developed for use in a specific group and can be

- disease-specific (e.g. MS, diabetes mellitus)
- function-specific (e.g. sexual or emotional)
- population-specific (e.g. geriatric, chronic diseases).

Due to the multidimensional character of QoL, a function-specific questionnaire which only addresses one aspect of QoL can hardly be called a QoL questionnaire.

General versus specific instruments

The Sickness Impact Profile,[12–14] the Nottingham Health Profile[15] and the Medical Outcome Study Short Form-36[16–18] are well-known examples of general QoL instruments. The Sickness Impact Profile is a behaviourally based measure, which consists of 136 items grouped into 12 categories (see *Table 22.1*). The categories ambulation, mobility, and body care and movement can be aggregated into a physical dimension. The psychosocial dimension consists of the categories social inter-action, alertness behaviour, emotional behaviour and communication. The Sickness Impact Profile is meant to be answered by the respondent about himself, either self-administered or interviewer-administered.

The items of the Nottingham Health Profile are based on patient-generated statements. The profile consists of two parts. Part I is concerned with problems of health and consists of 38 items which fall into six areas: sleep, physical mobility, energy, pain, emotional reactions and social isolation (see *Table 22.2*). The second part consists of seven statements relating to areas of life which are most often affected by health: paid employment, looking after the house, social life, home life, sex life, hobbies and interests, and holidays.

The Medical Outcome Study Short Form-36 (SF-36) (36 refers to the number of items) was developed to represent eight of the most important health concepts: physical functioning, role limitations due to physical problems, bodily pain, general health perceptions, vitality, social functioning, role limitations due to emotional problems, and mental health (*see Table 22.3*). Many items are derived from instruments which have been in use for more than 20 years. The eight health concepts were chosen from more than 40 health concepts studied in the Medical Outcome Study.

The scores of the Sickness Impact Profile, the Nottingham Health Profile and the SF-36 are reflected in a so-called profile. In a profile, information concerning the different domains of QoL is preserved, since each domain is assigned a summary score. The domain summary scores can be compared to each other on a metric.[9] Information concerning the separate attribution of single domains is lost in a single index number in which the scores of all QoL domains are transformed into one score.

In addition to the general QoL questionnaires, there are many specific (disease,

Categories*	Illustrative items
I. Independent categories:	
Sleep and rest (7)	I sit during much of the day I sleep or nap during the day
Eating (9)	I am eating no food at all, nutrition is taken through tubes or intravenous fluids I am eating special or different food
Work (9)	I am not working at all I often act irritable toward my work associates
Home management (10)	I am not doing any of the maintenance or repair work around the house that I usually do I am not doing heavy work around the house
Recreation and pastimes (8)	I am going out for entertainment less I am not doing any of my usual physical recreation or activities
II Physical dimension:	
Ambulation (12)	I walk shorter distances or stop to rest often I do not walk at all
Mobility (10)	I stay within one room I stay away from home only for brief periods of time
Body care and movement (23)	I do not bathe myself at all, but am bathed by someone else I am very clumsy in body movements
III. Psychosocial dimension:	
Social interaction (20)	I am doing fewer social activities with groups of people I isolate myself as much as I can from the rest of the family
Alertness behaviour (10)	I have difficulty reasoning and solving problems, for example, making plans, making decisions, learning new things I sometimes behave as if I were confused or disoriented in place or time, for example, where I am, who is around, directions, what day it is
Emotional behaviour (9)	I laugh or cry suddenly I act irritable and impatient with myself, for example, talk badly about myself, swear at myself, blame myself for things that happen
Communication (9)	I am having trouble writing or typing I do not speak clearly when I am under stress

*Figures in parentheses are the number of items in the category

Table 22.1
Subscales and illustrative items from the Sickness Impact Profile (SIP) (adapted from Bergner, 1981).[14]

Subscales*	Illustrative items
Physical mobility (8)	I have trouble getting up and down stairs or steps I can only walk indoors
Pain (8)	I'm in pain when I walk I have pain at night
Sleep (5)	I'm waking up in the early hours of the morning It takes me a long time to get to sleep
Energy (3)	I soon run out of energy Everything is an effort
Social isolation (5)	I'm finding it hard to make contact with people I feel there is nobody I am close to
Emotional reactions (9)	I'm feeling on edge I've forgotten what it's like to enjoy myself

*Figures in parentheses are the number of items in the subscale

Table 22.2
*Subscales and illustrative items from the
Nottingham Health Profile (NHP).*

function or population-specific) QoL questionnaires. Such scales have been developed in the specific group under study (e.g. MS patients, geriatric patients), and ask about problems or symptoms specific to that group. Therefore they are usually more sensitive. For example, the European Organization for Research and Treatment of Cancer has developed a questionnaire specifically for cancer patients[19] which includes items concerning adverse effects of chemo- and radiotherapy, such as nausea, vomiting and constipation; questions which are very relevant to people with cancer.

Proxies

An alternative way of measuring QoL is by using proxies. Proxies are people who are living in the direct environment of the patient, such as a spouse, significant other or a health care provider (in case the patient is living in an institution). Their opinion of the QoL of the patient is especially valuable when the patient is not able to give his own opinion. Information concerning the use of proxies in the QoL assessment in MS patients is not available.

Although few findings were unequivocal,

Subscales*	Items
Physical functioning (10)	The following items are about activities you might do during a typical day. Does your health now limit you in these activities? If so, how much? • lifting or carrying groceries • climbing one flight of stairs
Role-physical functioning (4)	During the past four weeks, have you had any of the following problems with your work or other regular daily activities as a result of your physical health? • cut down the amount of time you spent on work or other activities • accomplished less than you would like
Bodily pain (2)	How much bodily pain have you had during the past four weeks?
General health (5)	How true or false is each of the following statements for you? • I seem to get sick a little easier than other people
Vitality (4)	How much of the time during the past four weeks ... • did you have a lot of energy? • did you feel worn out?
Social functioning (2)	During the past four weeks, how much of the time has your physical health or emotional problems interfered with your social activities (like visiting friends, relatives, etc.)?
Role-emotional functioning (3)	During the past four weeks, have you had any of the following problems with your work or other regular daily activities as a result of any emotional problems (such as feeling depressed or anxious? • cut down the amount of time you spent on work or other activities • accomplished less than you would like
Mental health (5)	How much of the time during the past four weeks ... • have you felt calm and peaceful? • have you been a happy person?

*Figures in parentheses are the number of items in the subscale

Table 22.3
Subscales and illustrative items from the MOS SF-36.

Sprangers and Aaronson[6] identified five trends in the literature on proxy ratings. The first trend is that proxies, in general, tend to underestimate patients' quality of life. Secondly, proxy ratings of more observable domains such as physical functioning, and activities of daily living are highly correlated with reports from the patients themselves. Reports of psychological functioning and satisfaction with health, less observable domains, are more moderately correlated. Third, health care providers tend to underestimate the pain intensity of their patients. A fourth trend is that health care providers and significant others appear to evaluate patients' quality of life with a comparable degree of accuracy. Depending on the domain of QoL to be rated, health care providers or significant others may give the most accurate rating. Health care providers may be better raters of a patients' physical status, while significant others may be more accurate in assessing patient's psychological and social status. Finally, significant others' ratings tend to be more accurate when they live in close proximity to the patient. However, perceived burden of care-giving and the number of hours the significant other spends helping the patient has been found to affect adversely the proxy's ability to rate accurately the patient's functional status.

Studies concerning QoL in MS

Considering the prevalence of MS (in Western Europe 100 cases per 100,000 adults and in the USA 58 per 100,000) surprisingly little research has been done into the QoL in MS. In 1990 Brownscombe[20] published an abstract on the development of an MS-specific QoL measure. The instrument consisting of 155 items was tested in 50 MS patients. Since then no publications on this instrument have appeared in the literature.

Eighteen articles were retrieved in Medline (1992–October 1996) by using the MESH-Headings 'quality of life' and 'multiple sclerosis'. Fifteen articles were excluded from consideration: one article was written in Finnish, in six articles QoL appeared neither in the title nor in the abstract, and in eight articles QoL was not the main focus of the article. The remaining three articles focused on QoL in MS. Furthermore colleagues brought five recently published articles on the topic to our attention. Assessment of the quality of these eight articles was performed by using nine criteria based on the publications of Deyo,[21] Ter Riet *et al.*,[22] Van der Horst *et al.*[23] and Beckerman *et al.*[24]

- Is a research question or a hypothesis formulated?
- Is a definition of quality of life given?
- Are the variables clearly and unambiguously defined? (apart from the concept QoL)
- Are criteria for inclusion and exclusion reported?
- Is the sample described?
- Is the sample size given?
- Is there a statement about the reliability and validity of the measuring methods?
- Are the statistical methods used substantiated?
- Is the answer to the research question a logical conclusion of the research?

The assessment, which of course remains a matter of judgment, of the quality of the eight selected studies, is presented in *Table 22.4*. The content of these articles is described below. Within each description four parts can be distinguished. There is a description of the QoL instrument and its psychometric properties, the sample, the results of the study and our comments on the study.

Study	Assessment criteria								
	1	2	3	4	5	6	7	8	9
Rudick et al., 1992[3]	+	−	+	±	+	±	±	±	±
Vickrey et al., 1995[1]	+	±	+	±	+	+	+	+	±
Schwartz et al., 1995[26]	*	−	±	*	*	*	*	*	*
Brunet et al., 1996[28]	+	+	+	−	+	+	+	+	+
Cella et al., 1996[27]	+	+	+	−	+	+	+	+	+
Lankhorst et al., 1996[2]	+	±	+	±	+	+	±	+	+
Freeman et al., 1996[30]	+	−	+	+	+	+	±	+	+
Aronson, 1997[4]	+	+	+	±	+	+	−	+	+

Notes for assessment criteria
1. Is a research question or a hypothesis formulated?
2. Is a definition of quality of life given?
3. Are the variables clearly and unambiguously defined? (apart from the concept QoL)
4. Are criteria for in- and exclusion reported?
5. Is the population described?
6. Is the sample size described?
7. Is there a statement about the reliability and validity of the measuring methods?
8. Are the statistical methods used substantiated?
9. Is the answer to the research question a logical conclusion of the research?
+ Completely satisfies the assessment criterion
± Partly satisfies the assessment criterion
− Satisfies the assessment criterion hardly or not at all
* Not applicable

Table 22.4
Assessment of the quality of the studies concerning QoL in MS.

Rudick et al., 1992

Rudick *et al.*[3] used an instrument designed to evaluate QoL for persons with chronic illnesses, the Farmer QoL Index. By deleting six questions the instrument was modified for the study in MS patients. In its modified form it was administered as a structured interview consisting of 41 questions in four subscales: functional and economic scale (12 questions), social and recreational scale (14 questions), affect and life in general scale (11 questions) and a medical problems scale (4 questions). Reliability and validity data for the modified version are not provided. The psychometric properties of the original Farmer QoL Index were evaluated in patients with inflammatory bowel disease. It was found to have high test–retest and inter-rater reliability; correlation coefficients ranged between 0.75 and 0.95 for individual test items.

The results of 68 MS patients were compared to those of 162 patients with inflammatory bowel disease and 75 patients with rheumatoid arthritis. It was found that the QoL in MS patients was much lower than in inflammatory bowel disease and rheumatoid arthritis patients. The results of the MS patients show that Kurtzke's Expanded Disability Status Scale (EDSS)[25] correlated strongly with the medical problems score. Duration of MS appeared to be unrelated to QoL scores. Furthermore the results suggested that in MS patients vision is strongly negatively related to QoL. Since patients were included in the study if they had a definite diagnosis of MS and disease duration of at least 10 years, the results of the study are based on a subgroup of the MS population.

Vickrey et al., 1995

Vickrey *et al.*[1] developed the Multiple Sclerosis Quality of Life (MSQOL)-54 Instrument, an MS-specific QoL measure consisting of 54 items, based on the SF-36.[16–18] The items of the SF-36 were supplemented with 18 additional items in the following areas: health distress (four items), sexual function (four items), satisfaction with sexual function (one item), overall quality of life (two items), cognitive function (four items), energy (one item), pain (one item) and social function (one item). The psychometric properties of the MSQOL-54 were studied in a sample of 179 MS patients. Internal consistency reliability and test–retest reliability coefficients ranged from 0.67 to 0.96 which is considered moderate to high. The mean interval between test dates was 14 days. The construct validity of the MSQOL-54 was supported by the relationships between MSQOL-54 scale scores on the one hand, and self-reported disability and ambulation status, number of days unable to work or attend school, hospital admission, depressive symptoms and duration of MS, on the other.

As in the SF-36, the results of the MSQOL-54 are transformed scale scores ranging from 0 to 100, where high scores indicate better QoL. In comparison with the general US population the MS sample appeared to have worse scores on each of the scales. They have much lower scores on the two scales concerning physical functioning, a difference of 48 points. On the scales of pain and mental health there appeared to be just a small difference (less than 10 points); differences in the remaining scales vary from 20 to approximately 25 points. Standard deviations in the general US population varied from 34 and 33 for the role-physical functioning scale and the role-emotional functioning scale respectively to 18 for the mental health scale. Standard deviations for the remaining scales are between 20 and 24.

By using the SF-36 as a general core measure, comparisons of the QoL of MS patients to those of other patient groups and to the general population are possible. Norms are available among others for patients with hypertension, congestive heart failure, and diabetes type II. Another advantage is that the psychometric properties of the SF-36 have been well evaluated. For each scale, the median of the reliability coefficient (test–retest reliability or internal consistency) across studies equals or exceeds 0.80, with the exception of the Social Functioning scale. The validity of the SF-36 is studied by comparing it to other widely used survey forms, factor analytic tests, 'criterion-based' approaches (i.e. concurrent and predictive validity), and numerous correlational studies.[16]

Schwartz et al., 1995

Schwartz *et al.*[26] propose the use of the Q-TWIST methodology for MS. This methodology is meant for evaluating clinical interventions from the patient's perspective in terms of *Quality-adjusted Time Without Symptoms and Toxicities*. The methodology has not been fully developed at this moment. To extend the Q-TWIST methodology, which was originally developed for use in cancer patients, to MS the article proposes four steps. In step 1 *QoL dimensions have to be defined* which highlight specific aspects of the disease and treatment under study, and which consider the indirect costs of illness. The second step is to *develop sensitive measures* to assess the patient's status in each of the dimensions defined in the first step. The third step is to identify or develop *an instrument for assessing the importance of QoL dimensions* from the patient's perspective. The last step is to *determine appropriate time intervals* for administering these assessments. A range of values such as the resulting assessment data and importance weights are used to compute a Q-TWIST score for each treatment. In this method the emphasis seems to be on aspects of physical functioning, such as exacerbation and disease progression. In a hypothetical example described in the article, depression is the only variable concerning psychosocial morbidity. When applied in this way, the instrument does not fulfil the definition of QoL as described on p. 296. Furthermore, a precondition for this methodology is that *responsive* QoL instruments and instruments for assessing the *importance* of QoL dimensions are available. In summary, the Q-TWIST seems a promising methodology, but work remains to be done before it can be applied clinically.

Brunet et al., 1996

Brunet *et al.*[27] measured quality of life in a group of 97 MS patients using the SF-36. Compared to the general US population the patients scored low in three domains: physical functioning, role functioning due to physical functioning and energy/vitality. The relationship between patient characteristics, such as family history of MS, duration of MS, number of children, income, and assistance with the survey, and the subscales of the SF-36 was studied by means of regression analysis. A number of patient characteristics showed a relationship with the scores on the subscales of the SF-36. Of particular interest is a family history of MS which was associated with poorer physical and social functioning as well as more pain and less vitality.

In our view studying the relationship between patient characteristics and the quality of life in MS patients is very useful. It may indicate which patients will possibly have a low QoL and may be used to signal treatment needs.

Cella et al., 1996

Cella *et al.*[27] developed and validated a quality of life instrument consisting of 28 items from the general version of the Functional Assessment of Cancer Therapy quality of life instrument, plus 60 items generated by patients, care providers and literature review. The validation samples comprised a mail survey cohort ($n = 377$; response rate 74 per cent) and a clinical cohort ($n = 56$; response rate 100 per cent). By principal components and Rasch measurement model analyses the test length was reduced to 44 items, divided into six subscales: mobility, symptoms, emotional well-being (depression), general contentment, thinking/fatigue, and family/social well-being. The mobility subscale was strongly predictive of Kurtzke's EDSS. Reliability of the newly developed scale appeared to be good; internal consistency and test–retest coefficients varied respectively from 0.82 to 0.96 and from 0.85 to 0.91. Both sample cohorts provided evidence for content validity, concurrent validity and construct validity.

Lankhorst et al., 1996

Laman and Lankhorst developed the Disability and Impact Profile (DIP).[2,29] The DIP is a self-administered questionnaire covering a wide range of human activities which may be affected by a disabling disease. The DIP is based on the International Classification of Impairments, Disabilities and Handicaps and consists of 39 parallel questions about '(dis)ability' and 'impact'. It contains three symptom questions and 36 questions in five domains: mobility, self-care, social activities, communication and psychological status. The results are presented in a profile of weighted scores in which the 'disability' and 'impact' aspects of questions are taken into account. By using this profile of weighted scores it is possible to set priorities in the treatment of a patient which can be very useful in rehabilitation medicine. The reliability of the DIP was studied in 20 MS patients and found to be greater than 0.5 for 37 disability, 28 impact and 36 weighted scores. R is comparable to a measure of correlation. Concerning the validity, a close correlation between open-ended questions regarding the most negative consequences of the disease and low-weighted scores was found in rheumatoid arthritis and spinal cord injury patients.

In using the DIP in MS patients major disruptions of QoL (MD-QoL) defined as a loss on weighted score of more than 50 per cent were found. Group data from 73 MS patients showed an MD-QoL for 'clean home', 'work' and 'worry about deterioration'. In individual patients a median of 7 MD-QoL was found.[2] The DIP is used in MS, rheumatoid arthritis and spinal cord injury patients. Compared to rheumatoid arthritis and spinal cord injury, MS patients experience more problems in reading, memory, and concentration as measured by the mean weighted scores. Rating of the importance of a disability is viewed as a very positive point of the DIP, although in practice it may be difficult for patients to be precise in defining the importance of a disability.

Freeman et al., 1996

Freeman *et al.*[30] piloted the use of the SF-36 in 50 progressive MS patients. Assessment of disease severity, level of disability and the General Health Questionnaire were used for the evaluation of the SF-36. All participants in their study were admitted for a programme of inpatient neurorehabilitation. Results demonstrated that this specific group with moderate to severe disability has a low health-related quality of life compared to the general population, particularly concerning physical functioning and role functioning. Compared to four condition-specific groups – low back pain, menorrhagia, suspected peptic ulcer, and varicose veins – the MS patients showed lower scores in all subscales of the SF-36, except for pain. The SF-36 demonstrated marked floor effects in a number of dimensions, indicating that other scales, proven to be responsive to clinically significant change, are necessary in the evaluation of quality of life for this group. The authors acknowledge an important aspect of the measurement of outcome, i.e. responsiveness, which deserves more attention.

Aronson, 1997

Aronson[4] conducted a large survey in 697 MS patients and their care-givers in which questions concerning six components of QoL from a national survey in Canada were assessed: health, job or major activity, housing, finances, family and friendships, and QoL as a whole. Each component was measured by one item. These QoL questions were used previously in the General Social Survey conducted by Statistics Canada in 1985. No information on the reliability or validity of this instrument is provided.

Both health and job or major activity were rated as significantly less satisfactory by the MS patients compared to the care-givers. Employment status and household income were associated with QoL as a whole.

The results of the MS patients and their care-givers could be compared to the results of 1,692 disabled and 1,692 healthy persons who participated in the General Social Survey. In comparison with the disabled and the healthy group, persons with MS were less satisfied with health, job or major activity, and life as a whole. MS patients were more satisfied with housing and family relations than the disabled comparison group. Care-givers were less satisfied with finances and life as a whole, and more satisfied with housing, than the healthy persons. From the article it appears that each QoL component is measured by one question. In our view this can hardly be called a QoL questionnaire.

In summary in the last five years eight articles focusing on QoL in MS have been published. In a number of studies the SF-36 was used. The results of these studies with the SF-36 are fairly consistent and indicate that MS patients score poorly in a number of QoL domains, both in comparison with the general population and in comparison with patients with a different chronic disease. For the remaining studies, the diversity of instruments used makes it hard to compare their results. Much research concerning the QoL of MS patients therefore remains to be done. In the next section we provide some practical guidelines for future research to be conducted in this area.

Practical guidelines in measuring QoL in MS patients

The extensive ten-step schedule from Patrick and Erickson[31] is useful as a starting point for the assessment of QoL in general, consequently also for MS patients. Special notice will be given to steps 2, 3 and 6 which require particular attention in MS patients. The following paragraphs will describe the various steps.

(1) *Define the objectives of assessment.* Knowing the goal of the QoL assessment is important in the choice of a QoL instrument, since no instrument is suitable for all purposes. For most policy applications, or when two different patient groups have to be compared, general instruments are necessary. A disease-specific instrument may be more suitable and may give more information, e.g. when only MS patients are studied. Vickrey *et al.*[1] combined the advantages of both kinds of instrument in MS patients by using newly developed disease-specific questions in addition to the SF-36.

In measuring QoL three objectives can be distinguished: (*a*) discriminating among groups of persons at a single point in time; many QoL instruments have been designed and tested for this purpose; (*b*) predicting some future outcome on a 'gold standard'; in MS the EDSS might be the gold standard, although it has disadvantages like lack of sensitivity;[32] and (*c*) measuring changes over time, as is usually the case in a randomized clinical trial.[33] Since several new drugs, such as interferon and copolymer are currently being tested in MS, there certainly is a need for a responsive QoL measure (for 'responsiveness' see step 5).

(2) *Specify available resources* is a major practical consideration before selecting a QoL

assessment strategy. These resources include time, money and personnel. It is important to realize that the assessment of QoL generally requires more time than expected. In the case of MS, severely handicapped MS patients are often not able to complete a questionnaire without help. So, if one is interested in the QoL of the full spectrum of MS patients, one may need to assist severely handicapped patients in completing the questionnaires, either by filling in the questionnaire or by reading the questions aloud. This takes a lot of time and personnel (and thereby money).

(3) *Describe the population.* At least four characteristics of the population should be taken into account when selecting a QoL instrument. The first of these is the level of symptoms and disability. Healthy populations require different measures from ill populations. Several domains of HRQOL, such as physical functioning and self care may not be relevant for healthy people. When the level of symptoms and disability is very low, as can be the case in severely handicapped MS patients, it may be difficult to detect worsening health because of a floor effect. The reverse may happen for people with excellent health, which may be the case in recently diagnosed MS patients or patients with a benign form of MS, where a ceiling effect may arise. Secondly, age should be taken into account. Some questionnaires are developed for specific age groups, such as children or elderly people. Thirdly, the level of cognitive ability is important, especially in older or severely handicapped people. With such populations interviewer-administered questionnaires are recommended. Since in a community-based study and in a large clinic-based sample in MS patients 43 per cent and 59 per cent respectively appeared to be cognitively deteriorated,[34,35] it seems reasonable to make allowance for the level of cognitive ability in MS patients in the assessment of

QoL. A possible solution is to use a short screenings instrument, e.g. the Raven Progressive Matrices, for the detection of cognitive dysfunctioning.[9]

Finally, the ethnic or cultural identity should be considered. Beliefs, values and attitudes can influence answers on QoL questionnaires. It is important to study whether results gathered in different ethnic groups or different countries, as is the case in international clinical trials, are comparable. Much work on this topic remains to be done.

(4) *Conceptualize health-related QoL outcomes.* Treatment outcomes of the measurement have to be defined. They can be based on potential differences between two or more groups (as is the case in studies with a discriminative purpose), based on potential side effects of the treatment or outcomes of interest to patients, families, friends or clinicians. Since outcomes may be competing a main endpoint must be chosen. Generally a measure of disease or impairment (e.g. in the case of MS the EDSS) is chosen as a major endpoint, although QoL outcomes are increasingly used in combination with the major endpoint.

(5) *Assess methodological characteristics of potential measures.* A golden rule in choosing a QoL measure is that only validated and reliable scales should be used. For instruments which are used to measure change within subjects, as is the purpose of instruments used in clinical trials, it is important to look also at another psychometric property, i.e. responsiveness. Responsiveness is the property of an instrument to detect clinically important changes in the status of the patient.[36] This property of instruments is often overlooked.[37,38]

The chance that minor changes in the condition of a person will be detected when broad answer categories are defined is small. In the literature no clear recommendations for the optimal number of divisions in a rating scale are given. Research on the use of visual analogue scales is promising. They have been sensitive in the measurement of several subjective phenomena such as pain, well-being, mood, depression, and nausea.[39] Furthermore, they appear to have advantages like ease of administration, acceptance by respondents, and also perhaps more freedom to express a subjective experience than a set of restricted categories.[40] A visual analogue scale is a straight line, the ends of which are defined as the extreme limits of the sensation or response to be measured.[41] One responds to such a scale by placing a mark somewhere on the line.

(6) *Assess practical considerations and choose health-related QoL measures.* Aside from specifying resources such as the available amount of time, money and personnel (see step 2), other practical considerations should be taken into account. Acceptability of administration is an important issue. Three aspects can be discerned. One aspect involves how well an instrument satisfies research needs and resource constraints (research acceptability). At this moment three MS-specific QoL questionnaires are available: the MS Quality of Life-54,[1] the Functional Assessment of Multiple Sclerosis (FAMS)[27] and the Disability and Impact Profile.[2,29] If these instruments do not completely meet the needs requested, the development of a new assessment strategy can be considered. A second aspect relates to respondent burden, which is connected with length of response time and complexity of the questionnaire. Personal characteristics of respondents such as age and education level influence the length of response time. Respondent burden is a prominent issue in MS patients, since fatigue is a major problem in MS. In a recent study 40 per cent of MS patients listed fatigue as their most serious symptom.[42] A third aspect concerns the impact

of an instrument on an interviewer (amount and time of burden required).

(7) *Conduct a pre-test (5–25 administrations) or pilot study (>25 administrations).* This is a good opportunity to discover the practical problems of the study and the chosen QoL instrument, such as length of time the assessment takes to complete, respondents' reactions, and completeness of instruction. Furthermore, it is possible to gather some indicative data on reliability, validity and responsiveness.

(8) *Prepare data collection and analysis plans.* In the data analysis plans it should be described how each of the hypotheses is to be tested and which statistical tests should be used.

(9) *Collect data.* The major consideration in this step is to guarantee high quality of the data. Hopefully, many problems which were encountered in the pretest or pilot study will have been anticipated or eliminated. Standardization of procedures and monitoring of data collection are the major means to ensure the quality of the data.

(10) *Analyse and present findings.* Some QoL measures yield both an overall or summary score and component scores. Whenever possible, both kinds of scores should be presented to make clear the contribution of the individual components to the overall score.

Problems in measuring QoL in MS

At least three problems can be encountered in the assessment of QoL in MS patients. A major problem in the measurement is the lack of a clear definition of quality of life, as mentioned in the opening section. As a result, the many questionnaires which measure QoL differ in the number and the content of the domains they measure. The second and third problems occur mainly in longitudinal studies.[43] The second problem is called 'response shift'. This refers to the fact that the values and norms of a patient, which play a role in the judgment of QoL, can change in the course of time. For example, a wheelchair may be unacceptable for a person with MS who has minor walking problems. When this patient in the course of time develops major problems in walking a wheelchair may be seen as a very good and acceptable solution. Response shift can be a source of uncertainty: a change in scores can be attributed to a change in the status of the patient or to the response shift which took place. The third problem is that in the course of a study patients sometimes become too ill to complete the questionnaires. This is called selective patient drop-out. This phenomenon can be expected when severely disabled MS patients participate, which can be important in covering the whole range of MS patients, or persons with a fast course of MS participate. It can be compensated for by the use of proxy ratings. However, as mentioned before, proxy ratings have several disadvantages.

How to influence quality of life in MS

Since there is a lack of literature into QoL in MS patients, it is hard to say how the QoL of patients with MS can be influenced. Because in many of the studies described on pp. 299–301 a different QoL measure and different comparison groups are used the seven studies in which results concerning the QoL of MS patients are presented[1,3,4,27–30] are difficult to compare. Conclusions concerning how to influence the QoL cannot be drawn from these studies.

The availability of responsive measures for MS patients is a precondition for the measurement of effects. It might be that one of the recently available QoL measures is capable of measuring small changes in MS. With the exception of Vickrey *et al.*[1] and Freeman *et al.*[30] none of the studies mentioned above give an indication of the responsiveness of MS patients of the measure used. More research is needed in this field.

'Susan is 41 years old now. A lot has happened in the last ten years. The MS gradually worsened, but by being confronted day in day out with MS she accepted and integrated MS into her life. For the past five years she has been working three afternoons and this has resulted in more energy to meet and visit other people. John also learned how to live with a wife with MS.

Some of the friends of ten years before disappeared from their lives, others stayed, and new people whom they knew from the MS Society entered into their lives. In the last ten years her norms and values changed and she judges her physical functioning higher than ten years before, although her EDSS score increased from 2.0 to 5.5. Since she has learned how to handle MS, feelings of shame no longer limit her in her social contacts.'

References

1. Vickrey BG, Hays RD, Harooni R *et al*. A health-related quality of life measure for multiple sclerosis. *Qual Life Res* 1995; **4**: 187–206.
2. Lankhorst GJ, Jelles F, Smits RCF *et al*. Quality of life in multiple sclerosis: the disability and impact profile (DIP). *J Neurol* 1996; **243**: 469–474.
3. Rudick RA, Miller D, Clough JD *et al*. Quality of life in multiple sclerosis. *Arch Neurol* 1992; **49**: 1237–1242.
4. Aronson KJ. Quality of life among persons with multiple sclerosis and their care givers. *Neurol* 1997; **48**: 1–7.
5. Schipper H, Clinch JJ, Olweny CLM. Quality of life studies: Definitions and conceptual issues. In: Spilker B, ed. *Quality of Life and Pharmacoeconomics in Clinical Trials*, Philadelphia: Lippincott–Raven Publishers 1996; 11–24.
6. Sprangers MAG, Aaronson NK. The role of health care providers and significant others in evaluating the quality of life of patients with chronic disease: a review. *J Clin Epidem* 1992; **45**: 743–760.
7. Slevin MR, Plant H, Lynch D *et al*. Who should measure quality of life, the doctor or the patient? *Br J Cancer* 1988; **57**: 109–112.
8. Lankhorst GJ. Quality of life: an exploratory study. *Int J Rehab Res* 1989; **12**(2): 201–203.
9. Patrick DL, Erickson P. *Health Status and Health Policy*, New York: Oxford University Press 1993.
10. Patrick DL, Deyo RA. Generic and disease-specific measures in assessing health status and quality of life. *Med Care* 1989; **27** (suppl 3): S217–S232.
11. Guyatt GH, Jaeschke R, Feeny DH *et al*. Measurements in clinical trials: Choosing the right approach. In: Spilker B, ed. *Quality of Life and Pharmacoeconomics in Clinical Trials*, Philadelphia: Lippincott–Raven Publishers 1996; 41–48.
12. Bergner M, Bobbit RA, Kressel S *et al*. The Sickness Impact Profile: conceptual formulation and methodology for the development of a health status measure. *Int J Health Serv* 1976; **6**: 393–415.
13. Bergner M, Bobbit RA, Pollard WE *et al*. The Sickness Impact Profile: validation of a health status measure. *Med Care* 1976; **14**: 57–67.
14. Bergner M, Bobbit RA, Carter WB *et al*. The Sickness Impact Profile: development and final revision of a health status measure. *Med Care* 1981; **1**: 787–805.
15. Hunt SM, McEwen J, McKenna SP. *Measuring Health Status*, London: Croom Helm 1986.
16. Ware JE, Snow KK, Kosinski M *et al*. *SF-36 Health Survey. Manual and Interpretation Guide*, Boston: Nimrod Press 1993.
17. Ware JE, Sherbourne CD. The MOS 36-item short-form health survey (SF-36). I. Conceptual framework and item selection. *Med Care* 1992; **30**: 473–483.
18. McHorney CA, Ware JE, Raczek AE. The MOS 36-item short-form health survey (SF-36): II. Psychometric and clinical tests of validity in measuring physical and mental health constructs. *Med Care* 1993; **31**: 247–263.
19. Aaronson NK, Ahmedzai S, Bergman B *et al*. The European Organization for Research and Treatment of Cancer QLQ-C30: A quality of life instrument for use in international clinical trials in oncology. *J Nat Cancer Inst* 1993; **85**: 365–376.
20. Brownscombe I, Laupacis A, Rice GPA *et al*. Development of a disease-specific quality-of-life measure for multiple sclerosis. *Neurol* 1990; **40** (suppl 1): S142.
21. Deyo RA. Conservative therapy for chronic low back pain. Distinguishing useful from useless therapy. *J Am Med Ass* 1983; **250**: 1057–1062.
22. Ter Riet G, Kleijnen J, Knipschild P. De meta-analyse als review-methode [Meta-analysis as a review method] *Huisarts en Wetenschap* 1989; **32**: 176–181.
23. Van der Horst HE, Eijk JThM van, Schellevis FG. New insights into irritable bowel syn-

drome. A literature study. *Fam Practice* 1992; **9**: 405–414.

24. Beckerman H, Lankhorst GJ, Verbeek ALM *et al*. The effects of phenol nerve and muscle blocks in treating spasticity: review of the literature. *Crit Rev Phys Rehab Med* 1996, **8**: 111–124.

25 Kurtzke JF. A proposal for a uniform minimal record of disability in multiple sclerosis. *Acta Neurol Scand* 1981; **64** (suppl 87): 110–129.

26. Schwartz CE, Cole BF, Gelber RD. Measuring patient-centered outcomes in neurological disease. Extending the Q-TWiST method. *Arch Neurol* 1995; **52**: 754–762.

27. Cella DF, Dineen K, Arnason B *et al*. Validation of the Functional Assessment of Multiple Sclerosis quality of life instrument. *Neurol* 1996; **47**: 129–139.

28. Brunet DG, Hopman WM, Singer MA *et al*. Measurement of health-related quality of life in multiple sclerosis patients. *Can J Neurol Sci* 1996; **23**: 99–103.

29. Laman H, Lankhorst GJ. Subjective weighting of disability: an approach to quality of life assessment in rehabilitation. *Disabil Rehabil* 1994; **4**: 198–204.

30. Freeman JA, Langdon DW, Hobart JC *et al*. Health-related quality of life in people with multiple sclerosis undergoing inpatients rehabilitation. *J Neuro Rehab* 1996; **10**: 185–194.

31. Patrick DL, Erickson P. Assessing health-related quality of life for clinical decision making. In: Walker SR, Rosser RM, eds. *Quality of Life Assessment: Key Issues in the 1990s*, Lancaster: Kluwer Academic Publishers 1993; 11–63.

32. Willoughby EW, Paty DW. Scales for rating impairment in multiple sclerosis: A critique. *Neurol* 1988; **38**: 1793–1798.

33. Kirshner B, Guyatt G. A methodological framework for assessing health indices. *J Chron Dis* 1985; **38**(1): 27–36.

34. Rao SM, Leo GJ, Bernardin L *et al*. Cognitive dysfunction in multiple sclerosis. I. Frequency, patterns, and prediction. *Neurol* 1991; **41**: 685–691.

35. Heaton RK, Nelson LM, Thompson DS *et al*. Neuropsychological findings in relapsing–remitting and chronic progressive multiple sclerosis. *J Consult Clin Psychol* 1985; **53**: 103–110.

36. Guyatt G, Walter S, Norman G. Measuring change over time: Assessing the usefulness of evaluative instruments. *J Chron Dis* 1987; **40**: 171–178.

37. Guyatt GH, Deyo RA, Charlson M *et al*. Responsiveness and validity in health status measurement: A clarification. *J Clin Epidem* 1989; **42**: 403–408.

38. Pfennings L, Cohen L, Van der Ploeg H. Preconditions for sensitivity in measuring change: visual analogue scales compared to rating scales in a Likert format. *Psychol Rep* 1995; **77**: 475–480.

39. Cella DF, Perry SW. Reliability and concurrent validity of three visual-analogue mood scales. *Psychol Rep* 1986; **59**: 827–833.

40. Aitken RCB. Measurement of feelings using visual analogue scales. *Proc Roy Soc Med* 1969; **62**: 989–993.

41. Scott J, Huskinson EC. Graphic representation of pain. *Pain* 1976; **2**: 175–184.

42. Murray TJ. Amantadine therapy for fatigue in multiple sclerosis. *Can J Neurol Sci* 1985; **12**: 251–254.

43. Sprangers MAG, Aaronson NK, van Dam FSAM. Onderzoek naar de kwaliteit van leven [Studying the quality of life]. *Tijdschrift Kanker* 1993; **17**(6): 245–247.

23

Is inpatient rehabilitation effective in multiple sclerosis?

Jennifer A Freeman and Alan J Thompson

Introduction

Inpatient rehabilitation is advocated as an important intervention in the overall management of multiple sclerosis (MS).[1] Constant demands to increase service provision in this area are made by patients, therapists and the neurological charities. Inpatient rehabilitation is, however, costly its effectiveness has not been established, and little is known about the long-term carry-over of benefit. This information is fundamental in enabling evidence-based clinical decision making and ensuring continued improvements in patient management.[2]

Evidence about the effectiveness of interventions can be at different levels. The clinical experience of a wide range of doctors, nurses, therapists and patients provides some evidence to support the effectiveness of inpatient rehabilitation in MS. This is reflected by the large number of articles and textbooks which describe the rehabilitation process and provide anecdotal reports of its success.[3,4] Such evidence alone is inadequate. Effectiveness needs to be established in a scientifically acceptable manner.

This chapter addresses the question 'is inpatient rehabilitation effective in patients with MS?' The inpatient rehabilitation process is briefly described. Some of the methodological complexities involved in designing studies in this area are considered. A review of trials evaluating the effectiveness, and subsequent carry-over, of comprehensive inpatient rehabilitation is undertaken and suggestions for future studies are discussed.

The rehabilitation process

Inpatient rehabilitation is an integral part of the comprehensive health care management of MS. Its primary aim is to achieve the best possible quality of life for the person within the limits of their disease.[5] This is accomplished by:

- providing a comprehensive assessment of physical, social and psychological needs
- promoting physical, psychological and social adaptation to disability and handicap
- facilitating independence in daily activities
- preventing secondary complications such as contractures and pressure areas
- empowerment.

The process of inpatient rehabilitation has been described by a number of authors.[6–12] While no two centres appear to practise or deliver comprehensive care in an identical way, the literature demonstrates that a commonality of practice exists. The key elements are identified as:

- a multidisciplinary team approach
- interventions tailored to meet the individual's needs
- a patient-centred, functional, goal-setting approach.

Differences in service provision and delivery do exist, however. The structure and funding mechanism of individual health care systems appears to have a major influence on the model of care provided in each country. For example, in some countries patients with MS are routinely offered inpatient treatment on an annual basis,[13] whereas in others patients are selectively admitted according to current needs. Differences in the availability of specialist MS facilities (inpatient and outpatient) are also apparent. These were highlighted in a survey undertaken by the International Federation of Multiple Sclerosis Societies.[14] Of the 26 countries surveyed, 25 countries offered general consultation services, but only 16 provided specialty outpatient care, and 11 specialist inpatient care.

A further difference in service provision is the selection process for admission to inpatient rehabilitation. We believe that the selection process is critical to the efficacy of this service. In our view multidisciplinary assessment, to determine who will benefit from inpatient rehabilitation, underlies its success. Integral to this process is the identification of areas of potential improvement and the establishment of achievable goals, agreed by both the patient and the team, prior to admission.[15] Currently this practice is based on clinical judgement since no guidelines exist as to who benefits most from inpatient rehabilitation.

Methodological complexities in undertaking trials of rehabilitation in MS

A number of methodological problems are encountered when designing clinical studies both in the fields of rehabilitation[16–18] and MS.[19–23] Scientifically sound research which quantifies effectiveness, while remaining clinically relevant, is therefore particularly challenging. Some of these methodological difficulties are now outlined.

Measurement of change in a heterogenous population

Homogeneity of sample populations is recommended when designing outcome studies. This is difficult to achieve in MS, where a diversity of clinical manifestations is observed both in terms of disease course and clinical presentation. Furthermore, the chronic, progressive, variable and unpredictable nature of the disease course means that there is no stable point from which to make reference baseline measurements. This renders repeated assessments a formidable task. It is difficult to determine whether changes are a consequence of the intervention itself or the natural history of the underlying disease.

The nature of comprehensive inpatient rehabilitation

A clearly described and standardized intervention is required in order to conclusively attribute an outcome to a specific intervention.[24] Comprehensive inpatient rehabilitation, however, is an all-embracing concept with broad-ranging goals and varying interventions. Recognition of the diverse and ever-changing problems of people with MS means that programmes are tailored to the needs of individuals. Precisely defined standardized interventions are hence not only difficult, but often inappropriate, in a clinical context. In addition, unlike drug trials, no agreed selection criteria exist for admitting patients for inpatient rehabilitation.

Choice of appropriate outcomes and measurement instruments

The quality of outcome data is determined by the choice of appropriate outcomes and the quality of the measurement instruments used to produce it. The use of clinically relevant, psychometrically evaluated instruments, is essential to interpret study results confidently.[25,26] Choosing and measuring appropriate outcomes, which accurately reflect the broad aims of the multidisciplinary rehabilitation programme, is difficult, however.[27] Medicine has traditionally measured the effectiveness of interventions with outcomes such as mortality, presence or absence of disease, and length of disease-free interval. While these outcomes are easy to substantiate, they are not relevant for rehabilitation, where the aim is not to cure, but to make improvements in more subjective dimensions such as disability, handicap and quality of life. Currently few comprehensively evaluated instruments have been found suitable to measure these domains.[18]

Attributing the outcome to the intervention

The large number of variables involved in MS rehabilitation makes attribution of the outcome to the intervention extremely complex.[22] Controlling within a trial for these confounding factors is often difficult, and at times impossible.[17] For example, the accomplishment of many of the goals of rehabilitation depends on factors outside the control of the rehabilitation programme. These include: family support, access to community services, provision of aids and equipment, and economic considerations. If these influences are working against patients, even the best conducted programme is vulnerable to not meeting its goals.[28] The converse can also be true. This means attribution to the intervention is not always clear.

An added complexity is that the consequences of the service may take some time to become apparent. Knowledge of the carry-over of changes once the patient is discharged home, is crucial. Disregarding this can lead to a misinterpretation of the effectiveness of interventions, either suggesting the programme had not been effective when it had, or that it was effective when review in the longer term demonstrated otherwise.[28] No guidelines currently exist as to the appropriate times over which interventions should be evaluated.

These factors illustrate why research in the gold standard format of double-blind randomized placebo-controlled studies is extremely difficult to achieve in neurorehabilitation. It partly explains why relatively few studies have been attempted in this subject.

Studies evaluating comprehensive inpatient rehabilitation

Considering the widespread use and availability of inpatient rehabilitation in MS, relatively few studies have objectively evaluated its efficacy. Unfortunately the interpretation of many of these studies is limited by their design (*Table 23.1*). For example, most gathered data retrospectively from databases, using a single group, pre- and post-treatment design, with small sample sizes. In the main, assessments were undertaken on admission and discharge, with relatively little attention made to the duration of benefits. Despite these limitations, valuable information has been gathered, and improvements in methodology have been made.

Numerous questions arise when considering how effective the inpatient rehabilitation process is in MS. Some of these questions have been addressed more fully than others. The following is a review of these studies.

Reference	Trial method	Sample (n)	Main outcomes/instruments	Timing of assessments
Feigenson et al., 1981[29]	Prospective, single group, pre- and post study design	20	Impairment, disability and handicap: MS Functional Profile (a modified version of BUSTOP) Costs of intervention	Admission and discharge Costs were also measured at 12 months (by telephone interview)
Greenspun et al., 1987[31]	Retrospective, single group, pre- and post study design	28	Disability: CRDS	Admission, discharge, and three month review (by telephone if necessary)
Reding and La Rocca, 1987[37]	Retrospective study, using case matched analysis	20 pairs	Disability: ISS Hospital re-admission rate Cost of intervention The need for home help assistance	Review at 16 months (by telephone)
Carey and Seibert, 1988[30]	Retrospective multi-centre study assessing a range of conditions. Single group, pre- and post study design	6,194 of whom 196 had MS	Disability: LORS-II	Admission and discharge
Francabandera et al., 1988[38]	Prospective, stratified randomized study	84	Disability: ISS Need for home assistance (hours)	Admission, and at three monthly intervals for two years (three month results reported in this publication)
Kidd et al., 1995[32]	Prospective, single group, pre- and post study design	79	Impairment: DSS Disability: Barthel Index Handicap: ESS	Admission and discharge
Aisen et al., 1996[34]	Retrospective, single group, pre- and post study design	37	Impairment: FSS and EDSS Disability: FIM	Admission, discharge and telephone follow up (from between 6–36 months post discharge)
Kidd and Thompson, 1997[35]	Prospective, single group, pre- and post study design	47	Impairment: EDSS Disability: FIM Handicap: ESS	Admission, discharge and three month follow up
Freeman et al., (1997, in press)[33]	Stratified, randomized, wait-list controlled study design	66 (all in the progressive stage)	Impairment: FS and EDSS Disability: FIM Handicap: LHS	Baseline and six weeks
Freeman et al. 1997[36]	Prospective, single group, longitudinal study design	50 (all in the progressive stage)	Impairment: FS and EDSS Disability:FIM Handicap: LHS Quality of life: SF-36 Emotional well-being: GHQ-28	Admission, discharge and at three monthly intervals for one year

BUSTOP = Burke Stroke Time-oriented Profile; CRDS = Computerised Rehabilitation and Data System; DSS = Disability Status Scale; EDSS = Expanded Disability Status Scale; ESS = Environmental Status Scale; FIM = Functional Independence Measure; LORS-II = Revised Level of Rehabilitation Scale; FS = Functional Systems; ISS = Incapacity Status Scale; LHS = London Handicap Scale; SF-36 = Short Form 36 Health Survey Questionnaire; GHQ-28 = 28 item General Health Questionnaire.

Table 23.1
Summary of outcome studies of comprehensive inpatient rehabilitation in people with MS.

Is comprehensive inpatient rehabilitation effective in MS?

Feigenson and colleagues[29] were among the first to publish evidence about the efficacy of comprehensive inpatient rehabilitation in MS. They used a prospective, single group, pre- and post-treatment design. The sample consisted of 20 patients, with long-standing disability, all of whom had failed to respond to regular intensive multidisciplinary outpatient treatment; 19 of the 20 patients were female with a mean age of 44.8 years (range 22–62), and disease duration of 12.9 years (range 1–25 years). Following an average length of stay of 52.6 days, statistically significant improvements were noted in seven different functional areas: balance, self care activities, bed mobility, transfers, wheelchair management, homemaking skills and real-life activities. In addition the amount of help required to maintain patients at home was 'substantially decreased' for the entire year following rehabilitation. No significant change in any impairments was demonstrated, suggesting that spontaneous natural recovery (or deterioration) in neurological dysfunction had not occurred during the study period. Cost-benefit analysis was also undertaken. Following an initial assessment, crude estimates of the cost of care prior to rehabilitation were made by the treating team. The cost of rehabilitation was abstracted from invoices. One year following rehabilitation patients were surveyed by telephone to estimate their current levels of home assistance. Comparison of these figures showed a reduction in the annual cost of care following rehabilitation from US$25,909 to US$19,342. While acknowledging the crude method of cost estimation, the authors were confident that inpatient rehabilitation was cost-effective.

The largest published study was undertaken by Seibert and Carey.[30] This retrospective, single group, pre- and post-treatment study gathered data from 22 rehabilitation units. Its aim was to determine who made the most functional gains in inpatient rehabilitation. This study was not specific for MS, but studied eleven different diagnostic groups. Assessments of disability were made on admission and discharge. Comparisons were made with the MS patients and other conditions. On average, the MS patients were: less disabled on admission as measured by the Revised Level of Rehabilitation Scale (LORS-II), and had a shorter length of stay (22 days versus means ranging from 28 to 46 days). Patients with MS were younger than other diagnostic groups (mean 46 years versus means ranging from 49 to 70 years), apart from head-injured patients (mean 37 years). Neurological status was not monitored. Results showed that MS patients improved their level of performance on the LORS-II. These gains, however, were smaller than those of all other diagnostic groups.

Greenspun and colleagues[31] undertook a retrospective, single group, pre- and post-treatment study to investigate the effectiveness of inpatient rehabilitation on reducing disability. The Computerised Rehabilitation and Data System was used to evaluate disability on admission, discharge and at three months follow-up. Data was gathered on 28 patients (75 per cent female, mean age 42 years, mean disease duration 12.2 years), who participated in 33 episodes of inpatient rehabilitation over a four-year period. The average length of stay was 28 days (range 5–57). Neurological status was not monitored throughout the study period. Results were reported by describing the change in the percentage of patients improving their level of independence in mobility and self-care activities. Between admission and discharge, independence in ambulation improved from 18 to 76 per cent of patients, and in stairclimbing from 9 to 64 per cent of patients. Independence in self-care activities improved from 54 to 73 per cent in dressing; 39 to 70 per cent in bathing; 70 to 85 per cent in toileting; and 91 to 94 per cent in eating. At follow-up three months later, the majority of these improvements had been maintained.

The first study to distinguish patients by disease group, and to identify those recovering from a relapse or taking steroids, was undertaken by Kidd and colleagues.[32] They used a prospective, single group, pre- and post-treatment design to study 79 patients (49 females, mean age 48.8 years, range 17–61; mean disease duration 12.1 years, range 1–37). Assessments were made on admission and discharge using measures of impairment (Kurtzke's Disability Status Scale – DSS), disability (Barthel Index) and handicap (Environmental Status Scale – ESS). In terms of disease pattern, 15 patients were relapsing–remitting, 57 secondary-progressive, and 7 primary-progressive. The severity of disease was reflected by the relatively high scores on the DSS (median 7.0, range 4.0–9.0). The length of stay was short (mean 15 days, range 1–59). Following rehabilitation, statistically significant improvement was demonstrated by 65 per cent of patients in disability, and by 44 per cent in handicap. Improvement was most marked in those in whom a reduction in impairment had occurred, but was also seen in 63 per cent of those who had not changed neurologically.

The first controlled study was recently undertaken by Freeman and colleagues.[33] A stratified randomized wait-list controlled design was utilized to evaluate the effectiveness of a short period of inpatient rehabilitation. Sixty six patients, in the progressive phase of the disease, were randomly allocated to either immediate rehabilitation or a six-week delay before admission. Those in the treatment group participated in an individualized intensive multidisciplinary programme. All were assessed at 0 and 6 weeks with measures of impairment (Kurtzke's Expanded Disability Status Scale [EDSS] and Functional Systems [FS]), disability (Functional Independence Measure – FIM), and handicap (London Handicap Scale-LHS). At baseline assessment, both groups were comparable in terms of age, sex, disease duration and severity, disability and handicap. At the end of six weeks, although the level of impairment in both groups remained the same, those who participated in a short period of inpatient rehabilitation (average of 25 days) significantly improved their level of disability ($p < 0.001$) and handicap ($p < 0.01$) compared to those in the wait-list control group, who deteriorated slightly. It was concluded that despite unchanging impairment, inpatient rehabilitation resulted in reduced levels of disability and handicap in patients with progressive MS.

Do the benefits gained carry over in the longer term?

Each of the previous studies has looked at the short-term benefits of inpatient rehabilitation. It is of equal importance to determine how these benefits carry over once the patient has been discharged into the community. Aisen and colleagues[34] designed a retrospective, single group, pre- and post-treatment study to address this question. The authors reviewed the notes of 37 consecutive MS patients who were admitted to rehabilitation following a functional decline. Assessments of impairments (EDSS and FS scales) and disability (FIM) were reviewed on admission and discharge. In addition patients were followed up by interview (at nine months) and by telephone (once or twice somewhere between 6 and 36 months). Ninety per cent of subjects were female, with an average age of 47 years (range 24–68), time since diagnosis of 11.8 years (range 0.1–32), and EDSS score of 7.5. In terms of disease pattern, 6 patients were described as relapsing–remitting, 5 relapsing-progressive, and 26 chronic-progressive. The average length of stay was 32 days (range 12–77). Statistically significant improvements between admission and discharge were noted in all outcomes irrespective of disease pattern. Pyramidal and cerebellar functions improved particularly well. It is difficult to determine how long these benefits were maintained following discharge since the assessments were not performed at standardized points over the 6–36 month follow-up period.

Kidd and Thompson[35] used a prospective, single group, pre- and post-treatment design to assess 47 patients on admission and discharge (75 per cent female, mean age 40, median disease duration 13 years). Forty-four of these patients were followed up at three months. Assessments, at each time point, included impairment (EDSS), disability (FIM) and handicap (ESS). At discharge improvements were demonstrated by 17 per cent of patients in the EDSS score, 87 per cent in disability and 47 per cent in handicap. At three months, eleven patients had suffered new neurological symptoms, sufficient to cause a deterioration in the EDSS score in two patients. Gains in disability had been partly maintained in 86 per cent of patients. Handicap further improved following discharge with an additional 30 per cent of patients (total patients improved 77 per cent) improving their handicap score at three months. The authors suggested that the continued improvements in handicap were reflective of the work planned during the rehabilitation programme which had been subsequently carried out in the community.

Further attempts at determining the long-term benefits of inpatient rehabilitation have recently been undertaken by Freeman *et al.*[36] A prospective, pre- and post-treatment longitudinal design was used to assess patients on admission, discharge and at three monthly intervals for one year. Compared to previous studies, the outcomes measured were broadened to include patient oriented outcomes. Fifty consecutive patients, in the progressive phase of the disease, were assessed on impairment (EDSS and FS), disability (FIM), handicap (LHS), emotional well-being (General Health Questionnaire) and quality of life (Short-Form 36 Health Status Questionnaire). The sample was comprised of 29 females, with a mean age of 44.8 years (range 25–66), disease duration of 15.3 years (range 3–36) and median EDSS of 6.8 (range 6.0–9.0). Twelve month data was collected for 92 per cent of patients. Trends in both group and individual performance levels throughout the study period were plotted. Summary measures were calculated to determine the length of time taken for each individual to return to their baseline performance level. Results demonstrated that neurological status declined over the study period (median admission EDSS 6.8, EDSS at one year 8.0). Despite this worsening neurological status, improvements were maintained on average for approximately six months (range 0–365 days) in disability, handicap and emotional well-being, and for an average of ten months (range 190–365 days) in physical aspects of health-related quality of life.

How does inpatient rehabilitation compare to other forms of intervention?

This question has been addressed by two studies.[37,38] Reding and La Rocca[37] compared the outcome and cost of inpatient rehabilitation to acute hospital care using retrospective case matched analysis. Data from 20 pairs of patients, matched for sex and severity of MS, was reviewed. The level of disability (Incapacity Status Scale), rate of re-hospitalization, and need for home help assistance was determined by telephone review at 16 months follow-up. Costs of care were crudely estimated. Changes in neurological status were not monitored. At 16 month follow-up, no difference was demonstrated between the two groups in either their functional status or rate of re-hospitalization. Although the cost of inpatient rehabilitation was less per day than the acute hospital setting (US\$364 versus US\$625), the overall cost of admission was greater because of the longer length of stay (35 days versus 14 days). In his review of this study, La Rocca[10] suggested that if the average length of rehabilitation stay could be shortened, savings could be made without compromising patient care.

Francabandera and colleagues[38] compared inpatient to outpatient intervention. Following random assignment to either group, 84 patients were assessed on the level of disability (ISS) prior to admission and then at three monthly intervals for two years after discharge. The hours of home assistance required by the patient were recorded. On admission the two groups were comparable in terms of age, sex. EDSS scores, and hours of home assistance required. The initial level of disability between the groups, however, was statistically different; the inpatient group was more disabled than the outpatient group. Analysis of covariance was therefore used to control for this in the analysis. Comparison of discharge scores showed significant improvements in disability in the inpatient group, in contrast to the outpatient group where no improvements occurred. Preliminary results from the three-month follow-up demonstrated a statistically significant difference between the two groups.

The inpatient group had improved in terms of disability, whereas those in the outpatient group had deteriorated slightly. No impact on home care was shown. Neurological status was not monitored. A summary of results from the 12-month follow-up was reported by La Rocca and Kalb.[10] By twelve months both groups had reverted to pre-treatment levels of disability, with no statistically significant differences between them. They concluded that the initial advantage gained by inpatient rehabilitation appeared to be short-lived, and suggested that a periodic course of rehabilitation may therefore be necessary.

What aspects of rehabilitation are effective?

Little knowledge has been gained from these studies about what problems are most amenable to change and what elements of the rehabilitation programme are effective in achieving these benefits. These questions are probably best addressed by evaluating specific aspects of process and outcome rather than the comprehensive 'package' of care. Recently, two randomized controlled trials have been published which have investigated specific components of the rehabilitation package.[39,40]

Petajan and colleagues[39] evaluated the effectiveness of aerobic training on fitness and quality of life; 54 ambulatory MS patients were randomized to either continue their current lifestyle, or to include exercise three times weekly under supervision for 15 weeks. Physiological assessments were undertaken at baseline and at 15 weeks. Assessments on a range of psychological dimensions were undertaken at baseline, 5, 10 and 15 weeks. Compared with baseline ($n = 46$) the control group showed no significant changes over time for any variable. In contrast, the exercise group ($n = 21$) demonstrated statistically significant improvements in maximal aerobic capacity, isometric strength, body composition and blood lipid levels. Depression and anger scores were reduced at weeks 5 and 10, and fatigue was reduced at week 10. By week 15, however, these psychological benefits were no longer significant. Improvements in recreational management were maintained throughout. While acknowledging that some of these benefits may have resulted from the increased attention and social interaction,[41] this study concluded that exercise training resulted in improved fitness and had a positive impact on quality of life.

The effectiveness of a single inpatient admission for physiotherapy on improving mobility and related activities of daily living was investigated by Fuller and colleagues;[40] 45 MS patients, who had a recent history of deterioration in gait or transfer ability, were randomized to either 'early' (immediate physiotherapy) or 'late' treatment (physiotherapy delayed by nine weeks). Patients in the early group participated in physiotherapy for an average of 38 minutes per working day for 13.5 days. Assessments of mobility, activities of daily living, subjective visual analogue scores (patient and carer) and rating of randomized video clips of mobility were undertaken at baseline and at nine weeks. No statistically significant differences in change scores were detected in either group for disability, mobility, or video ratings. A significant reduction in mobility-related distress, as measured by the patient visual analogue scale, was noted in the treatment group. The authors suggested that improved patient selection or specific goal-directed intervention may improve the efficacy of the physiotherapy programme.

Studies such as these provide more specific information about which aspects of intervention are effective. This type of information helps to provide a more complete picture of the effectiveness of rehabilitation intervention.

What are the conclusions of these studies?

It is difficult to make meaningful comparisons between these studies due to the different sample populations and methodologies utilized. Few have described the sample population in terms of disease severity, many have failed to assess ongoing neurological status, and a wide range of outcome measures have been used. Unlike drug trials, where patient selection is an important feature of the study design, only a few of these studies have identified specific entry and exclusion criteria.[33,36,38]

It is notable, however, that every study demonstrated a reduction in the overall level of disability immediately following rehabilitation. Four also showed that it was associated with reduced levels of handicap.[29,32,33,36] Some notable differences in outcome are also evident. For example, whereas Feigenson *et al.*[29] reported that non-ambulators remained non-ambulators, Greenspun and colleagues[31] reported substantial gains in ambulation. Marked differences in the mean length of stay were also noted, varying from an average of 15 days[32] to 40 days.[29]

In terms of carry over, the limited evidence available suggests that the benefits gained are partly maintained in the longer term, although a return to initial levels of performance appears to occur by approximately twelve months.[34,36,38] Even preliminary conclusions about cost benefit cannot be made. In each of the two studies analysing this outcome,[29,37] costs were determined retrospectively, and were crudely estimated. Their findings should be interpreted with caution.

The future

More well designed research studies are required to establish the effectiveness of inpatient rehabilitation in MS. In our opinion, particular emphasis should be placed on evaluating the carry-over of benefits following discharge into the community, determining which aspects of rehabilitation are most effective and the cost benefits, since this information is especially scarce.

Differing opinions exist as to whether studies of inpatient rehabilitation should be extended to investigate the broader management of MS (for example assessment of inpatient and outpatient/community therapy combined as a 'package' of comprehensive care). Some argue that this combined package of care is reflective of current clinical practice and therefore should be evaluated. Others emphasize that these studies are fraught with methodological difficulties and that meaningful interpretation of their results may prove impossible.

Definitive studies will require larger numbers of patients. Given the relatively small numbers of specialist MS units, this will necessitate multi-centre participation involving a number of countries. To provide conclusive results a placebo group should be included in the study design. Attempts to address these issues are currently being planned by a co-ordinated network of task groups throughout Europe (RIMS – Rehabilitation in Multiple Sclerosis, and MARCH – MS and Rehabilitation Care and Health Services in Europe). It is acknowledged that the costs and practical difficulties of undertaking such studies are considerable, and perhaps prohibitive in an area where no vested commercial interests lie.

Conclusion

Methodologically sound study designs, which remain clinically relevant and practical, are essential for results to be convincing. These have proven difficult to achieve in the evaluation of MS inpatient rehabilitation. This is, in part, due to the complexity of designing studies in this area,[23,42] over and above those already recognized in drug trials.[43]

The evidence to date suggests that inpatient rehabilitation is effective in reducing disability in patients with MS, and that these benefits are partly maintained in the longer term. Benefits in terms of handicap and quality of life require further investigation before conclusions can be made. We stress the urgent need for further outcome studies of comprehensive inpatient rehabilitation in MS, to assess and predict outcomes more accurately. The methodologies used must apply rigorous scientific analysis and review to ensure that the results are scientifically credible.

References

1. *Multiple Sclerosis: A Working Party Report of the British Society of Rehabilitation Medicine*, London: Royal College of Physicians 1993.
2. Rosenberg W, Donald A. Evidence-based medicine: an approach to clinical problem-solving. *Br Med J* 1995; **310**: 1122–1126.
3. Mathew WB, Compston DAS, Allen IV *et al. McAlpine's Multiple Sclerosis*, 2nd edn. Edinburgh: Churchill Livingstone 1991.
4. Barnes M, Greenwood R, Barnes MP *et al.* eds. *Neurological Rehabilitation*, Edinburgh: Churchill Livingstone 1993; 485–504.
5. Schapiro RT, Langer SL. Symptomatic therapy of multiple sclerosis. *Curr Opin Neurol* 1994; **7**: 229–233.
6. Slater RJ. Comprehensive long-term care for MS patients. *Neurology* 1980; **30**: 37–38.
7. Scheinberg L, Holland NJ, Kirschenbaum M *et al.* Comprehensive long-term care of patients with multiple sclerosis. *Neurology* 1981; **31**: 1121–1123.
8. Erickson RP, Lie MR, Wineinger MA. Rehabilitation in multiple sclerosis. *Mayo Clin Proc* 1989; **64**: 818–828.
9. Schapiro RT. The rehabilitation of multiple sclerosis. *J Neurol Rehab* 1990; **4**: 215–217.
10. La Rocca NG, Kalb RC. Efficacy of rehabilitation in multiple sclerosis. *J Neurol Rehab* 1992; **6**: 147–155.
11. Mertin J. Rehabilitation in multiple sclerosis. *Ann Neurol* 1994; **36**: S130–S133.
12. Thompson AJ. Multiple sclerosis: symptomatic treatment. *J Neurol* 1996; **243**: 559–565.
13. Vaney C, Dubois S, Dehlinger A. Effectiveness of Inpatient Rehabilitation in Multiple Sclerosis. [Abstract]. *Multiple Sclerosis Consortium*, Atlanta 1996.
14. Paty DW. Overall summary of the survey of long term care strategies for patients with multiple sclerosis. *MS Management* 1994; **1**: 22–27.
15. Johnson J, Thompson AJ. Rehabilitation in a neuroscience centre: the role of expert assessment and selection. *Br J Ther Rehab* 1996; **3**: 303–308.
16. Tallis R. Measurement and the future of rehabilitation. *Geriat Med* 1989, January: 31–40.
17. Pollock C, Freemantle N, Sheldon T *et al.* Methodological difficulties in rehabilitation research. *Clin Rehab* 1993; **7**: 63–72.
18. Wade DT. *Measurement in Neurological Rehabilitation*, Oxford: Oxford University Press 1992.
19. Ellison GW, Myers LW, Leake BD *et al.* Design strategies in multiple sclerosis clinical trials. *Ann Neurol* 1994; **36**: S108–S112.
20. La Rocca NG, Schapiro RT, Scheinberg LC *et al.* Comprehensive care in multiple sclerosis: the whole versus the parts. *J Neurol Rehab* 1994; **8**: 95–98.
21. Whitaker JN, McFarland HF, Rudge P *et al.* Outcomes assessment in multiple sclerosis clinical trials: a critical analysis. *Multiple Sclerosis* 1995; **1**: 37–47.
22. Theriot KO, Brar S. Rehabilitation and physical therapy outcomes in multiple sclerosis. *J Neurol Rehab* 1993; **7**: 139–144.
23. Hobart JC, Thompson AJ. Clinical trials of multiple sclerosis. In: Reader AT, ed. *Interferon Therapy of Multiple Sclerosis*, New York: Marcel Dekker 1996, 398–407.
24. Wilkin D, Hallam L, Doggett M. *Measures of Need and Outcome for Primary Health Care*, Oxford: Oxford University Press 1992.
25. Hobart JC, Lamping DL, Thompson AJ. Evaluating neurological outcome measures: the bare essentials. *J Neurol Neurosurg Psychiatry* 1996; **60**: 127–130.
26. Hobart JC, Freeman JA, Lamping D. Physician and patient-oriented outcomes: which to measure? *Curr Opin Neurol* 1996; **9**: 441.
27. Jeffrey LIH. Aspects of selecting outcome measures to demonstrate the effectiveness of comprehensive rehabilitation. *Br J Occ Ther* 1993; **56**: 394–399.
28. Fuhrer MJ, Fuhrer MJ, eds. *Rehabilitation Outcomes: Analysis and Measurement*, London: Paul Brookes Publishing Co. 1987; 1–15.
29. Feigenson JS, Scheinberg L, Catalano M *et al.*

The cost-effectiveness of multiple sclerosis rehabilitation: a model. *Neurology* 1981; **31**: 1316–1322.

30. Carey RG, Seibert JH. Who makes the most progress in inpatient rehabilitation? an analysis of functional gain. *Arch Phys Med Rehab* 1988; **69**: 337–343.

31. Greenspun B, Stineman M, Agri R. Multiple sclerosis and rehabilitation outcome. *Arch Phys Med Rehab* 1987; **68**: 434–437.

32. Kidd D, Howard RS, Losseff NA *et al.* The benefit of inpatient neurorehabilitation in multiple sclerosis. *Clin Rehab* 1995; **9**: 198–203.

33. Freeman JA, Langdon DW, Hobart JC *et al.* The impact of rehabilitation on disability and handicap in progressive multiple sclerosis *Ann Neurol* 1997 (in press).

34. Aisen ML, Sevilla D, Fox N. Inpatient rehabilitation for multiple sclerosis. *J Neurol Rehab* 1996; **10**: 43–46.

35. Kidd D, Thompson AJ. A prospective study of neurorehabilitation in multiple sclerosis. *J Neurol Neurosurg Psychiatry* 1997; **62**: 423–424.

36. Freeman JA, Langdon DW, Hobart JC *et al.* Long term effects of neurorehabilitation in multiple sclerosis: a longitudinal study (abstract). *J Neurol* 1997; **244** (suppl 3): 510.

37. Reding MJ, La Rocca NG. Acute-hospital care versus rehabilitation hospitalisation for management of nonemergent complications in multiple sclerosis. *J Neurol Rehab* 1987; **1**: 13–17.

38. Francabandera FL, Holland NJ, Wiesel-Levison P *et al.* Multiple sclerosis rehabilitation: inpatient versus outpatient. *Rehab Nursing* 1988; **13**: 251–253.

39. Petajan JH, Gappmaier E, White AT *et al.* Impact of aerobic training on fitness and quality of life in multiple sclerosis. *Ann Neurol* 1996; **39**: 432–441.

40. Fuller KJ, Dawson K, Wiles CM. Physiotherapy in chronic multiple sclerosis: a controlled trial. *Clin Rehab* 1996; **10**: 195–204.

41. Johnson KP. Exercise, drug treatment, and the optimal care of multiple sclerosis patients. *Ann Neurol* 1996; **39**: 422–423.

42. Colville P. Rehabilitation management outcomes in multiple sclerosis. *MS Management* 1996; **2**: 55–57.

43. Noseworthy JH, Ebers GV, Vandervoort MK *et al.* The impact of blinding on the results of a randomised, placebo-controlled multiple sclerosis clinical trial. *Neurology* 1994; **44**: 16–20.

24

Models of care in progressive multiple sclerosis
Randall T Schapiro

Introduction

Viewed from any angle, managing a chronic disease is fraught with problems. There are many issues which never abate and must be constantly addressed. Progressive multiple sclerosis (MS), even without any management, eventually will stop progressing. Even though it may appear to be predictable, it is not. Nonetheless, the person with progressive MS faces a future with significant disability. Progressive MS management is directed towards decreasing disability with medical, rehabilitative, psychological, and other techniques. The goal of treatment is to allow function at its highest level. It is essential to develop techniques which allow a realization of each person's full potential. As a springboard for discussion what follows is a proposed ideal model of care for progressive MS.

There are many impediments to operationalizing this model. Following its presentation a discussion of some of those will ensue.

A model of care for progressive MS
Guiding principles

The great variability of MS, together with the numerous factors which influence the development of models of care leads directly to the major difficulties in the development of an ideal model of care for all with MS. This is also true if one limits the type of MS to the progressive variety. However, some axioms are clear when the word progressive is utilized:

- maintaining function despite neurologic progression should be considered a victory
- a good quality of life (including psyche) is necessary
- financial stability over a long time frame is a necessity
- the family as a unit must be considered
- hope must spring eternal.

The name 'progressive' MS implies that progression is prominent. As previously stated, all with progressive MS stop progressing at some point. The average age of death for those with MS is only slightly earlier than the average without.[1] Nonetheless increasing impairment is clearly a prominent feature of 'progressive' MS. As the World Health Organization (WHO) has made clear the neurologic impairment of an individual does not inevitably have to lead to decreased function (disability) and to decreased societal enjoyments (handicap).[2] However, losses are inevitable. To decrease this, the model of care for progressive MS must begin with the goal of allowing each person to continue to do as much as he or she can with what he/she has. The rehabilitation cannot only be restorative but must have a primary aim of maintenance. The neurologic rehabilitation of a function lost as a result of disease of the nervous system is intuitively understood. If a person loses the capacity to use an extremity because of stroke or MS, the rehabilitation team can work to restore function to that extremity. Failing that tactic, compensatory techniques may be utilized. This is described as *restorative rehabilitation* and is usually quite specific, with specific goals, and is easily measured.

In MS, restorative rehabilitation often occurs after an acute attack. It is relatively short in duration with success measured in terms of return to function of abilities to perform activities.

In progressive MS, rehabilitation is different. At times restorative rehabilitation is appropriate but it is difficult to restore that lost long before. Rehabilitation in a progressive disease must be directed towards preventing further loss or maintaining function. This is called preventative rehabilitation but is more often described as *maintenance rehabilitation*. Because progressive disease is generally misunderstood, this approach is often thought of as excessive and unimportant. An example of this is the lack of coverage for maintenance rehabilitation by the Medicare system in the USA. In reality, it can make the difference from simply existing to living a fulfilling life. The goal of maintenance rehabilitation is to attempt to keep ahead of the progression by slowly adapting to disability before and as it occurs. It is not time limited and must go on for the existence of the disease. It has a heavy emphasis on prevention of the secondary complications of disease including pressure sores, osteoporosis, and muscle atrophy. It also emphasizes the tertiary psychological and social aspects of disease.

The bulk of management of progressive MS revolves around this approach with an understanding of the spirituality of individuals, giving hope where none is apparent. This hope allows a bad prognosis to be less disturbing.

Essential components

In the progressive form of MS, patients have to work at keeping skills including activities of daily living (dressing, eating, toileting, etc.) despite the realities of increased weakness, ataxia, etc. Compensatory techniques must be encouraged and independence stressed as the desired goal.

Mobility must be emphasized. Spasticity management should include proper instruction in range of motion, stretching and aerobic exercises. Antispasticity agents including baclofen, tizanidine, clonazapam, dantrolene, and other appropriate medications should be prescribed with expertise. For those with intractable spasticity the programable baclofen pump and other surgical procedures should be available.

Transferring techniques to increase mobility and preserve safety for the care-givers should be taught. These include the pivot, sliding board, and Hoyer transfers.

The wheelchair must be prescribed properly with an understanding of the use and appropriateness of standard, three wheeler, and four wheel power chairs. The seating systems should be prescribed by properly educated professionals.

Tremor must be treated with exercises and medication. These include balance and coordination exercises with the Swiss ball, appropriate bracing and weighting, and the judicious use of medications including: propranolol, buspirone, clonazapam, isoniazid, and others.

Bladder and bowel continence concerns require proper evaluation with catheterization for residual urine or bladder ultrasound together with proper medication and/or catheterization techniques. Bowel programs must be practical and allow for convenience of those involved. Nurses are usually in the best position to follow through with these.

Other activities of daily living including dressing, grooming, eating, and general functioning need proper attention. This is best addressed with an appropriately educated occupational therapist.

Fatigue including normal fatigue, 'short-circuiting' fatigue, depression, and lassitude needs treatment with medication, counselling, and proper instruction in energy conservation (see Krupp, Chapter 21).

The skin should be inspected regularly for preventative and therapeutic measures allowing early detection and aggressive management. The skin is clearly more durable if proper nutrition is maintained. While there is not a proven 'MS diet', clearly good nutritional habits can decrease long-term complications in progressive MS. The diet must be low in fat with the proper balance of complex carbohydrates and protein. Learning the proper reading of nutritional labels is helpful.

Swallowing and speech inadequacies should be observed and appropriate compensatory techniques instituted before increased complications develop.

Sexual feelings and relationships are of importance in this young population of people. Appropriate counselling and adaptive techniques should be presented for those interested.

Transportation, public and private, is the lifeline for the progressively impaired individual. Any model of care for this population must concern itself with this need.

The model should consider a target of quality existence, not a vegetative end. Depression must be guarded against with experienced counsellors, appropriate medication and ongoing therapy. Cognitive problems should be understood and compensatory techniques utilized to lessen the effects. This is especially true in the progressive form of MS where cognition is of particular concern. Leisure time must be filled with planned activities which are both enjoyable and have a purpose of stimulation at the same time.

Preventative evaluations of skin, muscle, and bone may decrease future costs and lead to improved quality of life. However, all of this is expensive and because MS is a disease of relatively young people, who live long lives, it is very expensive. It is likely to be less costly in the long run to spend money on maintenance of health. This is directed towards preventing the secondary complications of chronic disease before the expensive problems occur. An appropriate model of care must be well funded, privately or federally, to work.

The model must consider the family of the patient and allow for respite, proper equipment for transfers, bathing, dressing and living. Clearly to make it function for an individual, the whole family must be involved. The family break-up surrounding MS is extremely high and is clearly a detriment to providing quality living. Thus the family needs protection with appropriate education, counselling, and services to diffuse the stress of any one person.

The stress of providing professional care must also be spread as no one professional can have all the skills and wisdom to provide the necessary services. The model necessitates a team of rehabilitation-oriented professionals who are expert at providing services for complicated problems. Because of practical considerations (money, time) all should not be involved at all times but their expertise should be available when the principal care director (physician) deems it appropriate. The principal director must be an expert to know and understand the skills available for consideration. He/she must have specific knowledge and skills to use the latest immune therapies for modulation of the disease along with specific knowledge of rehabilitation techniques.

As all this transpires the model must exude hope because without hope there is no reason for existence. The spirituality of an individual should be sustained within the model. This cannot be limited to a specific religious outlook but must generalize to all who wish to partake.

A single appropriate model of care for all persons with a disease as variable as MS is an impossibility. Each person's personality, background, and way of life determine what works for them. Practical economic considerations also play a large role in determining the specific model of care. This is more true today than ever before. Thus models of care in progressive MS include not only *practice* models but also *economic* models. Whether the model emphasizes the 'doctor–patient relationship' or is described as 'controlling managed care', it probably affects quality of life and has the potential to influence outcomes for those with this incurable disease.

The above model is a variation of the medical model. However, the last decade has changed the utilization of the medical model drastically.

Models of care
The medical models

The *medical model of care* is led by the physician. Each country looks upon the medical profession somewhat differently. In many countries the general physician cares for the general medical concerns of the populace. Whether the physician is called a generalist, family doctor, general practitioner, internist or some other term, he or she is the 'primary care' physician.

The image and the use of physicians have changed in the past 20 years. It was assumed 20 years ago that the old time general practi-

tioner was a thing of the past. Medicine had become too complicated for one physician to understand all the intricacies of chronic disease. Specialists and subspecialists were trained and the general physician appeared to be a relic. This left the person with common medical problems without a physician willing to be responsible for their routine management. That, together with the rising cost of medical care, led the way for the generalist to come back. Initially the 'come back' physician was labelled as a new kind of specialist: 'the family physician'. Currently this physician is often called a 'primary care' physician. The role of the primary care physician is to manage the general medical care of the patient. The person with MS is not immune to other, more common, diseases. Therefore it is logical for the person with MS to have a primary physician watching over the whole medical process. For efficiency the primary care doctor must work in concert with the 'MS physician' to provide total medical care. This team work is necessary because it is impossible for primary care physicians to manage progressive MS appropriately if they do not have enough experience with MS to understand the variability and complications of the disease.

Primary care physicians must understand the general aspects of disease and a person's reaction to disease. They must practise preventative health care and recognize the complications of disease to treat or triage them effectively.

In the 1990s, especially in the USA, the primary care physician has assumed a new role as the guardian of the budget. The term given to this MD is that of 'gatekeeper'.[3] In this circumstance, the physician moves from the position of patient advocate, watching over the person with disease, to that of financial overseer. In this role the primary care physician loses the advocacy function, often becoming an impediment to complicated management approaches.

The specialist often serves as a consultant, who becomes shielded from the patient by the primary care physician who has been put into a position to authorize each consult and follow-up visit. When the consultant is kept from direct patient contact, the model is consistent with the 'gatekeeper' philosophy. This may be carried to the point where approval for each recommended test or procedure is necessary. In these models, the patient's desires become suppressed to those of the primary physician. The numerous potential complications of progressive MS should alert all to the need of ongoing specialized care.

Thus for appropriate care a specialist must be involved in progressive MS management. While the specialist usually is the neurologist, not all neurologists are of the appropriate mindset to do the job well. Some neurologists conceive of themselves as diagnosticians. The diagnosis in progressive MS is self evident and needs no further elucidation. Apart from an in-depth knowledge of the nervous system's anatomy and physiology, the neurologist also needs to know how to manage symptoms, develop neurorehabilitation strategies, and have respect for other health professionals in the team. He/she must have a feel for the psychological problems of chronic disease and be able to develop treatment plans for such. Progressive MS needs management in all spheres, requiring specialized knowledge and leadership.

Physiatrists have specialized training in rehabilitation medicine and are also in a position to provide leadership in the arena of progressive MS. They may function in the MS doctor role or as a consultant to the team.

While highly regulated models of care are becoming popular because of the presumed cost savings, some models continue to empha-size cooperation of the physicians. The model changes with the primary care physician managing the general health problems of the person with MS and the specialist managing the MS without requiring permission from the generalist. The patient can then choose his/her physician team. The physician director is determined by the problems of the patient.

A different model of care recognizes that most people with MS are healthy apart from the MS. MS can dominate one's life. Thus the physician visited by most people with MS may be the 'MS physician', usually the neurologist. With these visits come familiarity and trust. In this model when the person with MS needs another physician, for a non-neurological problem, it is natural to turn to the neurologist for advice and triage. The MS doctor becomes the 'principal care' physician and is in a position to advise the general physician to deliver efficient care. This is *the principal care model* for a chronic condition. When the chronic condition dominates the health of the person, this model appears quite appropriate.

Because of the multiple potential problems of MS, it is impossible for one person to have the skills or time to manage all of them efficiently. To properly manage MS, the professional must treat the disease with the medications and expertise involving the immune system. Equally, if not more important, is management of the symptoms of MS with medication and rehabilitative principles. Of similar importance is the management of the person, understanding the psychological, vocational, marital, and social difficulties associated with the disease.

The MS team model

The *MS team model of care* gives the medical management of MS to the physician; the rehabilitation portion requires an experienced therapy team with experienced allied health professionals to maintain continuity.[4] This is closer in operation to the proposed model. However, in this model the physician may defer case management to a nurse or social worker who, with appropriate training, may keep in constant touch with the patient. Referrals then spring from that interaction with the case manager triaging as appears appropriate.

Progressive MS particularly necessitates professionalism in the components of the team because the medical management of the disease itself often falls short of the mark. Therefore the rehabilitation and symptom management have to be excellent allowing maintenance of function in the face of progressive disease.

Rehabilitation teams typically are composed of the patient, the physician, physical therapist, occupational therapist, nurse, speech pathologist, social service worker, neuropsychologist, home care nurse, and others, depending on circumstances. Physicians may include neurologists, physiatrists, psychiatrists, urologists, ophthalmologists, and others.[4]

Often these teams communicate via consultations, with a leader (physician) collating the information and developing a multidisciplinary plan. More efficient is the communication of the consultations face to face, with immediate feedback and the development of an interdisciplinary plan. This *team model of care* allows for numerous complexities of personalities (patient and team) to be taken into consideration.

In today's highly costly medical arena, it is not practical for a patient to be evaluated by a team at each visit of ongoing care. A skilled physician should be in a position to determine if and when a person requires the team approach. Much of the time no intervening rehabilitation professional will be necessary. Often only one of the group will be necessary. The neurologist in charge must have the skills

to triage the patient to the proper person. Sometimes that triage opens up unforeseen weaknesses which require other professionals and/or a full team evaluation. This results in far more efficient use of time and resources accomplishing the goal of allowing individuals to function at their highest levels. When the team is required for complex evaluation and treatment, each member of the team must remember that it is a team with cost and efficiency highlighted for effective, practical care. All must check his/her ego at the door and not be defensive of one's own profession. Together the various skills of the professionals work to maintain effective function of the patient.

Complicating the realities of the 1990s is the fact that there are many 'non-professional models' of care for MS and other chronic conditions.

The non-professional models

Any model of care begins with the person affected by the disease. Some individuals, for various reasons, manage their disease without professional interventions. This may occur for financial consideration but often comes from a distrust stemming from less than satisfactory professional interventions in the past. This model may be labelled as *the non-professional model of care.*

It is often believed that people who are active and questioning in their care may do better than those who do not question. There may be an open hostility directed towards professionals in this model which inspires an individual to do better than expected. However, there is an old adage in medicine that 'a doctor who treats him/herself has a fool for a patient'. This is based on being too close to a situation to view it objectively. This also applies to the 'non-doctor' trained patient who decides to direct his/her care without professional supervision. No one should question an 'independent' individual who wants to understand management strategies and participate in the decision making process but this model goes beyond that to no discussion, with decisions being made in a relative vacuum. Nonetheless independent attributes are helpful in chronic disease management and many utilize the non-professional model of care.

At what point personal responsibility for medical management and decision making to oneself becomes a negative is unclear. Certainly a 'take charge' attitude has many positives. Other helpful attributes, which are not professionally based but are important to 'healing oneself' include a sense of humor, spirituality, and an intense ethic to work towards 'wellness'.

Classical medicine has become very scientific. The 'art of medicine' has taken a back seat to medicine by fact. However, many, if not the majority, of people do not put as much stock in scientific medicine as the physician community desires. Uniformly, in countries around the world, the common person is turning to less scientific but more optimistic modes of treatment. This can be called *the alternative care* model.[5] There are many common threads. These often begin with a hands on physical orientation. This may include massage, manipulation, or simply touch. There is a mystical belief that through these modalities physiologic changes in the body can be stimulated. There is usually a tincture of meditation or spiritual touching. This may involve individuals or groups. Added to this is the belief that diet and vitamins are basically the answer to curing chronic disease. Despite little factual basis, this model often concludes that medicine actually is a negative towards managing chronic disease and that nature is the only way to truly eliminate discomfort.

The patients who choose this model frequently do so without trying the medical model but sometimes come from failures and lack of communication of the more classical approaches.

People who are considered experts in this model speak with conviction and appear to present opinions as facts when none are otherwise available. This intermingling of fact and opinion often involves the selling of a product. This may be a device or a food supplement.

As much as traditional science would like to see a medicine based only on thoughtful studies, alternative medicine is being accepted by the masses. The alternative practitioners usually believe in what they are advising.

In a disease with no known cause or definitive treatment protocol the door is left wide open for the development of less than ethical treatments. These may be called *quackery models* but for many are very believable. They often take advantage of the known placebo effect which is prominent in MS. They rely on testimonials and are often part of a pyramidal marketing process. They begin with a product or procedure which is usually innocuous in itself. The product is often given attributes which have nothing to do with any validated evidence. This product is then sold along with instructions which are usually more ritual than treatment.

Over time enough individuals feel strongly about the product or process that attention is drawn to the treatment. People who may or may not have MS but who have a prominent conversion reaction become 'cured' and the treatment protocol becomes a wonder for a while. This appears to have a half life of 3–4 years as evidenced by cobra venom, cow colaustrum, bee stings, hyperbaric oxygen, calcium oretate, and others.

Models of care can also be based on the funding of the model. If the varieties of competing models did not complicate the way towards an ideal model the administrative directors certainly do. There are models based on who is administrating the program.

The administrative models

These include *governmental models*, *public models*, and *private models*. Numerous *government models of care* for MS have been developed at various times. In the USA the Veteran's Administration has a series of hospitals which exist to take care of the veterans of military service. If one develops MS within seven years of the military association, one is deemed 'service connected'. This appears to blame the military for causing the disease even though most understand this is not the case.

If service connected the veteran is eligible for many services and treatments at no cost. This is very helpful for the destitute disabled but may take away motivation for rehabilitation and MS management.

The *public model* is for those who have no obvious resources and thus qualify for government aid. This provides services with little investment on the part of the patient. This may lead to frustration on everyone's behalf as the provider gets little reimbursement and the patient tends to think he/she should be eligible for more than the program allows. Usually this tends to have unhappy patients and unhappy providers with little satisfaction.

Fee for service, paid for either by the patient or by a third party, is the hallmark of the *private model*. The old saying 'you get what you pay for' is tested in this model. The patient is followed by a physician of his choice and services are ordered as thought appropriate by that physician. Rehabilitation services are provided upon physician order and are billed out as they are provided. This has the advantage of choice for the patient and the disadvantage of potential abuse of tests and services by the provider. All models have to face financial factors influencing them. Money

can be as important as medicine at any one time.

Money is said to be the root of all evil and it clearly is a driving force in healthcare. Its lack is prominent in every country and budgets determine models of care universally.

No matter which country is being examined, the federal government has a hand in determining the model of care. This is based not only on money but on the social and ethnic background of the country. Clearly, some countries are more caring of their constituents than others.

There are many preventative measures which help decrease infections, heart disease, lung disease, etc., but despite the best preventative efforts, disease happens. The belief that people can prevent most 'disease' is simply inaccurate. It should be replaced by an understanding of the need for a multi-pronged attack including prevention by decreasing risk factors and by decreasing the complications of disease.

This leads to spending money on new and improved technology when it is available, which in turn may drive the model of care whether in the transplant arena, antibiotic management or rehabilitative stage.

The model, to survive, must have funding, federal and local government support, populace support, and be appropriate for the targeted disease.

Economic factors are influencing the creation of models of care based on costs which may or may not have anything to do with the service and care of disabled individuals. The Disability Payment System is based on instituting a package price for the treatment of specific disease on a yearly basis.[6] Competition then develops over managing the person with that specific disease for a specific fee. The cost is developed from a snapshot of the fees billed for a year. Comorbidity clusters are factored into the price which comes from an amalgamation of these factors. People are categorized by their disability and eventually capitation (per head) costs are developed. These are dependent on utilization and take into account how many members there are with the specific disease per month in a population of otherwise normal people.

As capitation matures, the professionals recognize that they are given a set amount each year to take care of each individual in their population. If they spend less than that amount they may take home more money and if they spend more they will take home less in the following year. As previously noted this raises many ethical questions but brings about a sharp decrease in services offered. In a disease like MS where death due to the process is rare, the model affects quality of life rather than the actual medical outcome.

The reality is that while provider income goes down in this model, the cost of care does not change much as the overhead for the administration of the model is more than any cost savings. Eventually a provider, often the hospital, envisions cutting out the insurance carrier and offers the services of the enrolled physicians and the hospital, together with out-patient, and homecare services in one package called an 'Integrated Service Network (ISN)'.[7] ISNs then may compete on the basis of cost and 'quality' for patient populations but the profit is made by enrolling healthy people while treating the chronically ill enrolled efficiently and, in all likelihood, sparingly.

Conclusion

No clear present model is designed to manage progressive MS efficiently and effectively. However, the pieces are present in many. Government, practitioners, families, and patients need to band together to develop the future as it truly belongs to all of them.

References

1. Flachenecker P, Hartung HP. Klinische Forschungsgruppe fur Multiple Sklerose und Neuroimmunologie, Neurologische Klinik und Poliklinik (Course of illness and prognosis of multiple sclerosis). *Nervenarzt* 1996; **67:** 435–443.

2. World Health Organization International Classification of Impairments, Disabilities and Handicaps 1980.

3. Wachter RM. Rationing health care: preparing for a new era. *South Med J* 1995; **88:** 25–32.

4. Schapiro RT. Rehabilitation of multiple sclerosis. *MS Management* 1994; **1:** 31–33.

5. Furnham A, Kirkcaldy B. The health beliefs and behaviors of orthodox and complementary medicine clients. *Br J Clin Psychol* 1996; **35** (Pt 1): 49–61.

6. Reardon TM. Managed care contracting/capitation. *Ann Thorac Surg* 1995; **60:** 1500–1508.

7. Kralewski JE, de Vries A, Dowd B *et al.* The development of integrated service networks in Minnesota. *Health Care Management Rev* 1995; **20:** 42–56.

25

What can specialist nurses offer in caring for people with multiple sclerosis?

Jane Johnson

The user's perspective of service provision

In many ways this is an encouraging time in the development of knowledge, treatment and services for people with multiple sclerosis (MS).[1] The extent of the problem is starting to be recognized, and the cost to the individual and to the community is beginning to be acknowledged,[2,3] with the result that community care and rehabilitation initiatives are developing throughout the UK. However, knowledge about these developments is by no means universal, and while pockets of good practice in terms of treatment, management and support services are becoming more common, these have often served to highlight the inequality, confusion and fragmentation still experienced by many people with MS and their families. The British Society of Rehabilitation Medicine reports that 'the person with MS and their family often have to piece together the picture for themselves, partly from a neurologist who understands the disease but not their situation, and partly from those in the community who may understand their situation but not the disease.'[4]

Typical experiences reported by people with MS follow common themes and often differ significantly from the professional's more sanguine perspective.

Collections of symptoms, perhaps rather vague and transitory, may wax and wane over time but cause considerable concern. These may be attributed to stress or anxiety by professionals, family or the patient himself, but continue to cause distress. When a neurological referral does occur, this is often perceived by the patient as a fragmented and confused process involving numerous visits to the local hospital for blood tests, evoked responses, lumbar puncture and magnetic resonance imaging (MRI) scans. Whilst the professionals know that this is a logically planned process of elimination, patients may see no pattern to these investigations, often taking many weeks to complete and leading to many questions and considerable anxiety. Reluctance to discuss potential diagnoses can be taken as evidence of serious, life threatening disease, and vague descriptions of 'inflammation of the nerves' provide little reassurance. The patient may see several different doctors during this process and the eventual diagnosis of MS may come from a variety of sources. In one study 44 per cent learned the news from consultants, 6 per cent from junior hospital doctors, 38 per cent from a GP and 12 per cent from non-medical sources.[5] The ability of these individuals to give definitive responses to initial questions about prognosis, current research developments and treatment is obviously variable. After weeks of fear, anxiety and distress, other questions inevitably raise themselves in the patient's mind, but who can they discuss them with? They may not even have discussed it with their family yet.

In reality, the confusion often continues, as each person they discuss it with, either professionally or in a lay capacity, is likely to have differing views (and degrees of knowledge) about prognosis, possible treatment, including 'miracle cures', the benefit or otherwise of therapies and how they should view the future. Access to what could be a wide array of helpful services, from different providers at varying points in the disease progression, can seem impenetrable, even to the able bodied, without consideration of the added difficulty imposed by mobility or visual problems, poor memory or fatigue.

Dissatisfaction from the user's perspective is a common finding in numerous surveys into the perceived needs of people with MS.[5-7] This invariably focuses first on how the initial diagnosis was managed, an issue which often has serious consequences for how effectively the person with MS is able to face future challenges posed by the disease.[8] From diagnosis onwards, there is an intense need for information and knowledgeable advice which can empower people to take control of their current situation, and manage their lives to best effect. It is often the unpredictability and diversity of the disease, together with the lack of a common source of consistent information on which to base decisions which people with MS and their families find most distressing and debilitating[6] (MS Society and National Hospital for Neurology and Neurosurgery (NHNN) standards in health services, unpublished report).

Lack of specialist knowledge amongst some GPs and other community- and hospital-based professionals,[4] along with complex systems of referral, often lead to unidentified and unmet needs. In some cases this can lead to people with MS developing secondary complications following admission to hospital or nursing home care. Some professionals have been criticized for failing to understand the complexity of the lives of people with MS, and an extensive survey commissioned by the MS Society[6] identifies conflicting views between people with MS and some professionals as to what constitutes 'meeting needs' and appropriate attitudes to the disease.

In addition, professionals often do not communicate well amongst themselves. Discharge from hospital can be a particularly difficult time, when numerous hospital staff contact a variety of local authority or community staff with a view to setting up support services to continue care.[7,9,10] From a user's perspective it becomes clear that there is often no cross communication or key worker with responsibility for 'pulling the strands together' (one study reported between 10 and 60 workers from different sources coming into the homes of people with MS).[7] The advent of care managers for some people within the community is an obvious advancement, but again the patchy provision of this service, and the care manager's frequently limited knowledge of the special problems encountered by people with MS, can lead to further frustrations.

Numerous authors and surveys of people with MS have identified the need for continuity, co-ordination and easily accessible sources of information.[4,5,7,9,11] In addition, the issue of psychological support, both for people with MS and their carers, is an important recurrent theme which appears to have been poorly addressed at all stages in the past.[1,5,12]

What can specialist nurses contribute towards caring for people with MS?

These perceived gaps in service provision are beginning to be addressed in some areas, especially in the USA and the UK by a rapidly growing group of specialist MS nurses, often in association with neurological centres and/or local specialist multidisciplinary teams.[11] In addition, the recent development of beta-interferon treatment, with its associated need for patient teaching and ongoing support, has led to a commercially supported network of MS nursing posts.

As with all true nursing, the strengths of these posts lie in the nurse's ability to take an holistic, client centred view of needs, to 'get inside the skin' of patients or clients and discover what help they need and can use.[13] A major strength of nursing is its ability to 'mend the fragmentation in the system' so that the care experienced by the patient at the centre appears as meaningful and integrated as possible.[14] Despite specializing in the respect of caring for people with one disease process, MS nurses are able to bring their 'generalist' nursing skills to bear in helping address the wide range of physical, emotional and social problems typically experienced by people with MS.

What areas can be specifically targeted?

Initial and ongoing support

Providing an optimum start to the distressing realization of having a potentially disabling, progressive neurological disorder is essential. The often extended period of uncertainty, fear and confusion experienced before a firm diagnosis is made can be minimized by the development of focused MS diagnostic clinics. Here patients can complete a programme of investigations and return to see the same consultant neurologist to discuss the diagnosis within a minimal time frame. At this stage the need for

certainty of diagnosis whenever possible, honesty and clarity of communication, followed by support and information has been identified.[7,8]

It is well recognized that stress and anxiety limit an individual's ability to process information, and partially remembered discussions can lead to misunderstandings and further anxiety. The revelation of having an, as yet incurable, neurological disorder poses many questions about the future, but people are rarely able to formulate them in this initial clinic setting. What is needed is a reliable, knowledgeable contact point,[15] ideally without the formality of making repeated medical appointments. A useful model involves a specialist MS nurse accompanying the patient and family when the consultant discusses the diagnosis. The nurse then spends some time with the patient following the consultation, exploring and reinforcing what the patient and family have understood from the discussion, answering immediate questions and giving appropriate written information, including contact with the MS Society for them to study further. She may make another appointment to discuss issues raised following further consideration, or give them the opportunity to contact her themselves when they perceive the need. Set periods of telephone help-line availability can be useful, as well as regular drop-in clinics, but continuity and ongoing availability are key issues in helping to reduce anxiety.[10,16]

The psychological impact of the diagnosis of MS may be experienced over an extended period for some people and their families. Psychological support may include reassurance gained from occasionally checking out the significance of symptoms, or talking through the appropriateness of plans they are considering. There may be a recurrent need to revisit the issue of diagnosis or talk through their feelings and concerns for the future. In some cases there may be serious problems with adjustment and family dynamics which require referral for expert professional counselling beyond the skills of the MS specialist nurse, and a skilled nurse with ongoing patient and family contact is in an ideal situation to identify such needs, address them herself where possible, or refer and liaise appropriately.

Information, education and co-ordination

MS specialist nurses associated with neurological centres or multidisciplinary teams have access to a wealth of information and contacts, and can develop a comprehensive information service for people with MS, carers and professionals. A consistent point of initial contact can be invaluable in tracing specific services, and such a contact can be widely publicised in hospitals and the community. Many specialist MS nurses have a specific remit to provide education for other professionals or carers about the special needs of people with MS, so contributing more widely to improving the quality of care received. This may take the form of teaching sessions to ward nurses or nursing home and community staff, organizing study days or lectures of multidisciplinary interest, or merely working alongside other members of the multidisciplinary team, providing advice to ensure a co-ordinated hospital discharge for an individual with complex needs. The availability of an MS specialist nurse as an educational resource and knowledgeable link-worker is an important step in improving standards of care in many hospital and community settings and is a service development supported by the Department of Health.[17]

In the past, support for people with MS who are relatively well has not been a priority in many healthcare settings, with most interventions being aimed at managing existing problems.[18] The MS specialist nurse is in an ideal position to advise on potential problems such as the prevention of urinary infections, fatigue management, skin care, sexual dysfunction and simple principles of tone management which may help many individuals maintain their 'wellness' over time. Where more specialist advice is needed, prompt referral to appropriate members of the multidisciplinary team can be made, or in some cases joint multidisciplinary clinics may be held to assess and advise those at high risk of developing complications.[10,11] In addition, specialist nurses are able to monitor particularly vulnerable patients through home visits, regular telephone contact and liaison with community staff.[10]

Two patient education issues with specific need for nursing expertise involve continence management and beta-interferon treatment. Many studies have identified bladder dysfunction as one of the most troublesome symptoms experienced by people with MS[10,19,20] and one which is responsible for most acute and long stay admissions to hospital[21]. There is considerable scope for routine screening and assessment of risk factors for the development of urinary tract infections in this population, and for advice and education regarding the management of some existing problems. This can effectively be carried out by an appropriately experienced MS specialist nurse as part of an holistic review of potential problems. However, extensive and more complex intervention can only practically be carried out by a urology/continence service. Most MS nurses would work collaboratively with local continence services and, through the development of protocols, clarify the roles and relationships between the two services.[21]

The advent of interferon (IFN)-β as the first drug to have a distinct effect in reducing relapses in MS has brought with it a combination of optimism, ethical dilemmas and a real need for patient education, ongoing support and monitoring.[18] The media profile of IFN-β has been high, raising expectations and demands for treatment throughout the MS population. The high cost of treatment, potential side effects, restricted availability and strict clinical protocols have created a need for unbiased professional advice and help for patients to make informed decisions.[18] There is also a more practical need to teach the skill of regular IFN-β injection, either to the patient or in some cases their carers. This routinely brings specialist MS nurses in contact with relatively well people with MS, so increasing the valuable opportunity for health promotion.

Outcomes

In many progressive neurological conditions there is now considerable evidence to suggest that nurse-led initiatives aimed at providing consistent support, knowledgeable advice and multidisciplinary liaison, have a significant effect on the number of urgent outpatient referrals and hospital admissions for these groups.[10,16,21,22] A recent audit of the effectiveness of an MS nurse specialist post in Manchester found that regular medical outpatient appointments had decreased. In addition, the total number of 'MS inpatient days' with stays of longer than five days had decreased to 60 per cent, comparing equivalent six month periods before and after implementation of the service.[23] Reasons for acute or frequent admissions and extended hospital stays invariably involve urinary tract problems, with infections often leading to exacerbations of MS symptoms.[10,21] A study of the effectiveness of one nurse-managed MS clinic in the USA found that, before implementation, 43 per cent of hospitalizations of longer than seven days were due to urinary tract infections. In the year following active involvement from the MS nurse there were no such admissions.[21]

The importance of having easy access to a well informed link-worker who is able to discuss a wide range of concerns is not so easy to evaluate, although one UK study reported important improvements in the patient's knowledge of MS, coping, mood, confidence, life in general and family relationships, and a quarter contacted their doctor less often.[24] Many patients in this study emphasized how much easier it was to contact and talk to the MS liaison nurse than the doctor in an outpatient clinic, especially about sensitive matters such as incontinence or sexual dysfunction. In addition, the study found positive responses from GPs who reported reductions in their workload as well as improved knowledge about the management of MS through contact with the MS liaison nurse. Emerging evidence of the benefits of health promotion rather than treatment of existing problems therefore suggests that MS nurses are already making cost effective contributions to the management of MS in some areas.

If MS specialist nurses are to be effective what skills do they require?

Clinical nurse specialist posts, including those dedicated to MS management, require a significant degree of experience and seniority. Their mode of practice involves autonomous working in an independent role, making accurate assessments and problem-solving appropriately without the support of a nursing team. They need to be able to negotiate effectively with different disciplines and grades of staff on behalf of the patient, often acting on their own initiative, while maintaining a sensitivity and understanding of the roles and responsibilities of other members of the multidisciplinary team.

Working with people with MS experiencing complex problems requires a significant knowledge of neurology and neuroscience nursing, which may be developed through postgraduate courses and/or specialist experience. In addition, the considerable need for psychological support at all stages of the disease process, but especially around the time of diagnosis, requires well developed counselling skills and an empathic and supportive attitude towards patient and family.

Education and research awareness are also key issues. Teaching patients, carers and other health care workers is an essential part of the MS specialist nurse's role, and some understanding of the theory as well as the practice of teaching is invaluable. A degree of sensitivity is required in judging how much and what type of information a person with MS is ready for at any stage. Sensitivity is also needed in teaching other nurses and health care colleagues in circumstances which might suggest that their care could be improved. A sound understanding of research principles is valuable for several reasons. Research developments and the availability of clinical trials often become a preoccupation for some people with MS and therefore a recurrent source of enquiry. If the nurse is to provide sound information and help people understand the purpose and potential limitations of various clinical trials, she needs to have a working knowledge of these issues herself. The ability to appraise critically research findings which have implications for nursing practice informs future practice developments and provides a sound basis from which to teach. In addition, evaluation of the impact of an MS nurse specialist service or other topics of nursing enquiry require an understanding of research theory and practice, even if the MS nurse is not wholly responsible for the design of such studies.

In attempting to fulfil a co-ordinating flexible role, nurses can often be at risk of having their role eroded by multiple demands from various sources. The issue of taking on medical responsibilities in response to drives to reduce junior doctors' hours has been hotly debated.[25,26] In the field of MS it may be perceived by some that the nurse's organizational skills are best used in co-ordinating and administering a range of clinical trials, but the nurse must be able to justify and prioritize her involvement in terms of overall benefit to the patients she serves. To achieve and maintain this balance the nurse specialist needs to have a clear grasp of the 'essence of nursing'[13] and the confidence to assert her role when considering further developments in practice.

The need for higher education as well as considerable experience becomes clear. In recognition of this and the current trend towards increasing clinical nurse specialist posts, the United Kingdom Central Council for Nursing and Midwifery has developed guidelines for specialist practitioner's qualifications. These allow individuals to pursue formal developmental routes towards achieving this level of practice,[27] although it is likely that nurses will also continue to reach the required competence through their own combination of courses and experience. These nursing posts must be graded to reflect the seniority and skills required.

Conclusion

Despite the many encouraging recent developments in service provision and research, from a user's perspective, living with MS is often still perceived to be a struggle. The variability and unpredictability of the disease lead to a degree of insecurity and an associated need for consistency and clear information on which to base decisions in an attempt to plan for the future. However, recurrent themes of fragmentation and lack of continuity, difficulty in accessing information, poor communication, and lack of appropriate knowledge or expertise among some hospital and community staff, are still prevalent. Poor psychological support and lack of co-ordination over time are also cited, for people whose needs may be sporadic.

The identified need for centralized information, available from individuals with an understanding of neurological conditions, health and local authority provision and with collaborative links with a wide range of multidisciplinary therapeutic services, has led to the development of the MS nurse specialist's role. Nurses' skills in communication and co-ordination are being used to good advantage in empowering patients and their families to make better use of the services available, and feel more in control of their lives. Health promotion is an intrinsic part of nursing practice, and the MS nurse specialist role presents ideal opportunities to help individuals and their carers maintain healthy lifestyles where possible. Through educational initiatives, MS nurses are also able to contribute more widely to improvements in standards of care for people with MS. There is already a growing body of evidence to suggest that MS nurse specialists are providing a cost effective contribution to MS management, and the Department of Health supports increased involvement and co-ordination of specialist clinical and nursing input as a means of achieving greater consistency in hospital discharges.[17]

To achieve this level of service the special skills and educational requirements of nurses working in these independent roles need to be acknowledged, and appropriately rewarded. It seems likely that such roles will continue to increase, so allowing more people with MS and their families access to consistent support and information which may contribute towards improving their perception of the experience of MS.

References

1. McDonald I. What progress has been made on research? Report of the 1996 Richard Cave Memorial Lecture to the MS Society, National Conference Centre, Birmingham, reported in *Committed to a Better Future – MS Society Annual Report* 1996; MS Society.
2. Boulton A. British government highlights neurosciences. *Br Med J* 1996; **2**: 658.
3. Hatch J. The economic impact of MS. *MS Management* 1996; **3**: 40.
4. British Society of Rehabilitation Medicine. *Multiple Sclerosis (Working Party Report)*, London: Royal College of Physicians 1993.
5. McLellan DL, Martin JR, Roberts MHW *et al.* Multiple Sclerosis in the Southampton District. University of Southampton: Rehabilitation Research Unit and Department of Sociology and Social Policy 1989.
6. MS Society. Insight – Bridging the Gap of Misconceptions. Preliminary report of a commissioned study into the needs of people with MS by Brunel M.R. Research Unit. *MS Matters* suppl 7 1996, 5–8.
7. Thompson AJ, Johnston S, Harrison J *et al.* Service delivery in multiple sclerosis: The need for coordinated community care. *MS Management* 1997; **4**: 11–21.
8. Thompson AJ. Management of MS, towards defining a model of care. *MS Update* 1994; **8**: 36–38.
9. Association of British Neurologists. Neurological Rehabilitation in the United Kingdom – Report of a Working Party. London: Royal College of Physicians 1992.
10. Campion K. Meeting multiple needs. *Nursing Times* 1996; **92**: 28–30.
11. Winters S. A nurse-managed multiple sclerosis clinic: Improved quality of life for persons with MS. *Rehab Nurs* 1989; **14**: 13–16.
12. Kraft GH, Freal JE, Coryell JK. Disability, disease duration and rehabilitation service needs in multiple sclerosis: Patient perspectives. *Arch Phys Med Rehabil* 1986; **67**: 164–167.
13. Henderson VA. Preserving the essence of nursing in a technological age. *Adv Nurs* 1980; **5**: 245–260.
14. McWilliam CL, Wong CA. Keeping it secret: the cost and benefit of nursing's hidden work in discharging patients. *J Adv Nurs* 1994; **19**: 152–163.
15. Barnes MP. Multiple Sclerosis. In: Greenwood R, Barnes MP, McMillan TM *et al.* eds. *Neurological Rehabilitation*, London: Churchill Livingstone 1993; 485–504.
16. Grice H, Kilshaw J, Houghton E. Maintaining quality of life with a nurse-led care unit. *Nurs Times* 1995; **91**: 31–32.
17. Progress in practice: initial evaluation of the impact of the continuing care guidance, letter to H.A. Chief Executives, Directors of Social Services and Chief Executives of NHS Trusts, 30th October 1996; Department of Health.
18. Swales T. The need for specialist MS nursing for patients undergoing beta-interferon treatment in Lancashire and South Cumbria. *Europ J Neurol* 1996; **3**: 50 (abstract).
19. Betts CD, D'Mellow MT, Fowler CJ. Urinary symptoms and the neurological features of bladder dysfunction in multiple sclerosis. *J Neurol Neurosurg Psychiatry* 1993; **56**: 245–250.
20. Fowler C, Fowler C. Neurological bladder dysfunction and its management. In: Greenwood R, Barnes MP, McMillan TM *et al.* eds. *Neurological Rehabilitation*, London: Churchill Livingstone 1993; 267–277.
21. Walquist GI. Impact of a nurse managed clinic in multiple sclerosis. *J Neurosurg Nurs* 1984; **16**: 193–196.
22. Jahanshahi M, Brown RG, Whitehouse C *et al.* Contact with a nurse practitioner: a short term evaluation study in Parkinson's disease and dystonia. *Behav Neurol* 1994; **7**: 189–196.
23. Campion K, Cotton P, Moore CEG. Multiple sclerosis nurse specialists: a cost efficient service provider. *Europ J Neurol* 1996; **3**: 16 (abstract).
24. Kirker SGB, Young E, Warlow CP. An evalu-

ation of a multiple sclerosis liaison nurse. *Clin Rehab* 1995; **9**: 219–226.

25. Castledine G. Will the nurse practitioner be a mini doctor or a maxi nurse? *Br J Nurs* 1995; **4**: 938–939.

26. Cahill H. Role definition: nurse practitioners or clinical assistants? *Br J Nurs* 1996; **5**: 1382–1386.

27. UKCC. The Council's standards for education and practice following registration (PREP) transitional arrangements – Specialist Practitioner title/Specialist Qualification. London, UKCC 1996.

26

Building partnerships

Jan Hatch

Introduction

It is well known that multiple sclerosis (MS) is an incurable disease of the central nervous system; little is understood of its cause, there is no cure and there is little information about what may affect its course or how it will progress in an affected individual. It is a disease which affects people in the prime of life, with symptoms generally appearing between 20 and 50 years of age. It affects a significant number of people but it is not one which affects a high proportion of the population in comparison to heart disease, arthritis or cancer. However, it is the major cause of physical disability in people below retirement age in Europe, North America, Australia and New Zealand. Although the medical costs of the disease are not high, the social, economic and physical implications for people with MS and their families are significant.

Diagnosis is a difficult and often protracted process for people who have usually experienced a range of disturbing symptoms over a period of time. In many cases the diagnosis of MS is not given formally to an individual but is discovered following many years of distressing and confusing symptoms and tests. The disease progression is unpredictable and the course of MS is difficult to assess and monitor. Management of symptoms is more often than not a matter of trial and error, with some treatments or therapies working well for some

people but having no demonstrable effect on others; when symptoms are invisible and complex, often mingled with permanent disability, management and treatment can be complicated and demanding, with the burden often falling on the person themselves and their families.

In this book subjects dealt with include the pathogenesis and precipitating factors in MS, treatment trials and professional and medical management of aspects of MS. This chapter clarifies the perspective of the person affected by MS in comparison with that of the key professionals with whom they share the field. The role of people with MS as partners in care and treatment is explored in the light of the current context of service provision and treatment and management.

Perspectives on MS

MS presents a challenge to all of those affected by it. The complexity and variability of MS has given rise to many difficulties in its treatment and management for both professionals and individuals. It is difficult to find many professional staff, especially those working in the community, who have extensive experience and understanding of MS. The person with MS and the family often have to piece together the picture for themselves partly from a neurologist who understands the disease but not their situation, and partly from those in the community who may understand their situation but not their disease.[1]

The many different perspectives of those professionals and individuals concerned with MS give rise to many different approaches to the disease. Understanding these different perspectives is important in developing an understanding of the difficulties which people with MS experience in current approaches to its diagnosis and management. Improvements which are meaningful and beneficial to people with MS will only be made if researchers, clinicians and those who pay for care take into account the views of the people living with the disease.

In considering the perspective of those concerned with MS let us start with scientific researchers; their view of MS will be from the perspective of an explorer approaching a mystery requiring examination and scientific scrutiny. At present, MS is still an unsolved puzzle which intrigues and stimulates their investigations, particularly to find the causes and identify factors or features which may have an impact on the disease process.

This purely scientific approach does not have very much to do with the difficulties of individuals living with the disease but it is very important to people with MS that good scientific research of this kind is done. It can lift people's visions from the problematic and practical plane of their present troubles to the more promising plane of future medical success and thereby generates hope ... 'I never give up hope that some dramatic breakthrough will be made in the treatment of diseases of the nervous system.'[2]

Neurologists are another important group of professionals because they have the greatest general knowledge of the disease. They focus on the observation of a series of defined symptoms occurring over time; they examine, test and analyse these symptoms to make a diag-

nosis of MS and other neurological conditions and diseases. However, few of them will have a great deal of expertise and practical experience of managing the long-term course of their patients with MS as they are primarily concerned with the process of diagnosis. Although they do have a key role to play in treating severe relapses, they seldom have an input into the management of people with MS in the community. In some cases they will regularly monitor and assess their MS patients where a new treatment or therapy is on trial, but this generally focuses on the effects on neurological aspects of the disease process.

For most people with MS the role of the neurologist is potentially very important in their lives, not only because they are medically qualified personnel whose practises are largely concerned (from the person's point of view) with the differential diagnosis of MS, but because they represent in principle the main access to continuing specialist care and medical advice during the course of the disease. However, many people with MS do not have a very positive view of their neurologist. For almost all those in the groups studied, contact with the neurologist had been relatively brief, both at the point of diagnosis and later (I Robinson, unpublished work).

The next professional who has a vital role to play is the GP or family doctor. Most GPs will see MS as a series or multiplicity of symptoms and medical problems to be treated as they appear and disappear over a lifetime; however, their understanding of MS, its symptoms and effects will be limited by the small number of people with MS they will see in the course of their career. It is estimated that a general practitioner's list of 2,000 is likely to contain approximately 2 to 4 people with MS. Even in high risk areas a general practitioner's experience of the disease is likely, therefore, to be limited to a few cases.[3]

For most people with MS, their GP or family doctor will be the key professional to whom they turn throughout the course of their disease. The GP will be the one consulted about the first symptoms; he will make interim diagnoses of the cause and origin of those symptoms and will concern himself with the treatment of those presented. It would be a mistake, however, to conclude that the uncertainty and ambiguity which often characterizes the initial lay response to the early symptoms of MS is quickly resolved by this contact with the medical system.[4] For many people with MS the lack of quick resolution or diagnosis of the underlying condition causing their symptoms creates frustration and emotional upheaval as their mysterious symptoms come and go, sometimes over long periods of time, sometimes causing great disruption to their lives, with no satisfactory explanation. Their perception of the role of the GP is often affected by this experience and people will frequently begin to take a much more active role in seeking their own explanations for their condition and remedies for their difficulties.

Clearly, people with MS have a very different perception of the disease from that of professionals. It is also very individual depending on the person, his/her circumstances and experience. Many people with MS encounter it as a benign and infrequent visitor but for most people it is a disruptive and disabling demon living within them. For some, the disease appears to lie dormant for long periods of time, for others a progressive deterioration will take place with no remission. Most people will endure a lifetime of relapses and remissions eventually accumulating disabilities and deficits as the years go by, continually making adjustments to their lives and circumstances to adapt to their changing situation.

Very few people living with MS have been able to obtain the support and help that they have needed from the professionals on whom they have been dependent for assistance and treatment in meeting the challenges of their disease. The unpredictability and variability of the symptoms and course described above, and the unique needs of each person with MS, mitigate against any standard approach which may be taken to the provision of health and social care. People with MS cannot be cured and so many medical professionals dismiss the person who is diagnosed with the disease with the words 'there is nothing that can be done for you, so go home and try to live a normal life'. This perspective gives people diagnosed with MS the impression that nothing can be done to treat or alleviate symptoms or disabilities; it cuts them off from meaningful consideration of any treatment options and throws them back onto their own resources.

That is why it is so important to consider the experiences of people with MS in relation to the provision of medical services and treatments – in order to ensure more effective use of limited resources and to improve their general health through informed management. Promoting vigorous partnerships between people with MS and the professionals who care for and support them must increase in importance. Recognition of the role people have to play in their own care and management must become a key component of the professional perspective on all aspects of this disease. Only through such recognition can progress be made in ameliorating the consequences of MS for those who have it and who continue to struggle to live a purposeful and fulfilling life.

Pressure on resources affects treatment and management

Another important area for consideration is that of resources and how pressure on them affects the perspective and role of researchers, health and social care professionals and people with MS.

Today there is a growing problem in the provision of effective and economic health and medical services and treatments, and it is becoming increasingly clear that those who are the recipients of services have as much of a stake in that provision as anyone else. As taxpayers who are users of services provided by the State or as consumers purchasing services from an array of competing providers, patients are no longer passive recipients of care. They want and are demanding more say both about their treatment choices and the policies which affect health care overall.[5]

Involving the public more directly in decisions about priorities in the provision of health services has become a requirement for decision makers throughout Europe and North America due to increased consumer activity and pressure on limited financial resources for health and social care. In the UK the National Health Service has developed a collaborative strategy designed to encourage patient partnership, giving greater voice and influence to users of the services and their carers in their own care, the development and definition of standards set for services locally and the development of policy both locally and nationally (Priorities and Planning Guidelines 1996/97 EL(95)68). The document outlining this strategy states: 'there is some evidence that involving patients in their own care improves health care outcomes and increases patient satisfaction'.[6]

As shown above, there are sound reasons for people to begin to take a more active role in their own treatment and disease management. They must come to see themselves as active agents of their own well-being and care. They must assume responsibility for maintaining the best possible health status and dealing with the illness they face.[7] There is much evidence to show that people with MS are often forced to take on this role anyway because of the lack of professional knowledge and support they receive in the day-to-day management of the disease.

It is vital that professionals begin to develop beyond the traditional boundaries within their own practice and to do so in partnership with their patients, many of whom have achieved a high degree of personal knowledge and expertise in the course of living with MS. This personal experiential knowledge base needs to be backed up and reinforced with good, practical, professional research which is focused not only on professional interests but which includes an examination of the needs of people affected by the disease as they express them. People with MS must take their place at the centre of the health care team.

People with MS set their own agenda

It is clear that many individuals affected by chronic disease have a very personal investment and commitment to their own participation in treatment and management strategies. In common with others with long-term medical conditions, people with MS have taken action to help themselves and to make sure that the disease and its effects receive the attention of scientists, clinicians and those who make and influence health and social care policy.

Fifty years ago, the sister of a man diagnosed with MS placed an advertisement in the *New York Times* seeking information from anyone with MS who may have recovered from it. This was the beginning of a movement of people with MS and their families and friends whose aims were to find the cause of and a cure for the disease and to provide help and support to those living with it. Over the years, people with MS all over the world have created lay organizations to raise funds to stimulate and encourage medical and scientific research and to promote their own well-being.

This movement of people with MS and their families and friends initially focused their efforts on the search for the key scientific elements which feature in MS; over the past ten years the focus has shifted to include the development of programmes and applied research which will directly benefit people with MS in their struggle to live with MS and its symptoms and disabilities.

With no major breakthroughs in identifying the cause or finding a cure or effective treatment for MS and the realization that it is unlikely that there will be such a breakthrough, those living with it have begun to demand that more attention is paid to finding ways to manage their day-to-day needs and to improve their quality of life. This has given rise to an increased focus on the social and emotional consequences of living with MS and a demand for research into these aspects of the disease. The opportunities for professionals to work together with people with MS and their supporters in this field have never been greater. These lay people have developed a body of knowledge and experience in care and management which is rooted in the practicalities of daily life in the community. It is not bound by the conventions of professional education and training or the limits of institutionally based service provision and therefore offers the possibility of new insights and directions in care.

People living with MS

To a great extent, the increased public profile of all those individuals who are struggling to live with long-term medical conditions has stimulated new directions in research in the social sciences field where investigation into the effects of living with chronic illness on individuals and their families is a growing field. Gaining some insight into the experience of people with chronic medical conditions, gathering information about what they value and about their priorities, their expectations of care and treatment and their own management strategies and goals, has become an area of active research. This is associated with a reorientation of the focus for care from repairing damage caused by disease to education and understanding for living with chronic illness. In an age of changing consumer demands and expectations social research reflects the need for providers increasingly to offer choices not to make them.[8]

It is clear from the research carried out into the experiences of people with MS that most of them have not been and are not satisfied with the professional support that they receive in living with and managing their MS. They are frequently not offered even the most basic information about the disease and its action, let alone information about treatment or management options. This has resulted at best in a healthy independence from medical professionals among people less severely affected by MS and at worst devastating mismanagement and treatment of the disease in people most severely affected. In most cases, people with MS try to manage on their own or they seek the company and counsel of others with MS and struggle to find and provide themselves with remedies or therapies which provide some apparent relief, often despite any valid scientific basis or proof to support efficacy and safety.

Ignorance of the priorities and needs of people with MS can only lead to the development of unsuccessful treatments and management regimes which will waste precious and finite resources, time and energy. As pointed out above, this ignorance must be dispelled and professionals must begin to consider their patients as partners if any real progress is to be made. The findings of researchers studying the impact of the disease on individuals indicate that treatment and management should be centred on the individual's needs and not on the needs of practitioners or service providers. The health system has invested much time and energy in teaching doctors in all fields about human pathophysiology, the use of diagnostic tools and selecting the most appropriate drug. What has largely been missing is investment in teaching doctors how to communicate effectively with patients and their families about treating, managing and preventing crises related to the disease.[9]

Although treatments for relapses, symptoms and disabilities are available they have often been administered without reference to the overall effect of the disease and other treatments or management strategies already in place. In fact, on-going professional management of the disease and its overall physical, emotional and cognitive effects on the individuals has not been available for most people with MS. In most cases and in most places no one takes the lead role in disease and disability management except the person with MS him/herself and his/her family.

Conclusion

This isolation and fragmentation of treatment has had an enormous impact on the ability of people with MS and their families and friends to come to terms with living with the disease and to find ways of managing its effects on daily life practically and effectively. It has also had an effect on what medical professionals know about the disease, its impact on other aspects of health, how it varies within an individual and between individuals, how it affects physical and intellectual capabilities, how it affects family and social life, the lives of carers and children living with a parent with MS and how care and treatment should be approached to be of maximum benefit and effectiveness.

Professionals must guide the development of management programmes and strategies which integrate all the relevant disciplines that are so essential to the appropriate and effective management of all of the effects of the disease. People with MS must be at the centre of that process. They and their families and supporters must actively participate in the decisions that are made about treatment and management. Their need for information and involvement must be paramount in planning and implementing any programme of care. Their perspective must be taken into account if new treatment and management regimes are to be developed and implemented effectively.

References

1. Compston DAS, Evans CD, Feneley RCL *et al.* Introduction to British Society of Rehabilitative Medicine Working Party Report on Multiple Sclerosis. London 1993; 1–4.
2. Robinson I. *Multiple Sclerosis*. London: Routledge 1988; 126–127.
3. Compston DAS, Evans CD, Feneley RCL *et al.* Epidemiology and Possible Causes of MS. British Society of Rehabilitative Medicine Working Party Report on Multiple Sclerosis. London 1993; 5–6.
4. Robinson I. *Multiple Sclerosis*. London: Routledge 1988; 18–20.
5. From dependence to partnership: patients redefine their role in health care. *The Patient's Network* 1996; **1**: 1.
6. Quality and Consumers Branch. *Patient Partnership: Building a Collaborative Strategy*, Leeds: NHS Executive 1996; 2.
7. From dependence to partnership: patients redefine their role in health care. *The Patient's Network* 1996; **1**: 5.
8. Anderson R, Bury M. Introduction. In: Anderson R, Bury M, eds. *Living with Chronic Illness*, London: Unwin Hyman 1988; 1–4.
9. Assal JP. The role of patient education for people with chronic illnesses. In: Funnell C, van der Zeijden A, Ryser-Cseri M *et al. Patient-Centred Health Care – New Partnerships in Europe*, London: National Eczema Society 1996; 48–49.

Index